Operative Laparoscopy
Second Edition

The Masters' Techniques in Gynecologic Surgery

Operative Laparoscopy
Second Edition

with 44 contributors

Edited by

Richard M. Soderstrom, M.D.

Reproductive Health Specialists, P.S.
Clinical Professor of Obstetrics and Gynecology
University of Washington School of Medicine
Seattle, Washington

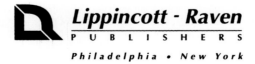
Lippincott - Raven
P U B L I S H E R S
Philadelphia • New York

Acquisitions Editor: Lisa McAllister
Developmental Editor: Emilie Linkins
Manufacturing Manager: Dennis Teston
Production Manager: Jodi Borgenicht
Production Editor: Rosemary Palumbo
Cover Designer: Betty Booker
Indexer: Susan Thomas
Compositor: Tapsco
Printer: Toppan Printers, Pte Ltd., Singapore

Printed and bound in Singapore

9 8 7 6 5 4 3 2 1

Library of Congress Cataloging-in-Publication Data
Operative laparoscopy: the masters' techniques/edited by Richard M.
    Soderstrom; with 44 contributors. — 2nd ed.
        p.   cm.—(The masters' techniques in gynecologic surgery)
    Includes bibliographical references and index.
    ISBN 0-397-51797-1
    1. Laparoscopic surgery.   2. Generative organs, Female—Endoscopic
surgery.   I. Soderstrom, Richard M.   II. Series.
    [DNLM: 1. Genital Diseases, Female—surgery.   2. Laser Surgery.
3. Surgery, Laparoscopic—methods.   WP 660 061 1998]
RG104.7.065   1998
618.1'45—dc21
DNLM/DLC
for Library of Congress

Care has been taken to confirm the accuracy of the information presented and to describe generally
accepted practices. However, the authors, editor, and publisher are not responsible for errors or
omissions or for any consequences from application of the information in this book and make no
warranty, express or implied, with respect to the contents of the publication.

The authors, editor, and publisher have exerted every effort to ensure that drug selection and
dosage set forth in this text are in accordance with current recommendations and practice at the
time of publication. However, in view of ongoing research, changes in government regulations, and
the constant flow of information relating to drug therapy and drug reactions, the reader is urged to
check the package insert for each drug for any change in indications and dosage and for added
warnings and precautions. This is particularly important when the recommended agent is a new or
infrequently employed drug.

Some drugs and medical devices presented in this publication have Food and Drug Administration (FDA) clearance for limited use in restricted research settings. It is the responsibility of the
health care provider to ascertain the FDA status of each drug or device planned for use in their
clinical practice.

Contents

Contributing Authors

Gregory T. Absten, M.B.A.
Executive Director
Professional Medical Education Association
943 30th Street
Marathon, Florida 33050

Ralph W. Aye, M.D.
Teaching Attending Physician
Swedish Hospital
Clinical Assistant Professor
Department of Surgery
University of Washington School of Medicine
801 Broadway, #901
Seattle, Washington 98122

Jonathan S. Berek, M.D.
Professor and Vice Chair
Chief, Gynecology and Gynecologic Oncology
Director, UCLA Women's Gynecologic
   Oncology Center
UCLA School of Medicine
Jonsson Comprehensive Cancer Center
CHS 24-127
Los Angeles, California 90095-1740

Philip G. Brooks, M.D.
Clinical Professor
Department of Obstetrics and Gynecology
UCLA School of Medicine
Attending Physician
Department of Obstetrics and Gynecology
Cedars-Sinai Medical Center
8700 Beverly Boulevard
Los Angeles, California 90048

Kim James Charney, M.D.
Assistant Surgical Professor
Department of Surgery
St. Joseph Hospital of Orange
1140 West LaVeta Avenue, Suite 620
Orange, California 92868

Joel M. Childers, M.D.
Clinical Associate Professor
Department of Obstetrics and Gynecology
University of Arizona
2625 North Craycroft Road, #201
Tucson, Arizona 85712

Stephen L. Corson, M.D.
Clinical Professor
Department of Obstetrics and Gynecology
Thomas Jefferson University School of Medicine
Women's Institute
815 Locust Street
Philadelphia, Pennsylvania 19107-6096

Theodore Coutsoftides, M.D., F.A.C.S.,
   F.R.C.S.(C)
Clinical Associate Professor of Surgery
University of California
101 City Drive
Orange, California 92668

James F. Daniell, M.D.
Clinical Professor
Department of Obstetrics and Gynecology
Vanderbilt University Medical School
2222 State Street
Nashville, Tennessee 37203

Michael P. Diamond, M.D.
Professor
Department of Obstetrics and Gynecology
Department of Physiology
Director, Division of Reproductive
   Endocrinology and Infertility
Wayne State University School of Medicine
4707 St. Antoine Boulevard
Detroit, Michigan 48201

John I. Fishburne, Jr., M.D.
James A. Merrill Chair, Professor and
   Chairman
Department of Obstetrics and Gynecology
University Hospital
920 S. L. Young Boulevard
Oklahoma City, Oklahoma 73104

Alan B. Gazzaniga, M.D.
Professor
Department of Surgery
University of California, Irvine
101 The City Drive
Orange, California 92868

Kenneth A. Ginsburg, M.D.
Associate Professor
Division of Reproductive Endocrinology
Department of Obstetrics and Gynecology
Wayne Styate University
Hutzel Hospital
4707 St. Antoine Boulevard
Detroit, Michigan 48201

Victor Gomel, M.D.
Professor
Department of Obstetrics and Gynecology
University of British Columbia
Vancouver Hospital & Health Sciences Centre
805 West 12th Avenue
Third Floor Willow Pavilion
Vancouver, British Columbia, Canada V5Z 1M9

Harrith M. Hasson, M.D.
Clinical Professor
University of Chicago
Chairman, Division of Obstetrics and
  Gynecology
Director, Gynecologic Endoscopy Center
Weiss Hospital
4646 N. Marine Drive
Chicago, Illinois 60640

Lucius D. Hill, M.D.
Professor
Department of Surgery
University of Washington School of Medicine
801 Broadway
Seattle, Washington 98122

Delbert Alan Johns, M.D.
Associate Professor
Department of Obstetrics and Gynecology
University of Texas Southwestern Medical
  Center at Dallas
Harris Methodist Fort Worth
1301 Pennsylvania Avenue
Fort Worth, Texas 76104

Jeffrey M. Johnsrud, M.D.
Private Practice in General and Vascular
  Surgery
1140 West LaVeta Avenue, Suite 470
Orange, California 92868

Ronald L. Levine, M.D.
Professor
Department of Obstetrics and Gynecology
University of Louisville School of Medicine
550 S. Jackson Street
Louisville, Kentucky 40202

Carl J. Levinson, M.D.
Clinical Associate Professor
Department of Gynecology and Obstetrics
Stanford University School of Medicine
845 Oak Grove, #220
Menlo Park, California 94025

Barbara S. Levy, M.D.
Clinical Assistant Professor
Department of Obstetrics and Gynecology
University of Washington School of Medicine
34509 Ninth Avenue South, #300
Federal Way, Washington 98003

Anthony A. Luciano, M.D.
Professor
Department of Obstetrics and Gynecology
University of Connecticut School of Medicine
New Britain General Hospital
100 Grand Street
New Britain, Connecticut 06050

Thomas L. Lyons, M.D.
Clinical Assistant Professor
Department of Obstetrics and Gynecology
Director, Center for Women's Care and
  Reproductive Surgery
Emory University Medical Center
1140 Hammond Drive, F-6230
Atlanta, Georgia 30328

Daniel R. Marcus, M.D.
Attending Surgeon
Department of Surgery
Swedish Medical Center
747 Broadway
Seattle, Washington 98122

John L. Marlow, M.D.
Clinical Professor
Department of Obstetrics and Gynecology
George Washington University School of
  Medicine
2440 M Street NW, #801
Washington, DC 20037

Dan C. Martin, M.D.
Clinical Associate Professor
Department of Obstetrics and Gynecology
University of Tennessee, Memphis
1717 Kirby Parkway, Suite 100
Memphis, Tennessee 38120-4331

Camran R. Nezhat, M.D.
Clinical Professor of Surgery
Clinical Professor of Gynecology and
  Obstetrics
Department of Gynecology and Obstetrics
Department of Surgery
Stanford University School of Medicine
900 Welch Road, Suite 403
Palo Alto, California 94304

Ceana H. Nezhat, M.D.
Clinical Associate Professor
Mercer University School of Medicine (Macon,
  Georgia)
Clinical Assistant Professor
Department of Gynecology and Obstetrics
Stanford University School of Medicine
900 Welch Road, Suite 403
Palo Alto, California 94304

Farr R. Nezhat, M.D.
Clinical Professor
Department of Gynecology and Obstetrics
Stanford University School of Medicine
900 Welch Road, Suite 403
Palo Alto, California 94304

Roger C. Odell
Electroscope, Inc.
4828 Sterling Drive
Boulder, Colorado 80301

Sanford S. Osher, M.D.
Department of Obstetrics and Gynecology
Bethesda North Hospital
10495 Montgomery Road, #14
Cincinnatti, Ohio 45242

Brian Palafox, M.D., F.A.C.S.
Assistant Clinical Professor
Department of Surgery
University of California, Irvine
St. Joseph's Hospital
1310 W. Stewart Drive, #502
Orange, California 92868

William H. Parker, M.D.
Clinical Professor
Department of Obstetrics and Gynecology
UCLA School of Medicine
Los Angeles, California

Resad P. Pasic, M.D., Ph.D.
Department of Obstetrics and Gynecology
University of Louisville
530 South Jackson Street, ACB—2nd Floor
Louisville, Kentucky 40292

James J. Perez, D.O., F.A.C.O.O.G.
Clinical Assistant Professor
Department of Obstetrics and Gynecology
Ohio University College of Osteopathic
  Medicine
Doctors Hospital West
Columbus, Ohio 43201

David B. Redwine, M.D.
Director, Endometriosis Institute of Oregon
St. Charles Medical Center
2500 NE Neff Road
Bend, Oregon 97701

Harry Reich, M.D.
Associate Professor, Clinical Obstetrics and
  Gynecology
Department of Obstetrics and Gynecology
Columbia Presbyterian Medical Center
161 Fort Washington Avenue, Atchley Building
New York, New York 10032

Jacques E. Rioux, M.D., M.P.H.
Professor of Obstetrics and Gynecology
Faculty of Medicine
Laval University
University Hospital
2705 boulevard Laurier
Sainte Foy, Quebec, Canada G1V 4G2

Marshall L. Smith, Jr., M.D., Ph.D.
Endoscopy Specialist
Good Samaritan Medical Center
926 East McDowell, Suite 125
Phoenix, Arizona 85006

Richard M. Soderstrom, M.D.
Reproductive Health Specialists, P.S.
Clinical Professor of Obstetrics and
  Gynecology
University of Washington School of Medicine
1101 Madison, Suite 580
Seattle, Washington 98104

Eugenio Solima, M.D.
Clinical Research Fellow
Department of Obstetrics and Gynecology
University of Rome Tor Vergata
Ple dell' Umanesimo
00197 Rome, Italy

Thierry G. Vancaillie, M.D.
Department of Obstetrics and Gynecology
Royal Hospital for Women
Sydney, Australia

Wendy K. Winer, R.N., B.S.N.
Adjunct Clinical Instructor
Emory University School of Nursing
Endoscopic Surgery Specialist
Center for Women's Care and Reproductive
  Surgery
1140 Hammond Drive, Suite F-6230
Atlanta, Georgia 30328

Christo G. Zouves, M.B.Ch.B., F.R.C.S.
  (England), M.R.C.O.G., F.R.C.S (Canada)
Medical Director
Pacific Fertility Center
500-55 Francisco Street
San Francisco, California 94133

Preface

In the early 1970s, gynecologic operative laparoscopy was confined to female sterilization, lysis of filmy adhesions, and electrocoagulation of endometriosis. By 1990, an array of sophisticated surgical techniques had been developed, which resulted in the relocation of many major surgical procedures to the realm of outpatient surgery. The techniques refined in gynecologic laparoscopy are now being transferred to non-gynecologic surgery—witness the development of laparoscopic cholecystectomy. The field of advanced operative laparoscopy is now developing explosively. There has been a proliferation of postgraduate, hands-on courses for surgeons. Entire endoscopic surgical teams are now responsible for a vast number of sophisticated procedures. Manufacturers have creatively answered the call for the custom-made endoscopy tools required by new procedures.

When I was first asked to edit and contribute to a book on operative laparoscopy as part of a series of surgery books, it was not clear how it should be organized. Gradually it became clear that a "how-to" book written by the masters of operative laparoscopy would be a help to all endoscopists in gynecology and general surgery. Each guest author was chosen because he or she is known as a master surgeon and teacher. Each was asked to diverge from the usual, formal style of a scientific periodical by writing in the first or the second person, in order to share more personally with readers their "pearls" of practical information, and to discuss indications or judgments as they might apply to a specific surgical approach.

This is a book for student surgeons, practicing laparoscopists, and operating room support staff. Though the experienced laparoscopist may be tempted to skip the chapters on basic physics and techniques, he or she should consult them to find alternatives to common problems.

Where there is more than one way to approach a surgical problem, such as myomectomy, more than one author was recruited. To attract the general surgeon and to cross-educate the gynecologist, several colleagues from general surgery contributed to the section on nongynecologic uses of operative laparoscopy. One such contributor, Dr. Alan Gazzaniga, is a true pioneer in general surgery, having developed his endoscopic skills decades before contemporary general surgeons took up the technique.

Surgeons without complications are either retired or liars! Complications are thoroughly discussed, from the nuances of technique to what to do if they occur. The master surgeons are well equipped, through their experience, to give guidance on proper management and care. Cogent advice is given on legal matters, with case examples of what to do and what not to do.

The final chapters carry the reader through the array of photodocumentation methods that can be used for records, professional teaching, and providing a pictorial record for the patient—an effective way to promote a bond between patient and surgeon.

The support and ingenuity of the manufacturers listed in the manufacturers' section is especially noteworthy. Their response to our needs over the past three decades has been remarkable, and without them this form of remote control surgery would be impossible.

Operative Laparoscopy
Second Edition

Operative Laparoscopy, Second Edition
The Masters' Techniques in Gynecologic Surgery
Lippincott–Raven Publishers, Philadelphia © 1998.

1

Equipment

1-1 Laparoscopic Equipment

Richard M. Soderstrom

A thorough knowledge of laparoscopic equipment makes the difference between a good laparoscopist and an excellent laparoscopist. There is no other gynecologic operation that can be more frustrating than a laparoscopic procedure done with defective or incomplete equipment. Unfortunately, because this operation is considered by many clinicians to be simple or minor, inexperienced personnel are frequently assigned to the care and feeding of laparoscopic equipment. If the operating technician (or the surgeon) is not familiar with the array of accessories for laparoscopy, the procedure can grind to a halt or, on occasion, be abandoned. It is ironic that only an hour or two of study will allow all who handle laparoscopic equipment to gain sufficient familiarity with all the accessories and adapters, which will help all to proceed with a smooth, uncomplicated laparoscopy.

In the beginning, manufacturers produced their own endoscopes, light sources, light cables, and accessories, each incompatible with those of other brands. Today, it is rare to find an endoscopic tool that does not have an array of adapters for compatibility—the problem lies in remembering which goes where and where they are stored. It is unreasonable for the surgeon to expect support personnel to know the names of all the accessories and adapters if he or she is not familiar with these devices. To say, "Bring me that gadget that fits on this thingamajig" evinces irresponsibility. However, a surgeon who knows his or her equipment well should insist that support staff be well informed, if for no other reason than that the patient expects it. An excellent way to achieve this goal is to have joint sessions with the operating room personnel, doctor, and manufacturer representatives when equipment is purchased. All should learn how to disassemble and reassemble instruments with moving parts and learn to identify parts that are worn, crushed, or broken before the defect leads to an operative complication. Defective equipment is one of the leading causes of laparoscopic complications, some of which are serious.

Laparoscopic equipment is expensive, delicate, and has a predictable amount of "down time." These facts should inform the replacement and repair program set in place at the time of initial purchase. After about 100 procedures, light cords will need to be replaced. Reusable trocars should be resharpened after 10 procedures; plan ahead—buy extra trocars to use while the dull ones are being sharpened. Instruments like graspers and scissors, used in most operative laparoscopies, will fail on occasion. To be without a spare is inexcusable. I was once asked to visit a hospital because of a rash of laparoscopic accidents (and an array of lawsuits). A quick perusal of this medical center's operating room uncovered broken equipment with missing parts and a 10-year hiatus since a new laparoscope had been purchased or an old one repaired. One laparoscope had only 10% of its fiber bundles intact; it was referred to as the "dim" laparoscope. There was no one person in charge of endoscopes, and the equipment was cleaned at the end of the day with standard surgical hardware, stacked in a pile to be sorted out later. My visit cost the hospital $60,000 in new equipment, a blow to the operating room budget that could have been prevented with a proper maintenance program.

LAPAROSCOPES

Optics

Most rigid endoscopes use the Hopkins rod lens system (Figure 1-1.1). Unlike the "lemon drop"-shaped glass lens used in binoculars, quartz rods with concave ends are aligned in tandem within the supporting shaft of the endoscope, creating a "lens of air." The Hopkins principle gives remarkable clarity and reduces the chance of dislodging a lens during handling.

The angle of view can be altered, as can the field of view (Figure 1-1.2). An oblique view is helpful when one wishes

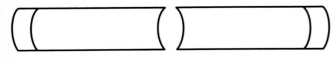

Hopkins System

Figure 1-1.1 The Hopkins rod lens system aligns quartz rods to form a lens of air.

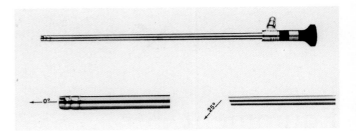

Figure 1-1.3 A diagnostic endoscope. (Courtesy of Richard Wolf Instrument Corp., Rosemont, Illinois.)

to explore a hidden recess such as the ovarian fossa or over the dome of the liver. Though the field of view may be limited to 120° when the endoscope is rotated the panoramic view may be 180° or more.

Because of the wide-angle field of view inherent in most endoscopes, a distortion of size and of peripheral view is inherent in the technology. Most laparoscopes provide a realistic image size when the end of the laparoscope is held 5 cm from the object. Moving the laparoscope closer creates magnification and a "zoom" effect. Withdrawing from the object shrinks its apparent size, but peripheral distortion is made minimal. In the beginning, the student struggles with this principle and can become easily lost or confused. When using operating accessories, the novice will frequently have problems with "past pointing," but practice will usually solve this problem.

Fortunately, most of the manufacturers have made the eyepiece of their endoscopes a standard size, which facilitates the attachment of photography cameras, television cameras, and teaching sidearms. The eyepieces are nonconductive to prevent electrical injury to the operator's eye, and some eyepieces can be focused for the operator who usually wears corrective glasses.

Types

There are two basic types of laparoscopes, one for diagnostic work, the other for operative laparoscopy (Figures 1-1.3 and 1-1.4). The lens system is the same in both, but the image size is usually smaller in the operating laparoscope of the same diameter. This difference is influenced by the size of the operating channel built into the shaft of the laparoscope or the amount of fiberoptic bundles contained within the shaft. If one wants a large operating channel, one must sacrifice the size of the lens system or the number of fiberoptic bundles (Figure 1-1.5). Thus a diagnostic operating laparoscope of equal size provides a larger image, less distortion, and the most light—an ideal instrument for quality photographs or television. Of course, one can increase the diameter of the operating laparoscope to reduce these restrictions.

I am frequently asked, "What laparoscope should I buy?" My answer is "Several types," but that may not be practical. The most versatile is a 10-mm diameter operating laparoscope, with a 3- or 5-mm channel and a 0° or 5° lens.

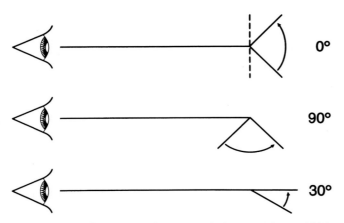

Figure 1-1.2 The angle of view can help to explore a hidden recess. As the telescope is rotated, the field of view is enhanced with an oblique lens.

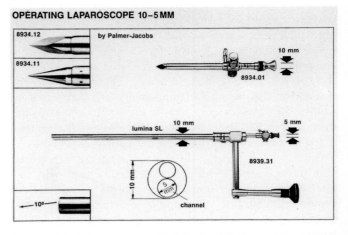

Figure 1-1.4 An operating laparoscope with a 5-mm operating channel. Most prefer the pyramidal tip as the conical tip requires more force during insertion. (Courtesy of Richard Wolf Instrument Corp., Rosemont, Illinois.)

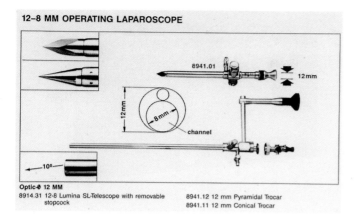

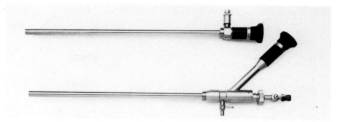

Figure 1-1.6 A versatile laparoscope set: a 10-mm diagnostic endoscope and an operating 10-mm endoscope with a coupler that will accept standard 5-mm operating instruments or a CO_2 laser attachment. (Courtesy of Olympus Corp., Lake Success, New York.)

Figure 1-1.5 A large-channel laparoscope. This is used for mechanical sterilization techniques. Because of the reduced area for fiber bundles and a smaller lens, the available light is less than that of a diagnostic scope of similar size, and the field of view is reduced. (Courtesy of Richard Wolf Instrument Corp., Rosemont, Illinois.)

With this instrument you can diagnose, have the convenience of the operating channel, and take reasonable photographs or use television. But for the purist, there is nothing better than a diagnostic laparoscope for a bright, clear view (Figure 1-1.6).

During the seventies, friendly debates would rage between the "one-hole" and the "two-hole" laparoscopists. Today an accomplished laparoscopist is one who, with equal ease, can use a diagnostic or operative laparoscope and is familiar and comfortable with "multiple-hole" laparoscopy. In fact, the latest operative techniques in laparoscopy require an operative laparoscope combined with the use of multiple secondary puncture sites and secondary accessories.

photography. This size of laparoscope shows promise for office laparoscopy under local anesthesia.

INSUFFLATION

The Veress Needle

The Veress needle is the most popular instrument for intraabdominal insufflation (Figures 1-1.7 and 1-1.8). By design, a blunt cannula is contained within the shaft of a sharp, 6- to 12-cm 16-gauge needle. In the hub of the needle is a spring that allows the blunt inner cannula to retract inside the needle shaft when pressure is placed against the tip of the blunt cannula (the cannula in its passive state protrudes about 4 mm beyond the needle tip). When the needle is thrust into the abdominal wall, the blunt tip retracts to allow the cutting edge of the outer shaft to penetrate the layers of the abdomen. Once the instrument has traversed the abdominal wall, the spring forces the blunt tip out ahead of the sharp needle to protect against laceration

Sizes

Any rigid endoscope, regardless of size, can be used for laparoscopy provided the trocar sleeve for the endoscope is compatible. A 4-mm cystoscope will fit nicely through a 5-mm trocar sleeve placed into the abdominal cavity. You should remember this if the laparoscope is dropped and broken during a procedure; don't panic—a cystoscope may save the day.

Most often, the sizes used are 5-mm (diagnostic) and 10 mm (diagnostic and operative). Other sizes are available for special procedures. At present a 2.7-mm fiberscope is under evaluation. Instead of a rod lens system, the image is passed through flexible fibers similar to those used in flexible colonoscopes and gastroscopes. By encasing these fibers in a rigid sheath, the diameter can be kept small because twice as much light is transmitted. The image seen through the fibers has a gridlike appearance but is satisfactory, even for

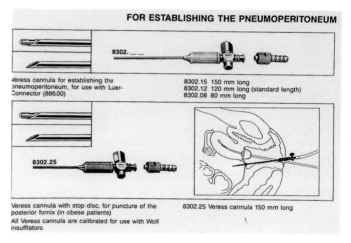

Figure 1-1.7 Veress cannulas. (Courtesy of Richard Wolf Instrument Corp., Rosemont, Illinois.)

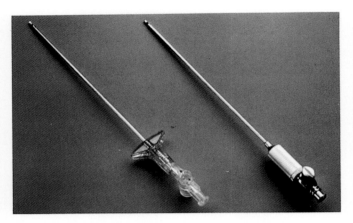

Figure 1-1.8 The disposable Veress needle on the left has the advantage of always being sharp. It does not need to be cleaned, and its internal parts cannot be lost. (Courtesy of U.S. Surgical Corp., Norwalk, Connecticut.)

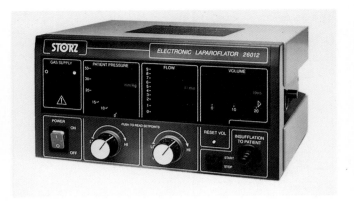

Figure 1-1.9 A high-flow insufflator for operative laparoscopy. (Courtesy of Karl Storz Co., Los Angeles, California.)

of an intraabdominal viscus. A stopcock on the needle hub controls the flow of gas when the insufflation tubing is attached. Maintenance of the Veress needle is important. It needs to be disassembled, flushed, and cleaned after each use. A bent Veress needle is worthless and dangerous.

A standard Touhey needle, frequently used for spinal anesthesia, is a good alternative to the Veress needle. Some surgeons have used a blunt cannula alone and report success.

Insufflators

Insufflators are available in a variety of sizes and configurations. They can all be used to deliver CO_2 or N_2O, but adapters are necessary if these two gases are to be interchanged with the same insufflator. The basic function of an insufflator is to control the *pressure* of gas being delivered to the abdominal cavity. This can be governed by the flow rate and volume delivered, but the physiologic concern surrounds intraabdominal pressure. A "high-flow" insufflator is just as safe as a "low-flow" insufflator provided the in-line pressure does not exceed 20–30 mm Hg (Figure 1-1.9). In such a system, once the intraabdominal pressure reaches this maximum, flow of gas will cease. When leakage occurs, during the removal of instruments for instance, the flow will resume as the intraabdominal pressure falls. Thus the volume of gas or the flow of gas that passes through an insufflator is of little concern; it is pressure that must be controlled.

Most insufflators have a flow meter, but those that do not are equally safe. So-called low-flow insufflators (i.e., 1 L/min) may create significant problems when leakage occurs, especially during complex operative maneuvers where good distention is mandatory.

Gas

Three gases have been used for laparoscopy—CO_2, N_2O, and room air. Room air is not absorbed well, leaving the patient with days to weeks of postoperative shoulder pain from diaphragmatic irritation. Room air is not soluble in blood, raising the risk of air embolism should the gas enter a blood vessel.

CO_2 is the gas most commonly used for laparoscopy; N_2O is favored by many. The arguments of the proponents and opponents are usual ones of theory. However, with laser laparoscopy, CO_2 is recommended; N_2O seems preferable for laparoscopy under local anesthesia.

LIGHT

Light Sources

The development of a remote light source was a turning point for endoscopy. Miniature light bulbs placed at the

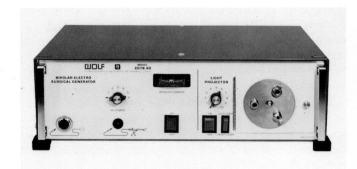

Figure 1-1.10 A standard light source built into a bipolar electrosurgical generator. The rotating turret female connector accepts several brands of fiberoptic cables. (Courtesy of Richard Wolf Instrument Corp., Rosemont, Illinois.)

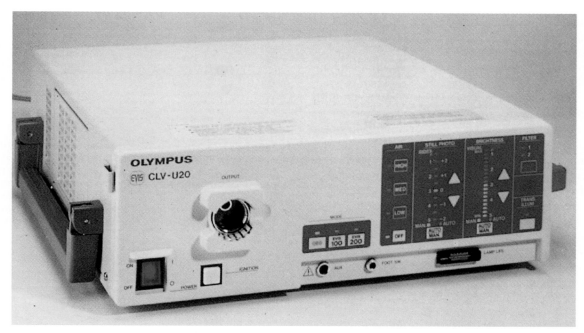

Figure 1-1.11 This xenon light source has automatic sensors to prevent flashback from light tissues when one uses a television camera. The strobe flash feature of this unit sets the proper exposure, making still photography simple. (Courtesy of Olympus Corp., Lake Success, New York.)

distal end of an endoscope were dim, hot, and had a short lifespan, frequently blowing out in the middle of the procedure and frustrating the endoscopist. Once the technology of fiberoptic light transmission entered the scene, this ''cold'' system opened new horizons for endoscopy; the spread of light is more uniform, the candlepower enhanced, and the life of the light bulb in the light box is many hours.

Today, most light sources have interchangeable connectors to adapt to different light bundles or cords (Figure 1-1.10). The standard light sources use a halogen bulb similar, if not identical, to the light bulbs used in photographic slide projectors. For photography, a color-corrected halogen or xenon light source is frequently used (Figure 1-1.11). Most light sources have two bulbs, one for backup should the main bulb fail; a few have a standard photographic bulb and a xenon bulb. Where the halogen or xenon bulb is best for movies and television, distal strobe light units are the best for still photographs. Each year, amazing developments in automation of contemporary cameras and flash units are applied to endoscopic photography.

Though maintenance for a light source is minimal, over time the light bulbs lose their brilliance; they should be changed before they burn out. For the standard halogen light bulb, a new bulb should be installed after 25 hours of use. Beware—read the manufacturer's recommendations for bulb replacement, for a severe electric shock can occur if the bulb is incorrectly removed or replaced.

Light Bundles

Light bundles or cords are of two types, coherent and incoherent bundles. Coherent bundles have organized fiberglass strands that tend to carry the light through each bundle in a columnated or ''focused'' arrangement. These fiber strands are usually thicker in diameter than those used in incoherent bundles. A quartz lens at the distal end of the light source helps to focus the transmitted light; thus there is less light lost than with incoherent bundles (Figure 1-1.12). Coherent bundles are used in flexible endoscopes to transmit the visual image.

Incoherent bundles are packed in a random fashion within the sheath of the flexible light card. Because the transmitted light is scattered as it travels through the light bundle, the available light to the endoscope may be reduced to 15% of the origin. Increasing the diameter of the cord and adding more fiber bundles helps increase the available

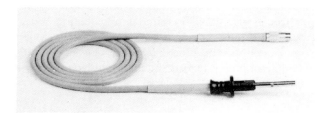

Figure 1-1.12 A coherent light bundle with a quartz rod lens at each end, which enhances light transfer. (Courtesy of Olympus Corp., Lake Success, New York.)

light, but larger cords are less flexible and are heavy. However, incoherent light cords are inexpensive, making the replacement cost more palatable.

In recent years an alcohol light cord was introduced for photography and television. The increased amount of available light is substantial, but some of the red spectrum is lost, and the peripheral spread of light is poor, creating a central hot spot. Should the cord be broken, the alcohol in it is lost, and a new cord is necessary.

Unfortunately, when the fiberoptic cord is connected to an endoscope (which contains fiberoptic glass bundles to transmit the light through the endoscope), it is impossible to line up the fiber bundles. This reduces available light to the operating field unless the laparoscope is manufactured with the fiberoptic cord as an integral part of it. For general use, such an expensive laparoscope is not necessary, and its maintenance requires the utmost of care. Most light cords have adapters to fit a variety of endoscopes; the trick is remembering to buy the adapters and have them handy.

TROCARS AND SLEEVES

Primary

Trocar sleeves used for the introduction of the laparoscope are usually 0.5-mm wider than the outside diameter of the laparoscope. A flap valve or trumpet valve is necessary to contain the intraabdominal gas during the insertion and removal of the laparoscope (Figure 1-1.13). The flap valve type is convenient, but it does not allow the operator to pull an object out of the abdomen (i.e., an intraabdominal intrauterine device), for the spring-loaded flap valve will close on the object during removal.

On the other hand, a trumpet valve is controlled manually by the external valve stem. Thus the valve can be kept in the open position as long as desired. Trumpet valves are harder to disassemble and clean than flap valves and must be replaced properly or they will freeze in their housing. All trocar sleeves require a flexible gasket to seal against leakage of gas between the laparoscope or secondary accessory and the inner wall of the trocar sleeve. Mismatched gaskets can create havoc during a laparoscopy. If the open-

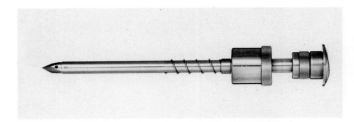

Figure 1-1.14 A secondary trocar and sleeve. This metal trocar sleeve with its flap valve reduces gas leakage while introducing secondary instruments. The spiral threads on the outside prevent undesirable movement of the sleeve when one removes secondary instruments. For electrosurgery use the all-metal sleeve to reduce the risk of a capacitance effect (see Chapter 3). (Courtesy of Karl Storz Co., Los Angeles, California.)

ing in the gasket is too small, it will tear during the introduction of the laparoscope or accessory tool, and leakage of gas may be beyond control. The problem of a gasket that is too large is obvious.

Several trocar sleeves use ''O'' ring gaskets. These have the advantage of long wear, and they cannot be mismatched once they are installed. A hub for tightening is used to hold the O ring in place; however, if the hub is tightened too much, flattening of the O ring will occur, which in effect reduces its inside diameter. When this happens the shaft of the laparoscope will not slide freely within the trocar sleeve; leave the O ring hub loose.

In the early 1970s, because of the reported electrical burns to the abdominal wall (owing to the use of high-voltage, high-wattage generators), fiberglass or Teflon laparoscope trocar sleeves were manufactured. By 1990, the generators manufactured for laparoscopy were much less powerful, and the nonconductive trocar sleeve became unnecessary. Because of the risk of capacitance (see Chapter 3), the Food and Drug Administration issued a regulation that all trocar sleeves larger than 7 mm should be metal.

Secondary Trocars and Sleeves

Secondary trocars and sleeves are available in a variety of diameters and lengths, most being made of nonconductive materials (Figure 1-1.14). Some have valves, others do not. The above comments about gaskets also apply to secondary trocar sleeves. The trocars have either pyramidal or conical tips on which pyramidal tips are usually used for larger trocar insertions. Pyramidal tips require repeated sharpening, or the thrusting power needed to penetrate the abdominal wall can become dangerous. Once again, this is an example of how proper maintenance in laparoscopy improves safety.

Disposable Trocars

In 1986 a disposable trocar and sleeve was introduced. Its advantage is a sharp pyramidal tip, a controllable flap

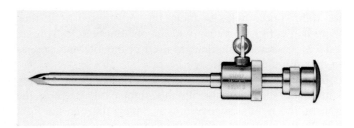

Figure 1-1.13 A metal laparoscope trocar and sleeve with a flap valve. (Courtesy of Karl Storz Co., Los Angeles, California.)

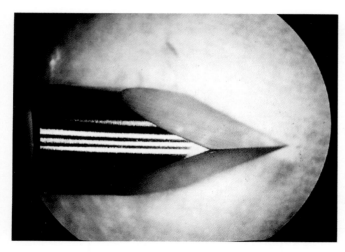

Figure 1-1.15 The disposable trocar tip is always sharp, which reduces the pressure needed to penetrate the abdominal wall. This allows for better control of entry and a margin of safety. (Courtesy of U.S. Surgical Corp., Norwalk, Connecticut.)

valve, and a protective sheath that springs out over the trocar tip after the abdominal wall has been penetrated (Figures 1-1.15 and 1-1.16). Another feature is the availability of interchangeable gaskets in assorted sizes, so smaller instruments can be placed through larger trocars without excessive loss of the distending gas. Though the cost of these instruments may seem high, the increased margin of safety and the elimination of the manpower hours for cleaning makes them an attractive addition to the cafeteria of laparoscopic accessories. In theory, the protective sleeve may reduce the incidence of bowel perforation and large vessel injury. After ten years of extensive use, there does not appear to be a reduction in intra-abdominal perforation because of the presence of a protective, retractable sheath. In fact, the term "safety shield" may lull the laparoscopist away from the strict protocols developed to prevent injury to intra-abdominal organs during the insertion of these sharp instruments.

SECONDARY INSTRUMENTS

There are a variety of diagnostic and operating secondary instruments. Many of the designs are being changed, and new instruments are being developed each year. Many of the secondary instruments have been redesigned for the 3-mm or 5-mm operating channel of the operating laparoscope.

In any basic set, an instrument for palpating and displacing the mobile viscera is necessary (Figure 1-1.17). Some type of grasping instrument is imperative. Insulated instruments are available for electrosurgery. The choice between

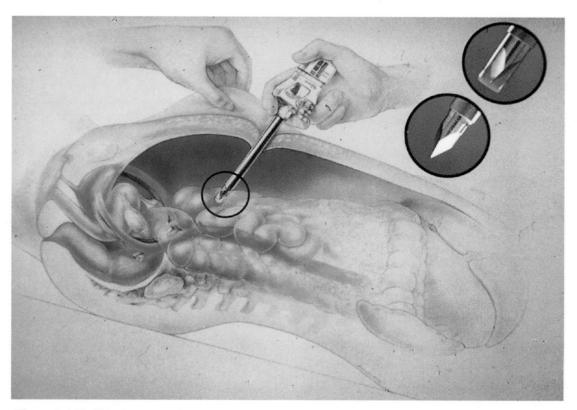

Figure 1-1.16 This disposable trocar and sleeve has a retractable, protective sleeve that will lock in place once the abdominal wall has been penetrated. (Courtesy of U.S. Surgical Corp., Norwalk, Connecticut.)

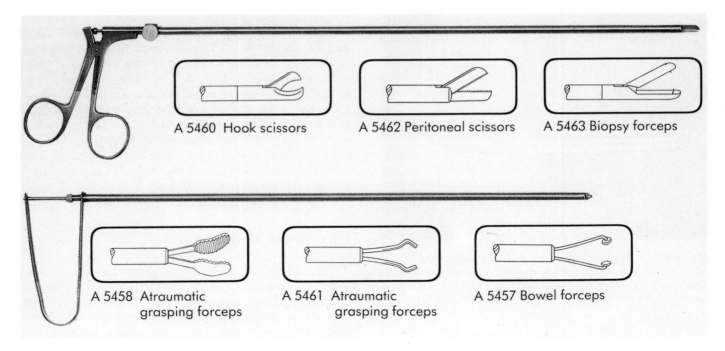

A 5460 Hook scissors

A 5462 Peritoneal scissors

A 5463 Biopsy forceps

A 5458 Atraumatic grasping forceps

A 5461 Atraumatic grasping forceps

A 5457 Bowel forceps

Figure 1-1.17 These are only a few examples of the vast and varied choices of secondary instruments for manipulation and active surgery. (Courtesy of Olympus Corp., Lake Success, New York.)

specialized instruments—such as scissors versus a knife—is an individual one, and those who are enthusiastic and knowledgeable about operative laparoscopy feel that all the instruments, with few exceptions, have a place in laparoscopy and should be available in the surgical suite.

A word of caution: Always read the instructions accompanying any secondary instrument. An example is the biopsy drill of Palmer; there are several different versions, and the mechanics can confuse the operator, thus raising a potential risk for the patient.

A special comment should be made about bipolar electrosurgical instruments. First, they can be used only with lowvoltage coagulators. They work best using a *cutting* waveform. These forceps are designed primarily for coagulation and are not meant to be effective against large bleeders. Thus unipolar systems must always be available in the operating theater.

UTERINE MANIPULATORS

In gynecologic laparoscopy, a ''must'' is some instrument placed into the endometrial cavity of the uterus that

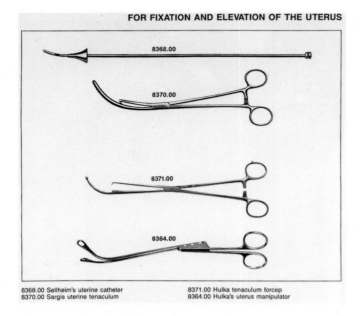

FOR FIXATION AND ELEVATION OF THE UTERUS

8368.00

8370.00

8371.00

8364.00

8368.00 Sellheim's uterine catheter
8370.00 Sargis uterine tenaculum
8371.00 Hulka tenaculum forcep
8364.00 Hulka's uterus manipulator

Figure 1-1.18 The top uterine manipulator can also be used for chromotubation. The bottom manipulator is designed for postabortion tubal sterilization procedures. (Courtesy of Richard Wolf Instruments Corp., Rosemont, Illinois.)

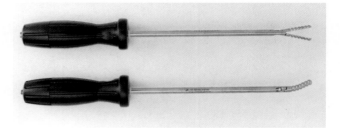

Figure 1-1.19 The Soderstrom uterine manipulator permits a 180° rotation to the uterus to help place the infundibular ligament on stretch for easy applications of instruments used in LAVH.

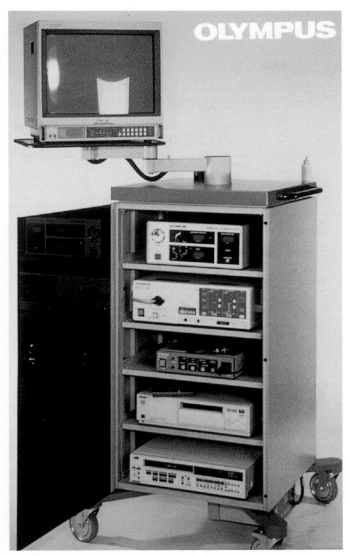

Figure 1-1.20 A mobile storage cart for laparoscope accessories and energy sources promotes good service and low maintenance requirements.

will extend far enough through the vaginal introitus to allow the operator and/or assistant to manipulate the uterus manually during the procedure (Figure 1-1.18). Many operators wish to include tubal insufflation in their procedure. The acorn-tipped tubal insufflation cannula has been redesigned specifically for laparoscopy. Melvin Cohen, MD, has introduced a springloaded channel into the shaft of his cannula, which attaches to the single-tooth tenaculum placed on the anterior lip of the cervix so that the cannula is self-sealing, thus preventing dye instillation leakage.

Stephen Corson, MD, has designed a similar acorn cannula, with the addition of a weighted handle, which is helpful in displacing the uterus anteriorly away from the small bowel, which might be contained in the pelvic cavity. It is particularly advantageous during tubal sterilization procedures using electrosurgery.

Because uterine perforation occurs occasionally with rigid uterine manipulators, H. Hasson, MD, has designed a balloon catheter for placement in the endometrial cavity. A semirigid metal tube inside the lumen of the catheter gives sufficient rigidity for uterine manipulation and allows the instillation of dye for tubal insufflation. The distended balloon prevents dye leakage.

For advanced laparoscopic procedures several uterine manipulators have been designed to increase the mobility of the uterus; they are especially helpful during laparoscopic assisted vaginal hysterectomy (LAVH). One such manipulator permits a 180° rotation of the uterus to help place the infundibular ligament on stretch for easy application of hemostatic clips or precise placement of electrical forceps (Figure 1-1.19).

TELEVISION EQUIPMENT

The introduction of small television cameras for use in laparoscopy has opened new opportunities for advanced laparoscopic procedures. Because of this, an entire chapter is devoted to this technology (Chapter 22–2). Complications during the training phase of laparoscopy were reduced markedly when television became an integral part of laparoscopic procedures.

CONCLUSION

In general, all kinds of laparoscopes perform their tasks well. Some can now be autoclaved—a debatable advantage since it has been shown after thousands of laparoscopies that gas sterilization every 24 hours, with cold sterilization (i.e., Cidex) between cases, is quite safe. As is true with any other fine optical instrument, proper maintenance is mandatory, and if possible, special personnel should be assigned to the care of laparoscopic equipment (Figure 1-1.20).

Unfortunately many parts—i.e., trocars and additional instruments—are not interchangeable from one company to another, so a hospital operating theater may be forced to use only one manufacturer's instrument and accessories. The laparoscopist must define his or her needs and goals, examine all instruments in coordination with surgical personnel, and finally review the existing equipment before making a purchase decision.

Operative Laparoscopy, Second Edition
The Masters' Techniques in Gynecologic Surgery
Lippincott–Raven Publishers, Philadelphia © 1998.

1-2   Endoscopy Equipment: Maintenance and Management

Wendy K. Winer

Gynecologic endoscopy has changed dramatically during the past two decades, due to changes in techniques made possible by new levels of technology in instruments and equipment. Nurses and physicians play an enormous role in the selection and use of these new items. This chapter describes maintenance and management of the newest hi-tech equipment now available or becoming available as operative endoscopy advances.

One of the key ingredients in providing the patient with optimal care is using quality instrumentation and equipment. All endoscopy team members must be properly trained in selection and use of this hi-tech instrumentation and equipment before, during, and after surgery, so that patients receive maximum benefit from advanced operative endoscopic procedures.

During the selection and purchase process, the initial focus should be on the videocamera and laparoscope. The adaptation of the camera to the scope enables surgeons and nurses to work together as an ''endoscopic team.'' Each member of the team: the surgeon, surgical assistant, surgical tech, circulating nurse, laser nurse and anesthesiologist, must be able to follow and anticipate as each observes the procedure on videomonitor.

Several things need to be addressed so everyone can benefit from this hi-tech environment. During the process of selecting instrumentation and equipment, all items that the operating room currently has for endoscopic procedures in all specialties must be evaluated. If at all possible, equipment that may be useful should be set aside and used. Since most hospitals and/or surgery centers have limited funds, establish a priority list, keeping quality and safety in mind. Several specialties may be able to share items, which could require some creative scheduling until all specialties have their own complete sets of instrumentation and equipment. Until the proper instrumentation and equipment is in place, and the entire ''endoscopic team'' has been thoroughly trained and credentialed for operative endoscopy, advanced procedures should not be done.

Effective selection of new equipment and instrumentation to complement what may already exist in the facility is the next step toward organization of an efficient setup and layout of these items. (Figure 1-2.1) A thorough evaluation and an understanding of these procedures must be done to make appropriate selection of materials. Begin by attending professional meetings to learn more about these procedures. Choose a meeting where a broad assortment of quality instrumentation and equipment is represented by many companies involved in manufacture of laparoscopic armamentarium, for example, the annual meeting of the American Association of Gynecologic Laparoscopists (AAGL). Physicians as well as operating room personnel should attend; I recommend a selection committee made up of physicians, nurses, and materials management people who work specifically with endoscopic procedures.

The Association of Operating Room Nurses (AORN) or The American College of Obstetrics and Gynecology (ACOG) are large meetings but are not as specialized as the AAGL for laparoscopy, although they do offer a wide array of all types of surgical instrumentation and equipment in the exhibit areas. Local AORN or surgeon meetings get multitudes of exhibitors, giving one the opportunity not only to see the equipment, but to make contact with local representatives. Smaller meetings may have an advantage by including laboratory sessions where the instrumentation and equipment can be used in a simulated ''hands-on'' session. After your selection team has narrowed down the possibilities, arrange for the company representatives to bring in the equipment and instrumentation on a trial basis.

Watching surgery performed by surgeons and surgical assistants who are recognized experts in this area may help a great deal in the selection process. In this way, one might be able to observe and see what they're using or learn why they like it. At the same time, one can get ideas of what setup and layout is used effectively by an experienced endoscopy team, to serve as a helpful guide in designing an efficient setup for your setting.

Ask colleagues what equipment has been successful for them. Scan and read pertinent medical journals and current books to learn more about these procedures and the material used. Meet the local representatives who cover your area to see how responsive and knowledgeable they are. *Once again, always attempt to get companies to bring the equipment to the operating room for everyone to try before a final decision on purchasing is made.* Select equipment from a company that not only has the best product but also has representatives who are the most attentive and responsive to proper training and use of the equipment. Before you purchase, investigate the company's maintenance policy. Speak with others who have purchased the same items to see how they've fared. Ask questions about the repair

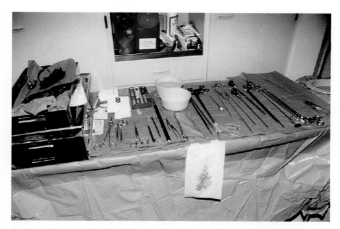

Figure 1-2.1 An effective setup, layout, and organization of instrumentation helps to promote optimal efficiency intra-operatively.

policy, turnaround time for repairs, warranty, and whether the firm will supply a comparable loaner when yours is being repaired or replaced. Find out where the manufacturer is located and how accessible replacement parts are. The selection committee needs to identify and make a checklist of criteria for what constitutes good equipment, according to your institution's needs. These criteria may include the quality of equipment, how well it functions, how often it breaks down, service and/or maintenance provided, whether it can be upgraded if it becomes obsolete or outdated, what type of training will be provided, and, of course, cost. It is important to know whether a piece of equipment offers flexibility: how many things can be done with the equipment and how much crossover between different specialities is possible, to make it financially more feasible?

Preferences may vary among surgeons in the same specialty. For example, in gynecology the selection may be based on an instrument or piece of equipment that the majority of gynecologists prefer, such as a particular manufacturer's videocamera, laparoscope, high flow insufflator, high intensity light source, videomonitor, and carts. After everyone has had an opportunity to evaluate and/or test the equipment, the selection committee makes a final decision. To avoid controversy over the choice, everyone who will be using these items should be given an opportunity to evaluate and comment on the equipment before purchase. Remember, cost should not be the only deciding factor; patient safety should always be the number one priority when final selection is made.

Once the equipment is ordered, the next step is to plan for education and training; the importance of this cannot be overemphasized. This should include proper use of the new equipment and correct care and maintenance. It works best when physicians and nurses are trained simultaneously. Ongoing education should be set up and regulated through the surgery's credentials committee. Proper maintenance should be taught by the company which manufactures the equipment. This includes proper care, handling, cleaning,

disassembly and assembly and how to troubleshoot the equipment if a malfunction occurs. Information about when and how to contact the company should be readily available with each piece of equipment, in case a malfunction occurs. Note: Many manufacturers have a phone number or emergency hotline that is answered 24 hours a day.

Below is a suggested list that one might use to serve as a guide during evaluations and in developing a checklist of key hysteroscopic and laparoscopic instrumentation and equipment made by some of the leading manufacturers who are responsive to gynecological surgeons' needs. Please keep in mind that this is only a guide based on this author's experience in endoscopy, and inherently subjective to what may be available in a particular locale.

Laparoscope

Evaluate what the desired degree is (i.e. zero degree), length, diameter (i.e. 10 mm is most often used, 5 mm may be desired in some instances, and 3 mm may be used for diagnostic procedures under minimal or IV sedation, to evaluate pain), straight or operative scope (operative is desired when using something through the operating channel, i.e., laser), monopolar or bipolar and/or scissors or grasper (length of these 5 mm instruments is generally 45 cm).

Videocamera

One-chip vs. three-chip—consider clarity, sharpness of picture, lines of resolution, and sufficient light.

Insufflator

A high flow insufflator is strongly recommended for advanced procedures, to maintain an abdominal pressure of approximately 15 mm HG. Maintaining the pneumoperitoneum is of paramount importance when suctioning fluid, laser plume or electrosurgery smoke. Extra gas tanks should be kept on hand (upright and stored at the proper temperature), as well as proper tubing with an in-line filter. Note: Never use a laparoscopy insufflator for hysteroscopy.

Electrosurgery Generator

Always have a backup generator, foot pedal, cord, and bipolar instrument. Use a generator that allows both monopolar and bipolar. Newer generators supply more power for bipolar as compared to older microbipolar generators. Note: Always be sure the patient has been grounded when using monopolar. A curved bipolar dissecting forcep is quite helpful during these procedures to increase efficiency during surgery. It can function as an excellent bipolar as well as an effective grasper.

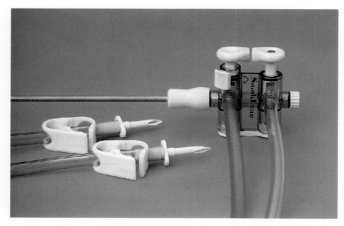

Figure 1-2.2 An excellent irrigation system which has the capacity to deliver a minimum of pressure of 300 mm Hg is used. (Photo courtesy of Davol, Inc., Cranston, RI.)

Suction/Irrigation

An efficient irrigation system is of paramount importance for good visibility (Figures 1-2.2 and 1-2.3). A pressurized system is recommended with a disposable trumpet valve system that is easy to handle, and should have nonsticking trumpet valves with no leakage. Irrigation probes vary in length and diameter. Most common is 28 cm or 33 cm length, 5 mm diameter with holes around the atraumatic tip. A probe 10 mm in diameter with holes (pool tip) may be helpful for use when a large amount of irrigating and suctioning is done, i.e. dermoid cyst or large leiomyomata. It is worthwhile to keep a set of sterile, reusable tips, because the disposable probe may only come in a 5 mm diameter as well as in one particular length (Figure 1-2.4). Suction canisters should have a built-in filter, to keep the central in-wall suction system from clogging. Large canisters may be helpful when large amounts of fluid are used, as they are in operative hysteroscopy and advanced operative laparoscopic procedures.

Laser-Carbon Dioxide (CO₂), Neodymium YAG (Nd: YAG)

With the Nd:YAG laser a contact tip, ERP6 or ERP4, is preferable for laparoscopy (11 mm fibers are recommended to be used through the operating channel of the scope) or a KTP laser. No one should operate the laser who has not been properly trained and earned credentials. Proper laser safety guidelines should be established by the laser-credentialling committee of the hospital or surgery center, and followed by all members of the endoscopy team. This will vary depending on the laser wavelength used, and could include items like proper protective eye wear for the patient and everyone in the operating room, ''laser in use'' sign on the operating room door, and goggles hanging on

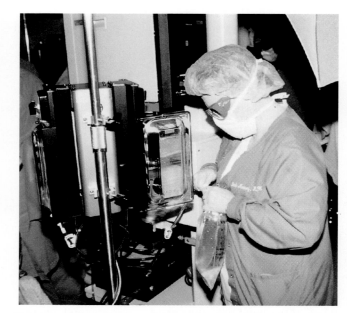

Figure 1-2.3 A disposable hand-held system with trumpet valves to irrigate easily and to suction, is used as part of this pressurized system. (Photo courtesy of Davol, Inc., Cranston, RI.)

the door for anyone who enters. A fire extinguisher should always be kept in the room or just outside the door.

Hazardous Waste Machine

It is helpful to purchase a hazardous-waste machine for safe disposal of fluids and/or sharps. This will help to reduce the risk to health care workers.

Warming Device

By maintaining the temperature of the irrigation (bags of fluid) a warming device may help in maintaining patient's

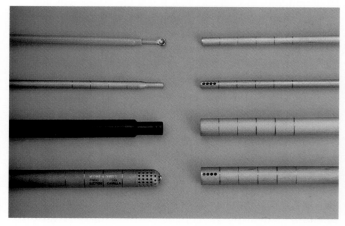

Figure 1-2.4 A set of reusable irrigation probes may be desired.

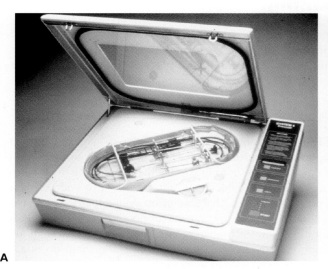
A

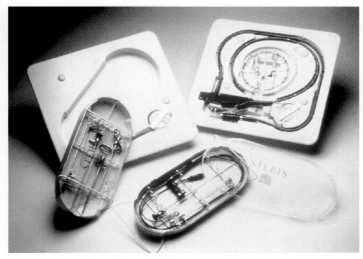
B

Figure 1-2.5 A. The Steris I system of liquid sterilization of cameras and endoscopics with paracetic acid has proven to be an effective sterilizer in many institutions. **B.** Many various trays are available depending on the type of scopes being sterilized, i.e. flexible, rigid or scopes with an operating channel. (Photos courtesy of Steris Corporation, Mentor, OH.)

body temperature, as well as decreasing laparoscope fogging during the procedure.

Light Sources

High-powered Xenon-type light source. The best picture may occur when the laparoscope, camera, light source, and light cord are all manufactured by the same company. Always keep a back-up light bulb and light cord. Label the light source with the date a new bulb has been installed. These bulbs generally should be changed by someone who has been instructed by the manufacturer in the proper way to do this (preferably a biomedical engineer); otherwise, this machine should not be opened.

Hand-held Instruments

Reusable 5 mm grasper (atraumatic and traumatic) and scissors are advisable, to reduce the cost of disposable scissors and reusable scissors which need to be sent out frequently for sharpening. There are reusable scissors with a tip that is reused for numerous procedures until it becomes dull. When this occurs, the tip is detached from the reusable handle and replaced. In addition, it is useful to have a 10 mm claw-type grasper for tissue removal, and 10-mm scissors for morcellation of large pieces of tissue. Note: Be sure all handheld instruments that are used with electrosurgery are properly insulated. Instruments that are labeled as disposable by the manufacturer should not be reused. In many cases, these instruments cannot be safely resterilized, and their insulation is often damaged during autoclaving. Before each use, all instruments must be checked for insulation, and must be op-

erating properly with all screws intact. Some companies are refurbishing disposable instruments and testing them to ensure their level of safety and integrity. To ensure safety, the user should carefully read the manufacturers' warranty and any instructions accompanying the instrument.

Sterilization of Endoscopes—Autoclave vs. Liquid Sterilization

Camera manufacturers recommend draping of cameras to prolong their life expectancy. Many new scopes are being made autoclavable (Figure 1-2.5). This may vary from one country to another due to variations in temperatures and lengths of steam sterilization. When in doubt, never steam-autoclave a scope without checking with the manufacturer first.

Hanging Orbiters vs. Carts

Orbiters offer many nice features, but they are expensive and may be difficult to move. If you select a cart, be sure it is accessible from the back, and is the proper height for the surgical team (Figure 1-2.6).

Suturing Instrumentation

Needle drivers, knot pusher, and needle grasper are essential for endoscopic suturing needs.

Patient Warming Device

The equipment is used intraoperatively and/or postoperatively to maintain patient's body temperature.

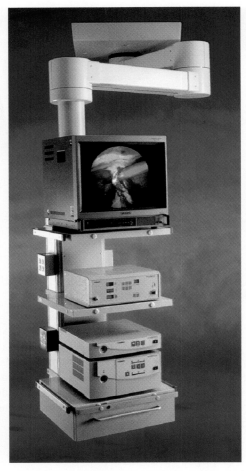

Figure 1-2.6 Hanging orbiters can save room and get the cords off the floor. (Photo courtesy of Heraeus Surgical, Inc., Milpitas, CA.)

Bipolar Instrumentation

Bipolar graspers that are multifunctional may save operating time by being as versatile as an efficient grasper and an excellent coagulator. Note: A disposable bipolar forceps may be preferable because of fewer malfunctions and easy assembly. Always keep a backup forceps and cord (sterile).

Trocars and Veress Needle

Reusable vs. Disposable trocars (diameter i.e. 5 mm, 10/11 mm and/or 12 mm with or without stabilizers and with a reducer) and a Veress Needle. If using a reusable Veress needle, be sure it is properly cleaned. The opening of these two shafts should line up correctly. The spring mechanism and valve must work smoothly.

Stirrups

These should be padded so the patient is protected from nerve damage and/or tissue damage and should be easy

to position and readjust preoperatively as well as intra-operatively. The patient's heel should be seated in the stirrups without pressure on the calves. All Velcro straps should be loose enough to place 2 fingers between the patient's leg and the straps.

Videomonitors

High resolution Videomonitors (the 19″ size is the most popular), should have at least as many lines of resolution as the videocamera to maximize the benefit of a good camera. In addition, cables to monitors should be wide enough to provide the amount of resolution available in many newer cameras and monitors. Whenever possible, use at least two monitors, one for the surgeon and one for the surgical assistant. The rest of the team can position themselves accordingly to be able to view the procedure. Important note: Assistant's monitor should be the same size and as close as possible to the quality of the surgeon's monitor in order to provide optimal assistance during the procedure.

Videorecorders

There are several available: VHS, 8 mm, and Betacam.

Morcellator: Harmonic Scalpel or Laparosonic Coagulating Shears (LCS)

The 5 mm hook of the harmonic scalpel or 10 mm LCS coagulates, and is an efficient cutter and/or morcellator (Figure 1-2.7).

Uterine Manipulator

This instrument is reusable, and has a variety of tips. It offers versatility, i.e., for dye injection and is a good manipulator for a large uterine myomectomy or hysterectomy.

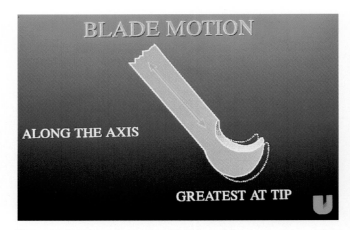

Figure 1-2.7 The 5 mm hook probe of the harmonic scalpel is an efficient way to morcellate tissue, cut, and coagulate. (Photo courtesy of Ethicon Endosurgery, Inc., Cincinnati, OH.)

Hysteroscope

Types include both flexible and rigid 4 to 6 mm diameter (Figure 1-2.8).

Cystoscopy

Because more and more gynecologists who are doing laparoscopic bladder neck suspensions (laparoscopic Burch procedure) are doing cystoscopy at the end of the procedure, a 30° and/or 70° cystoscope may be considered.

Additional Items to Consider

Videoprinter, endoscopic organizer pouch, 16 French foley catheter with drainage bag, an under-buttocks drape for hysteroscopy and/or cystoscopy, suture at least 27″ to 30″ in length to be used laparoscopically, 5 mm atraumatic dissector (Kittner or 10 mm cherry dissector), foam rubber padding for patient's arms and neck, laparoscopy pack, wide hysteroscopy and/or cystoscopy tubing and 1 back table, 2 mayos (vaginal and laparoscopic), and an additional back table for operative hysteroscopy or laparoscopic-assisted vaginal hysterectomy. In addition, a sterile D&C setup is often used on the vaginal mayo. Note: Always have a sterile laparotomy setup in the operating suite, in case a laparoscopy must be converted to a laparotomy. Materials such as Interceed (an absorbable adhesion barrier), mesh (i.e. Vicryl, Proline, Gortex, or Mersilene), and hemostatic agents (Instat, Surgical or Thrombin) may be used during laparoscopic procedures. These should be available in the operating room suite in case the surgeon desires to use them.

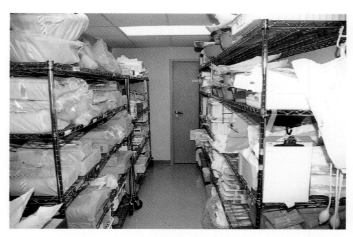

Figure 1-2.9 Instrumentation should be properly packaged and labeled for easy recognition.

Maintenance of Equipment

In addition to having the "endoscopic team" specially trained by the manufacturer, a "maintenance team" should be organized that focuses on endoscopic instrumentation and equipment.

The same group of technicians should regularly care for these items. In that way, they will be familiar with the specific "do's" and "dont's," and proper disassembly and assembly. It is important that all items be carefully packaged, labeled and kept together (Figure 1-2.9). Each instrument or piece of equipment often has specific screws, adapters, seals, and parts that, if misplaced, could prevent it from being used; this could, potentially, cause a case to be canceled. Because of this potential problem, purchase and store backup parts in a convenient location, in case one is misplaced, broken, or lost. All items that are not disposable must be carefully handled at the end of each procedure so they are not inadvertently discarded. All equipment should be properly turned off at the completion of the procedure, and gas tanks securely closed. Careful handling and transfer of the patient to the recovery room, followed by the careful handling and cleaning of instrumentation and equipment, is vitally important upon completion of the procedure.

Proper cleaning and sterilization instructions are also critical for all items. Most disposables are not meant to be re-sterilized. Whether a scope or instrument may be safely steam-autoclaved is important. Many of these items cost thousands of dollars and if they are inappropriately sterilized, it not only may ruin the instrument, but also could present an unsafe environment for the patient. When in doubt, do not steam-autoclave. Being sure screws are tightened and seals are in proper working order is extremely important, particularly in videocameras. A torn seal may make the difference between a clear picture and a foggy one if moisture penetrates the camera seals. The proper tools to fix these things must be kept readily available and

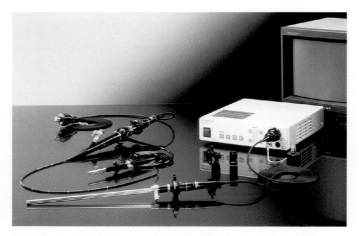

Figure 1-2.8 Office hysteroscopy with a flexible hysteroscope, videocamera, small 8″ or 13″ monitor and light source can be quite useful for diagnostic procedures in the office, with the patient experiencing little or no discomfort. This saves the patient from having a general anesthetic in surgery.

clearly labeled, so everyone knows where they are. If the seals of the scope or camera need to be replaced, this should be done by the manufacturer.

Preference cards should be kept for all surgeons, that correspond with each endoscopic procedure they do. A diagram should be included which shows such things as how they prefer the position of the patient's arms and legs. In addition, the cards should list and diagram the placement of all equipment, monitors, and the energy sources the surgeons prefer. This helps operating room personnel when a circulating nurse or surgical technician is absent, or when a case is done during the night. A notebook should be kept with the step-by-step instructions on how to operate all equipment, and on proper maintenance and care of endoscopic instrumentation and equipment.

Operative endoscopy has the potential to be extremely beneficial to the patient. The single most important thing the entire endoscopy team can do to help ensure that this occurs safely and efficiently is for everyone to be properly trained in these advanced procedures. This in turn promotes the proper selection, care, and maintenance of the entire range of endoscopic instrumentation and equipment. Through continued training and education, patients will have the opportunity to benefit from this new high-tech endoscopic environment, evidenced by improved surgical outcomes.

SUGGESTED READING

Amsco's *Positioning patients for surgery*. AMSCO Education Services, 1987:1–3, 12.

Association of Operating Room Nurses 1996. *1996 Standards & Recommended Practices*, 95–125, 163–9, 191–211, 233.

Association of Operating Room Nurses. New sterilization technology. *Surgic Serv Mgmt* 1995;2:4–44.

Carter J. A new technique of fascial closure for laparoscopic incisions. *J of Laparoendosc Surg* 1994;4:143–8.

Corfman R, Diamond M, DeCherney A. *Complications of Laparoscopy and Hysteroscopy*. 1993.

Deprest JA, Cusumano PG eds. Posterior pelvic floor repair. In: *Advanced Gynecologic Laparoscopy*. New York: The Parthenon Group; 1996; 175–83.

Gomel V. Operative laparoscopy: time for acceptance. *Fertil Steril* 1989;52:1–11.

Gomel V, Taylor PJ. Diagnostic and operative gynecologic laparoscopy. St. Louis: Mosby Year Book; 1995.

Gruendenmann B. *Positioning plus*. Education Department, Devon Industries, Inc., May, 1984.

Hulka JF, Reich H eds. *Textbook of Laparoscopy*, 2 ed, Philadelphia: W.B. Saunders, 1994.

Hulka JF, Reich H, eds. *Textbook of Laparoscopy*, In 3rd ed, Philadelphia: W.B. Saunders, in press.

Kadar N. Randomized trials involving laparoscopic surgery: valid research strategy or academic gimmick? *J Gynecol Endosc* 1994;3:69–73.

Kelly HA. *Operative Gynecology*, New York: Appleton, 1988.

Liu CY. *Laparoscopic Hysterectomy and Pelvic Floor Reconstruction*, Blackwell Science, 1996.

Lyons TL. Laparoscopic resection of rectovaginal endometriosis using the contact ND: YAG laser and primary closure with suturing techniques. *J Pelv Surg* 1996;2:8–11.

Lyons TL, Winer WK. The Nolan-Lyons modification of the Burch procedure. *Journal of the American Association of Gynecologic Laparoscopists* 1995;2:95–9.

Lyons TL, Winer WK. Vaginal vault suspension. *Endosc Surg & Allied Tech* 1995;3:88–92.

Lyons TL. Laparoscopic treatment of urinary stress incontinence. *Atlas of Laparoscopic Techniques for Gynecologists*. Tulandi; 1994:131–6.

Martin DC, Diamond MP. Operative laparoscopy comparison of lasers with other techniques. *Curr Probl Obstet Gynecol Fert* 1986;9:656–8.

Meeker M, Rothrock J. *Alexander's Care of the Patient in Surgery*, St. Louis: Mosby Year Book; 1995;3:211, 1263.

Nezhat C, Winer WK, Cooper JD, *et al.* Endoscopic infertility surgery. *J Reprod Med*. 1989;34:127–34.

Nezhat F, Winer WK, Nezhat C. Salpingectomy via laparoscopy: a new surgical approach. *J Laparoendosc Surg* 1991;1:91–5.

Nezhat F, Winer WK, Nezhat C. Fimbrioscopy and salpingoscopy in patients with minimal to moderate pelvic endometriosis. *Obstet Gynecol* 1990;75:15–7.

Nezhat F, Winer WK, Nezhat C. Laparoscopic removal of dermoid cysts. *Obstet Gynecol* 1989;73:279–81.

Nezhat C, Winer WK, Nezhat F. A comparison of the CO_2, argon and KTP 532 lasers in the videolaserscopic treatment of endometriosis. *Colposc Gynecol Laser Surg* 1988;4:4–47.

Nezhat F, Winer WK, Nezhat C. Is endoscopic treatment of endometriosis and endometrioma associated with better results than laparotomy? *Am J Gyn Health* 1988;2:10–6.

Nezhat F, Winer WK, Nezhat C. Videolaparoscopy and videolaseroscopy: alternatives to major surgery? *Female Patient* 1988;13:46–53.

Nezhat F, Winer WK, Crowgey S. Videolaseroscopy for treatment of endometriosis and other diseases of the reproductive organs. *Obstet Gynecol Forum* 1987;1:2–5.

Schmaus D, Nelson S, Davis D. Association of Operating Room Nurses. Positioning the Surgical Patient. 1986:1–6, 40–4.

Semm K. Instruments and equipment for endoscopic abdominal surgery. In: *Operative Manual for Endoscopic Abdominal Surgery*. Semm K (ed). Chicago: Year Book; 1987:46–123.

Soderstrom R. *Operative Laparoscopy, The Masters' Techniques*. New York: Raven Press, Ltd; 1993:1–15, 47–86.

Sutton & Diamond. *Endoscopic Surgery for Gynaecologists*, 2nd ed. Role of the operating room nurse. London: Philadelphia: W.B. Saunders, in press.

Thompson JD, Rock JA. *Te Linde's Operative Gynecology*. Philadelphia: JB Lippincott; 1993:1–12.

Winer WK. A laparoscopic approach to rectocele repair. *Today's Surg Nurse* 1996;18:37–40.

Winer WK. Thorough patient followup encouraged for all cases, not just research and booklets help prepare patients for laparoscopy, ensure informed consent. *Laparoscopic Surg Update* 1996;4:28–31.

Winer WK. Operating room personnel. *Operative Gynecologic Endoscopy*. In 2nd ed., Sanfilippo JS, Levine RL, eds. New York: Springer-Verlag; 1996:412–22.

Winer WK. New procedures for women that are being done endoscopically. *Min Inv Surg Nurs* 1995;9:87–9.

Winer WK. Nursing aspects of gynecologic endoscopy. In: McLucas B, ed., *Endosc Surg and Allied Tech* 1995:109–11.

Winer WK. Why the use of lasers in gynecological laparoscopy has declined. *Min Inv Surg Nurs* 1994;8:138–9.

Winer WK. Harmonic scalpel. What it is, is it better than laser, electrosurgery or scissors for advanced operative laparoscopic procedures? *Lasers and Advanced Technology Specialty Assembly Newsletter for AORN*. 1994;2:2.

Winer WK. Minimal access surgery for nurses and technicians. *Gynaecology*. Hall FA, ed. Oxford: Radcliffe Medical Press; 1994:94–109.

Winer WK. A comparison of the CO_2 laser and the harmonic scalpel. *Min Inv Surg Nurs* 1993;7:54–6.

Winer WK. The role of the operating room staff in operative laparoscopy. *J Am Assoc Gynecol Laparosc* 1993;1:86–8.

Winer WK. The set-up for operative endoscopy. *Laser Nurs* 1991;5:139–145.

Winer WK, Lyons TL. Suggested set-up and layout of instrumentation for advanced operative laparoscopy. *JAAGL* 1995;2:117–20.

Yuzpe AA. Television in laparoscopy. *Laparoscopy*. Phillips JM, Corson SL, Keith L, *et al.*, eds. Baltimore: Williams & Wilkins; 1977:306–25.

APPENDIX 1-2A

Equipment—Review of Responsibility

I. Instruments
  A. Remove instrument tray.
  B. Check contents for:
    1. Laparoscopic optics
    2. Laparoscopic sleeve with trumpet valve (10-mm: check valves to make sure they operate)
    3. Trocar
    4. Veress needle
    5. Fiberoptic cable
    6. CO_2 tubing
    7. 6-mm fiber sleeve, red rubber gasket
    8. Atraumatic and traumatic forceps
    9. Electrical cable
    10. Electrosurgical instruments, i.e., proper insulation
    11. Irrigation/suction. Note: verify no broken or malfunctioning instruments. Always have a backup sterile bipolar or monopolar as well as a card (peel pack sterile cards).
  C. Autoclave tray contents for 10 to 20 minutes.
  D. Sterilize endoscopes and light cord in steris (liquid sterilizer). Average cycle takes 30 minutes.
II. Gas regulator
  A. Check main gas tank. Open valve. Needle in gauge on left should rest in colored zone. If below this area, tank will need replacement soon.
  B. Open "fill" valve. Middle gauge needle should rotate from 5 L (or 10 L) to 0 L. The ball in the ball valve cylinder should rise to the top.
  C. Close off the gas outlet. The ball in the ball valve cylinder should drop to the bottom. The needle in the right-hand (pressure) gauge should rise to the colored area.
  D. If the above do not occur as indicated, check to see whether the flow knob is on "automatic." If so, it should be replaced to its regular ("hand") position.
III. Light source
  A. Plug-in light protector
  B. Turn dial on; make sure light bulbs are working. Keep light off until surgeon requests; light.
  C. Have spare bulb available.
  D. **NEVER** leave a light cord unattached lying on the drapes, because they may catch fire.
IV. Electrosurgical source
  A. Plug in apparatus. Check to make sure it is operating.
  B. Check functioning of foot switch.
  C. Check electrical integrity of base place (return electrode) and its plug.
  D. Use disposable ground plate.
  E. Set coagulating current on low setting.
  F. Turn instrument off.
  G. Turn instrument on *only* when surgeon requests it, and off during the procedure when he or she requests it.
V. After the procedure (to be the responsibility of the surgical tech)
  A. Disassemble and wash all instruments in cool soapy water and rinse in clean water at temperature less than 100°F.
  B. Dry all instruments and replace them in large tray as they were found. Be sure no adapters or small pieces are lost.
VI. Nursing staff
  A. Turn off main CO_2 valve.
  B. Open flow regulator valve gently until no flow registers.
  C. Replace instrument tray on top shelf.
  D. Allow light projector fan to run for 5 minutes, then turn off.
  E. Store auxiliary instruments on lower shelf and lock.
  F. Place laparoscopy stirrups on shelf.
VII. "Laparoscopy set"—Autoclave:
  A. 1 sponge forceps for prep.
  B. 1 4-inch basin for prep material.
  C. 1 urethral catheter (or Foley).
  D. 1 single-hinged Graves speculum (or 2 Sims).
  E. 1 controlling tenaculum (9-inch).
  F. 3 towel clips.
  G. 1 scalpel holder (for No. 15 or 11 blade).
  H. 1 long metal boat.
  I. Suture or clips (do not open until you're sure the surgeon will use this—RNFA can help with this).
  J. 1 needle holder.
  K. 1 Mouse-tooth pickup forceps.
  L. After suitable distention of the abdomen with gas, the doctor will withdraw the Veress needle. The patient is placed in 15° to 30° Trendelenburg position.
  M. The umbilical incision may be widened with the knife blade.
  N. The larger trocar and cannula are inserted. (A prior check is made by the scrub nurse to determine that the trumpet valve on the cannula is working properly.)
  O. The laparoscope itself has been soaking in warm (not hot) saline; it is handed to the doctor and connected to the light table. Using an antifog agent may help if placed on the tip of the scope 15 minutes prior to insertion.
  P. After viewing the pelvic organs, the doctor may wish to insert ancillary instruments, either
    1. Through the operating laparoscope, or
    2. Through a second incision.
  Q. In cases of tubal sterilization, the coagulating equipment will be turned on and attached to the appropriated instruments.

R. If the patient has a fertility problem, the doctor may want to ascertain tubal patency. A dye (methylene blue or indigo carmine), diluted in 10 ml of saline, should be available to be injected through the cannula in the cervix.

S. At the conclusion of the procedure, the gas is allowed to escape from the abdomen; all of the instruments are removed. (Remember the instruments in the vagina.) The skin incisions are closed, usually with a subcuticular stitch, occasionally with clips or Steri-Strips.

T. *Important:* Be sure that the laparoscopy equipment is handled carefully and turned over to responsible personnel for proper cleaning and sterilization.

APPENDIX 1-2B

Nurses' Instructions

I. Instrument preparation
   A. Instruments are to be taken apart and thoroughly cleaned, i.e., by hand and then ultrasonic cleaner.
      1. Gas sterilized or
      2. Steris (liquid sterilization for endoscopes and cord) for a single cycle of 30 minutes.
      3. Autoclave (do not autoclave scopes or cord unless authorized by the manufacturer).
   B. Have warm sterile saline available, not over 100°F.
   C. The following should be present in the room:
      1. Fiberoptic light source.
      2. Insufflating apparatus (CO_2 or N_2O), preferably high flow.
      3. Apparatus for coagulation.
      4. Laparoscopy equipment and instrumentation.

II. Patient preparation
   A. If possible, the intravenous line is to be placed in the patient's arm opposite to where the surgeon stands.
   B. Patients are catheterized after abdominal prep. Have catheterization equipment available, including material for a perineal prep. Attach catheter to a drainage bag for calibration throughout the procedure.
   C. The patient need not be shaved (unless requested by the surgeon). An abdominal and vaginal prep is done, unless nothing is to be used in the vagina intraoperatively.
   D. The patient is placed on the operating table with both arms tucked in at her side.
   E. The doctor will indicate whether he wishes to use
      1. The dorsal position with the instruments in the vagina extended beneath the table, or
      2. Leg holders, or
      3. Knee stirrups (positioned at approximately 45°).
   F. The coagulator ground plate is placed in contact with the patient if monopolar is to be used; not necessary with bipolar.

III. Procedure
   A. The anesthetic is begun.
   B. The patient is catheterized (French or Foley, no. 16); the catheter is left in place and attached to the thigh with adhesive tape. Caution: be sure there is no tension on the catheter.
   C. The doctor inserts a uterine manipulator or cannula utilizing a single-tooth tenaculum.
   D. The nurse performs the abdominal prep and paints with Betadine (cleaning the navel thoroughly: use Q-tips when necessary).
   E. The patient is draped with a routine lap sheet.
   F. The insufflation apparatus is checked to determine that
      1. There is CO_2 in the tank.
      2. The valve is opened.
   G. The light apparatus is checked to be sure that
      1. The bulb is in working order.
      2. The fiberoptic cord is attached to the light source after it is securely attached to the scope.
   H. The coagulator machine should be readily available, the ground plate attached to the patient, and the cord to the machine, and the foot pedal in proper position. (Broad plate is not necessary if only bipolar coagulator is used.)
   I. The doctor makes the umbilical incision (no. 15 or no. 11 blade).
   J. The Veress needle is attached to the insufflator tubing to check the intrinsic pressure and to be certain the needle is patent. Then the needle is inserted into the peritoneum. (Have a 10 mL Luer-Lok syringe available, with normal saline.)
   K. The tubing from the insufflator is connected to the Veress needle. The doctor will direct the nurse as to the adjustment of the flow gas.
   L. After suitable distention of the abdomen with gas, the doctor will withdraw the Veress needle. The patient is placed in 15° to 30° Trendelenburg position.
   M. The umbilical incision may be widened with the knife blade.
   N. The larger trocar and cannula are inserted. (A prior check is made by the scrub nurse to determine that the trumpet valve on the cannula is working properly.) After the trocar is placed, the abdomen is insufflated through the trocar insufflation port followed by the placement of the laparoscope through the trocar sleeve.

Operative Laparoscopy, Second Edition
The Masters' Techniques in Gynecologic Surgery
Lippincott–Raven Publishers, Philadelphia © 1998.

2

Technique

2-1 Physiologic Considerations during Anesthesia for Laparoscopy

Richard M. Soderstrom

There are two major debates in the anesthesia literature on proper technique for laparoscopic surgery. The first regards whether intubation is always necessary. Neophytes in anesthesiology for laparoscopy would be well advised to start out by intubating all of their patients, providing assisted ventilation. Avoid assisting or controlling respiration by mask so as not to inflate the stomach. If one chooses not to intubate, extreme care should be taken to provide a clear airway, and if any question of stomach distention is raised, a Levine tube should be passed. Though it has been shown that the risk of gastric regurgitation is minimal during laparoscopy, adequate suction and intubation equipment should be readily available. There is general agreement that intubation is mandatory for the obese, in all cases.

INSUFFLATION COMPLICATIONS

It has been shown that carbon dioxide retention plus halothane anesthesia increases the chance of cardiac arrhythmias. Since cardiac arrhythmias are the first sign of impending problems, a precordial or esophageal stethoscope is recommended. Bradycardia is associated with increased abdominal pressure and impaired venous return, produced by insufflation.

The second controversy regards the choice of nitrous oxide or carbon dioxide as the anesthetic agent. The following is a brief outline of the pros and cons of each gas:

- Carbon dioxide
  1. pro
     - (a) does not support combustion or explosion
     - (b) is rapidly absorbed from the abdominal cavity, reducing chances of postoperative shoulder pain
     - (c) is rapidly soluble in blood, so the chance of gas embolism is reduced unless large volumes are insufflated
  2. con
     - (a) is not readily available in most operating rooms
     - (b) hypercarbia a threat if assisted ventilation is not adequate
     - (c) causes peritoneal discomfort when using local anesthesia
- nitrous oxide
  1. pro
     - (a) readily available in most operating rooms
     - (b) hypercarbia not a threat, particularly in the non-intubated patient
     - (c) is not explosive
  2. con
     - (a) supports combustion at the same kindle point as common room air
     - (b) is absorbed slower than carbon dioxide from abdominal cavity and following accidental intramuscular insufflation (i.e., 68% the absorption rate of carbon dioxide gas.)

The basic problems with carbon dioxide insufflation are possible hypercarbia and abdominal discomfort. To prevent this, intubate and use hyperventilation. I am among the minority who use and favor nitrous oxide over carbon dioxide. The usual concern with nitrous oxide is its ability to support combustion; in Seattle, Washington, over 20,000 cases of laparoscopy with electrocoagulation have been performed without a combustion complication.

Of the deaths associated with laparoscopy, anesthetic complications lead the list of causes. The following outline should be familiar to the laparoscopic surgical team.

I. General anesthesia
  A. Respiratory complications

- Airway pressure rises, with decrease in compliance due to increase in abdominal pressure and head-down position.
- Pulmonary shunt increases, with decrease in arterial oxygen tension.
- Arterial carbon dioxide tension rises from peritoneal absorption of carbon dioxide and hypoventilation.
- Regurgitation and pulmonary aspiration of stomach contents occur due to increase in gastric pressure, gas (usually oxygen) in the stomach, or from bagging before intubation and head-down position.
- Sore throat occurs due to traumatic intubation.
  1. Prevention and management
     (a) Use minimum amount of inflating gas (2 to 3 L).
     (b) Maintain good muscle relaxation with no bucking or straining in order to reduce abdominal and airway pressures.
     (c) Avoid extreme head-down position and utilize intrauterine cannula for manipulation and exposure of pelvic organs.
     (d) Employ mild controlled hyperventilation (not excessive) to avoid hypercapnea.
     (e) Increase inspired oxygen concentration to prevent hypoxia.
     (f) Intubate trachea to secure clear airway, to control ventilation without pushing air into the stomach, and to prevent aspiration.
     (g) Use semilithotomy position to reduce abdominal pressure.

B. Cardiovascular complications
- Venous return is reduced, with decrease in cardiac output from pneumoperitoneum and positive-pressure ventilation (partially compensated by Trendelenburg and lithotomy position).
- Arrhythmia from hypercapnea is induced by peritoneal absorption of carbon dioxide or hypoventilation.
- Pulse pressure narrows due to cardiac compression caused by pneumoperitoneum.
- Bradycardia is induced by peritoneal stretching.
  1. Prevention and management
     (a) Use minimum amount of inflating gas to avoid excessive intraperitoneal pressure.
     (b) Employ slow rate and large tidal volume ventilation, to reduce mean airway pressure, to promote better venous return, and to decrease shunting.
     (c) Use anticholinergic drug to block vagal hyperactivity.

C. Gastrointestinal complications
- Stomach distends with gas, induced by bagging for oxygenation before intubation.

- Gastric perforation occurs due to passage of a needle or a trocar through a distended stomach.
- Regurgitation and aspiration occur.
  1. Prevention and management
     (a) Avoid bagging (controlled ventilation) before intubation. (Occlude esophagus with cricoid pressure if bagging is necessary.)
     (b) Obtain oxygenation before intubation with patient's spontaneous respiration.
     (c) Deflate distended stomach with nasogastric tube before insertion of a needle or a trocar.
     (d) Use endotracheal anesthesia to prevent distention of stomach and aspiration.

D. Neuromuscular complications
- Postfasciculation muscle pain is experienced, due to use of succinylcholine.
- Brachial nerve palsy occurs due to stretched-out arms.
  1. Prevention and management
     (a) Pretreat patient with small dose of curare (3 mg) or Pavulon (0.5 mg) 2 to 3 minutes before succinylcholine injection.
     (b) Tuck in one arm on the surgeon's side and avoid any pressure on major nerves.
     (c) Turn patient's head to the side where the arm is out to avoid overstretching of plexus.

II. Local anesthesia
A. Complications from intravenous analgesics
- Phlebitis may occur with use of diazepam.
- Respiratory depression (apnea) may occur with use of narcotic analgesics.
- Arterial carbon dioxide may rise from carboperitoneum and respiratory depression induced by analgesia.
- Inadequate analgesia or sedation is possible.
  1. Prevention and management
     (a) Dilute intravenously given drugs by selecting a large-caliber vein, and use rapid infusion of intravenous fluid during injection to reduce the local concentration of drugs and thus the incidence of phlebitis.
     (b) Avoid excessive dose of analgesic to prevent respiratory depression.
     (c) Have anesthetist stand by for ventilatory assistance and airway management. Consider using nitrous oxide.

B. Complications from local anesthetic
- Anaphylaxis
- Seizure due to overdose
- Bradycardia
- Bruising at site of injection
  1. Prevention and management
     (a) Take careful past history of local anesthetic reaction, and use amide-linked agents.
     (b) Limit the amount of local anesthetic.
     (c) Avoid intravenous injection by moving and

aspirating the needle constantly while injecting local anesthetic.

(d) Avoid hitting major vessels to prevent hematoma.

(e) Treat systemic local anesthetic overdose reaction with a small amount of ultrashortacting barbiturate (such as pentothal 50 mg), midazolain, or diazepam given intravenously; oxygen; and other supportive measures.

Operative Laparoscopy, Second Edition
The Masters' Techniques in Gynecologic Surgery
Lippincott–Raven Publishers, Philadelphia © 1998.

2-2   Office Laparoscopic Sterilization under Local Anesthesia

John I. Fishburne, Jr.

Laparoscopic sterilization may be accomplished under local or general anesthesia. In the United States most procedures have been performed under general anesthesia, as indicated by the 1990 membership survey of the American Association of Gynecologic Laparoscopists (AAGL), which reported that only 8% of survey respondents utilized local anesthesia for laparoscopic sterilization.

Local anesthesia, however, offers several significant advantages. For one, the well-known risks of general anesthesia are avoided. Rapid recovery and decreased anesthesia time are also features of the local anesthetic technique, and the cost tends to be less than for general anesthesia, largely because of reduced recovery time. Furthermore, the technique is convenient for use in the outpatient setting and has even been adapted to the outpatient office environment. Because the patient is awake and able to complain when complications occur, early awareness of these is the rule. Nausea and vomiting also are less common. Furthermore, through the use of television technology, it is possible to permit the patient to observe the procedure directly, a factor that certainly enhances understanding of the procedures involved and may reduce medicolegal risks.

Laparoscopic surgery under local anesthesia also has several disadvantages. This approach requires precise and gentle surgical technique, and there may be increased patient anxiety. Discomfort may also occur, particularly if the surgeon does not employ sedative and analgesic drugs appropriately, or uses rough surgical technique. Another disadvantage may be related to the use of the office environment. In this situation there may be delayed treatment of complications while the patient is transported to an operating room. Also, pain may occur during coagulation or manipulation of pelvic organs, and this may lead to movement, which increases the risk of thermal injury during electrocoagulation. Some consider it a disadvantage that the surgeon operating under local anesthesia must maintain close verbal contact with the patient so as to provide ''vocal analgesia'' and to remain constantly aware of the patient's condition.

Almost all patients are candidates for outpatient laparoscopy under local anesthesia. The exceptions are those of American Society of Anesthesiologists (ASA) class II or greater, the very obese, those with a history of multiple intraabdominal procedures and/or peritonitis, those in whom the likelihood of laparotomy is great, and especially those who manifest extreme anxiety.

PRE- AND INTRAOPERATIVE MEDICATION FOR LAPAROSCOPY UNDER LOCAL ANESTHESIA

The patient should be given a nonsteroidal antiinflammatory agent such as ibuprofen 800 mg 30 minutes prior to surgery, to reduce the incidence of uterine cramping associated with insertion of instruments and manipulation of this organ.

Intraoperative medication should include atropine 0.4 to 0.6 mg given intravenously, for partial vagal blockade; midazolam (Versed) 2.5 mg given intravenously in divided doses, as a tranquilizer/sedative; fentanyl 0.05 to 0.1 mg given intravenously, for narcosis; and a local anesthetic agent such as bupivacaine 0.5% or lidocaine 1%. A narcotic antagonist (naloxone 0.4 mg/mL) must be available in the operating room.

Clinical Pharmacology

Midazolam

Midazolam (Versed) is a potent tranquilizing agent. It is three times as potent as diazepam but is formulated in an aqueous solution so that it does not precipitate when mixed for administration with intravenous fluids. The onset of its effect is more rapid than that of diazepam, and it is metabolized in the liver with an elimination half-life of 1 to 4 hours. Its adverse effects include respiratory depression and apnea, anterograde amnesia, and hypotension, which are additive with large doses of fentanyl. It should be remembered that cimetidine may increase serum levels of midazolam and may delay its elimination.

Fentanyl

Fentanyl (Sublimaze) is a synthetic narcotic analgesic that is 100 times more potent than morphine (0.1 mg = 10 mg of morphine). It has less emetic activity than morphine and does not release histamine. Its elimination half-life is 3 to 4 hours. Its adverse effects include respiratory depression, chest wall rigidity, bradycardia, hypertension or hypotension, and nausea and vomiting.

Bupivacaine

Bupivacaine (Marcaine or Sensorcaine) is a potent local anesthetic agent of amide linkage. It has a pKa of 8.1 and is highly soluble in lipids. It is also tightly protein bound (95%) and is a preferred agent for laparoscopy.

Bupivacaine has a rapid onset and a prolonged duration of action. Peak blood levels are achieved in 60 minutes. The major side effects are cardiotoxicity and convulsions. The convulsive blood level is 4.5 to 5.5 μg/mL. The maximum safe dose is 3 mg/kg (150 mg).

Bupivacaine is administered as a field block around the umbilicus. Five milliliters of a 0.5% solution is infiltrated subcutaneously, followed by 10 mL of the same concentration above and below the fascia, to produce a field block. Five milliliters of the same concentration is flowed over each tube, yielding a total dose of 25 mL or 125 mg. Spielman et al. (1985) described transperitoneal absorption of bupivacaine as compared to lidocaine. Peritoneal administration of bupivacaine yielded a serum concentration of 0.44 μg/mL compared with blood levels of 1.5 to 2.5 μg/mL when the same drug was administered peridurally. Mean pain ratings for trocar insertion, fallopian tube manipulation, and postoperative discomfort were slightly lower with bupivacaine than with lidocaine, although these differences were not statistically significant.

Nitrous oxide is preferred as the insufflation agent when performing laparoscopy under local anesthesia. Carbon dioxide produces excessive abdominal discomfort, presumably due to peritoneal irritation. This is obviated by the use of nitrous oxide. A study by Minoli et al. (1982) indicated that pain scores during laparoscopy were significantly less when nitrous oxide was used as the insufflation agent.

TECHNIQUE OF OFFICE LAPAROSCOPY UNDER LOCAL ANESTHESIA

Careful patient selection is critical to a successful program of outpatient laparoscopic sterilization under local anesthesia. The operating surgeon should see the patient preoperatively and perform a physical exam, including a careful pelvic examination. During this visit a thorough informed consent should be given, and the patient should be provided the opportunity to have her questions answered satisfactorily. At this preoperative visit, the excessively anxious patient can be identified and encouraged to undergo laparoscopic sterilization under *general* rather than *local* anesthesia.

On the day of surgery, the patient is admitted to a preoperative area where a nonsteroidal antiinflammatory agent is administered. She dons a hospital gown, an intravenous line is inserted, and baseline vital signs are obtained. At this time the patient is given the opportunity to have additional questions answered.

The operating instruments should have been previously sterilized. Before beginning the procedure the surgeon should inspect them to ascertain that the inventory is complete and that all instruments are in proper working condition. The patient is administered atropine 0.4 mg and midazolam 1 mg intravenously. After 4 to 5 minutes her mental status is assessed, and an additional 1.5 mg of midazolam is usually administered. The abdominal-perineal preparation is then begun, using a prewarmed antiseptic solution such as povidone iodine. After this has been accomplished, fentanyl 0.05 mg (1 mL) is administered intravenously. A single-hinged vaginal speculum is inserted, and the vagina and cervix are prepared with the same prewarmed antiseptic solution.

The cervix is grasped with a single-toothed tenaculum, and a Hulka uterine controlling instrument is inserted into the uterine cavity and attached to the anterior lip of the cervix. The surgeon then changes gloves and properly drapes the abdominal operative site. The diamond-shaped field block is then initiated, and 3 to 5 minutes are allowed to elapse to ensure adequacy of analgesia. With a scalpel equipped with a no. 11 blade, a small infraumbilical transverse incision is made. The Veress needle is passed through this into the peritoneal cavity, and 2 to 3 L of nitrous oxide gas is insufflated.

The needle is withdrawn and the laparoscopic trocar inserted. I prefer a pyramid-pointed or disposable trocar, which is maintained in extremely sharp condition. The laparoscope is then inserted, and the pelvic organs are visualized. The uterus is gently maneuvered using the Hulka instrument so as to expose to view the left fallopian tube. A cannula is then passed through the operating port of the laparoscope and approximately 5 mL of 0.5% bupivacaine solution is allowed to flow gently over all surfaces of the fallopian tube and the broad ligament, up to the round ligament. Application of local anesthetic solution to the ovary and uterine fundus may further enhance the analgesia. A similar procedure is carried out upon the right adnexal structures.

After the operation, the instruments can then be withdrawn from the abdomen and the nitrous oxide gas evacuated with the aid of the patient, who is urged to cough so that residual gas can be expelled. At this time care should be taken to avoid passage of atmospheric air into the peritoneal cavity. Should this occur, postoperative shoulder discomfort is more pronounced and long-lasting. The laparoscope trocar should be withdrawn under direct vision, with the laparoscope in place, so as to minimize the risk of herniation of abdominal contents through the small fascial incision. The subumbilical incision can be closed easily with a single subcuticular suture of absorbable material, such as 4-0 Dexon.

At the conclusion of the procedure the vital signs are again obtained, having been monitored every 5 minutes during the procedure by the circulating nurse. The patient is then encouraged to stand and walk to the nearby recovery area, where she is given light food (soda crackers) and drink (cola or coffee). Discharge usually takes place within 20 to 30 minutes, once the vital signs have been judged to be stable.

A patient who has received systemic sedation should be discharged in the company of an adult. She should not be permitted to drive an automobile for 24 hours.

SUGGESTED READING

Fishburne JI Jr. Anesthesia for the outpatient: sterilization and other procedures. In: Symonds M, Zuzpan FP, eds. *Clinical Diagnostic Procedures in Obstetrics and Gynecology, Part B: Gynecology.* New York: Marcel Dekker, Inc.; 1984;255–84.

Fishburne JI Jr. Anesthesia for laparoscopy, considerations, complications, techniques. *J Reprod Med* 1978;21:37–40.

Fishburne JI Jr. Office laparoscopic sterilization with local anesthesia. *J Reprod Med* 1977;18:233–4.

Hulka JF, Peterson HB, Phillips JM. American Association of Gynecologic Laparoscopists' 1988 membership survey on laparoscopic sterilization. *J Reprod Med* 1990;35:584–6.

Mercer JP, Lefler HT Jr, Hulka JF, Fishburne JI Jr. An outpatient program for laparoscopic sterilization. *Obstet Gynecol* 1983;41:681–4.

Minoli G, Terruzzi V, Spinzi GC, Benvenuti C, Rossini A. The influence of carbon dioxide and nitrous oxide on pain during laparoscopy: a double-blind, controlled trial. *Gastrointest Endosc* 1982;28:173–5.

Peterson HB, Hulka JF, Spielman FJ, Lee S, Marchbanks PA. Local versus general anesthesia for laparoscopic sterilization: a randomized study. *Obstet Gynecol* 1987;70:903–8.

Poindexter AN III, Abdul-Malak M, Fast JE. Laparoscopic tubal sterilization under local anesthesia. *Obstet Gynecol* 1990;75:5–8.

Spielman FJ, Hulka JF, Ostheimer GW, Mueller RA. Pharmacokinetics and pharmacodynamics of local analgesia for laparoscopic tubal ligations. *Am J Obstet Gynecol* 1985;146:821–4.

Operative Laparoscopy, Second Edition
The Masters' Techniques in Gynecologic Surgery
Lippincott–Raven Publishers, Philadelphia © 1998.

2-3 Basic Operative Technique

Richard M. Soderstrom

INSUFFLATION

Many experts feel that mastering proper insufflation technique of the abdomen is the most important step to ensure successful laparoscopies. The insufflation needle should puncture the peritoneum with ease, and the needle tip should come to rest in a space free of vital structures, allowing a free flow of gas. Fortunately, those organs with great motility, i.e., the bowel, are resistant to needle puncture except when fixed by some pathologic process. Situations that may impede proper needle placement include patient obesity, extensive pelvic adhesions, fixation of intraabdominal organs, and large pelvic or abdominal masses. Each of these impediments can usually be thwarted by choosing an alternate insufflation site.

Sites

Umbilical

In the United States, many surgeons use the umbilicus for needle insufflation. A short Touhey needle placed vertically through the center of the umbilicus has been a popular technique at the Johns Hopkins Medical Center. The abdomen must be relaxed and lifted, by hand or with towel clips, away from the great vessels located several centimeters below the umbilicus. This technique eliminates the possibility that the needle will transect the thick abdominal fascia and reduces the chance of improper insufflation into an extra peritoneal space. As with most insufflation methods, anesthesia should be adequate to allow proper elevation of the relaxed abdominal wall.

Subumbilical

The subumbilical needle insertion into the hollow of the pelvis is practiced by most gynecologists. A few experienced surgeons insert the Veress needle directly into the abdomen without abdominal wall elevation; however, this technique requires a keen appreciation for the spatial relationships of the abdominal wall, the sacral promontory, and the bifurcation of the great vessels. It should not be used by novices without close supervision. Lifting the lower abdominal wall prior to needle insertion is favored by most. The needle is inserted at a 45° angle to the plane of the abdominal wall and directed at the uterine fundus at the midline (Figure 2-3.1). When the lower abdominal wall is elevated, the axis of the needle path is lifted away from the sacral promontory, giving the inserter a sense of security during insertion. Unfortunately, on occasion the peritoneum sags away from the overlying fascia, and the needle tip may not puncture the peritoneum. If this is not appreciated by the operator, the properitoneal space may be inadvertently insufflated.

At this point, a fact of physics should be mentioned. There is no space in the abdominal cavity, only a potential space. When one lifts the abdominal wall prior to needle insertion, the bowel does not "fall away." Only after air enters this potential space will the bowel drop away from the anterior abdominal wall. Thus, when inserting the needle, leave it open, not closed.

Left Upper Quadrant

Inserting the needle in the left upper quadrant of the abdomen was employed by Raoel Palmer in France. A cross-section of this level of the abdominal cavity will reveal the deep space available for safe needle insertion. The stomach and transverse colon are resistant not only to needle puncture but also mobile. The spleen lies high above the lower level of the rib cage and is located in its posterior fossa, safe from accidental puncture.

The needle is inserted at a point 3 cm from the midline and 3 cm below the left rib cage (Figure 2-3.2). The needle is directed 15° *cephalad* after the abdominal skin has been stretched taut by pulling the skin caudally. The operator can feel it when the needle "pops" through each layer of the abdominal wall (Figure 2-3.3). You will find this method invaluable when the patient is obese or if the properitoneal space is accidentally insufflated.

Vaginal

A culdocentesis insufflation can be employed in patients with a cul-de-sac free of adhesions. It, too, is helpful in the obese patient and may be considered an efficient means of insufflation while the abdomen is being prepared.

Suprapubic

On occasion, the properitoneal space may be insufflated to an excessive degree, making proper reinsertion of the

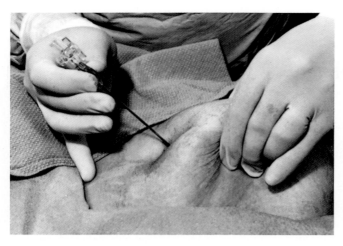

Figure 2-3.1 Inserting the Veress needle (U.S. Surgical Corporation) at a 45° angle to the plane of the abdomen, directed at the uterine fundus. The stopcock should be left open.

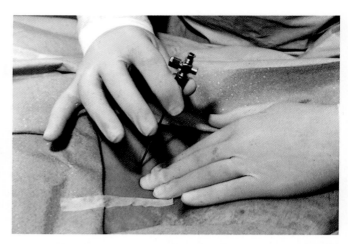

Figure 2-3.3 Inserting the needle at a 15° angle cephalad, the insertion point being 3 cm below the left costal margin and 3 cm to the left of midline. With the skin held taught, the needle traverses the layers of the abdominal wall. At each layer a popping sensation is felt.

needle difficult. When this happens, an alternate needle placement to consider is the suprapubic insertion of the needle into the dome of the uterus. The operator stabilizes the uterine manipulator and pushes the uterus up against the anterior abdominal wall (Figure 2-3.4). After careful palpation of the fundus, the needle is inserted through the abdominal wall and punctures the uterine fundus. If the fundus has been impaled, the needle will move as the fundus is moved with the uterine manipulator. The surgeon then holds the needle steady with one hand while the other hand withdraws the fundus to a caudal position; the fundus is thus disengaged from the needle (Figure 2-3.5). This guarantees intraabdominal placement of the needle tip, and the fundus will bleed for only a brief period.

Postplacement Procedures

After placing the needle, regardless of technique, flush the needle with 20 mL of saline to ensure patency (Figure 2-3.6). If the needle should puncture a viscus such as the bowel, enough saline will have been instilled to alert you when the needle is then aspirated (Figure 2-3.7). Should the aspirated contents suggest bowel contents, repeat the needle insertion with a clean needle. If the saline returns clear and clean, the needle is probably in the properitoneal space, and you can start the insufflation process again. If this happens, it may be helpful to insert the Veress needle with the inner cannula retracted to increase the odds of adequate peritoneal puncture.

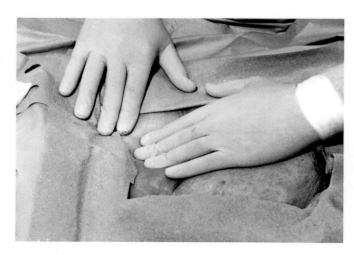

Figure 2-3.2 Palpating the left costal margin and the upper abdominal midline to locate a point for needle insertion in the left upper quadrant.

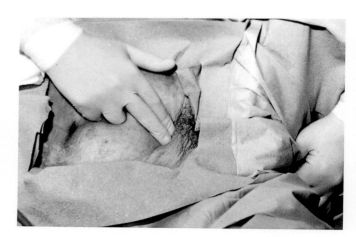

Figure 2-3.4 Pushing the fundus against the abdominal wall with a uterine manipulator permits it to be easily palpated.

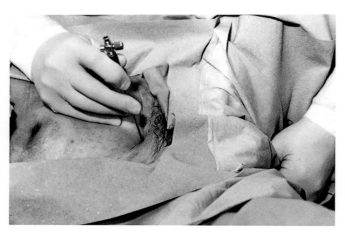

Figure 2-3.5 Impaling the dome of the fundus with the Veress needle while stabilizing the uterus with the manipulator. Once the fundus is impaled, the uterus is drawn away from the needle tip before attempting insufflation.

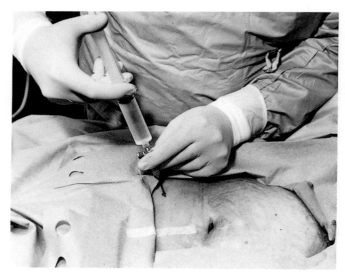

Figure 2-3.6 Flushing the needle with saline prior to insufflation (the upper quadrant technique).

Physiology of Insufflation

Three gases have been used for laparoscopy—room air, CO_2 and N_2O. Room air is readily available and can be instilled with simple hand pumps; however, after the procedure, should some residual air be left behind (this usually happens), absorption is so slow that referred shoulder pain from diaphragmatic irritation will persist for days.

CO_2 is the most common insufflation gas used in laparoscopy. It is delivered through an insufflator designed for that purpose and is supplied worldwide in heavy-duty tanks under 2000 pounds of pressure. CO_2 is rapidly absorbed by the peritoneum and will not support combustion. Cardiac arrhythmias can develop if the procedure is long and hyperventilation is not maintained during the period of abdominal distention. Under local anesthesia, some patients complain of peritoneal pain if the procedure is lengthy. Some postulate that fine droplets of carbonic acid are formed on the peritoneum, which then cause an inflammatory reaction.

N_2O has the same molecular weight as CO_2 and is also rapidly absorbed but is less soluble than CO_2. It neither creates hypercarbia nor causes peritoneal irritation during long procedures. It is supplied in tanks or is frequently available in modern operation rooms through in-line ceiling supply systems. N_2O is not combustible, but it does support combustion, as does room air. For this reason, CO_2 is preferable for laser laparoscopy.

During insufflation the flow of gas should be monitored. With an in-line pressure of 20 mm Hg, the average Veress needle will permit about 1000 mL of gas per minute to flow through its cannula. Though flow meters indicate how much gas has passed through the system, they do not measure the intraabdominal content of gas. Leakage, a common problem in laparoscopy, prevents such a measurement. In reality, the physiologic phenomenon of intraabdominal pressure is the most important ingredient in safe insufflation, *not* the number of liters instilled. For example, a pediatric patient may require less than 1 L of gas to reach a proper insufflation pressure, and a woman who, in the recent past, has delivered triplets, may require 10 L of gas before the laparoscope trocar can be inserted safely.

Percussion during insufflation only confirms that the gas is flowing somewhere below the fascial plane. Gas in the properitoneal space will dissect readily under the fascia of

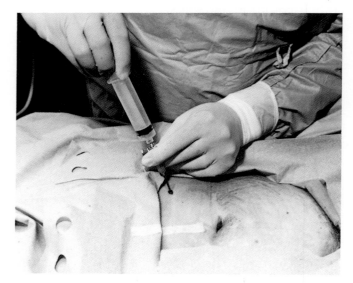

Figure 2-3.7 After flushing the needle with 20 mL of saline solution, the needle is aspirated (the upper quadrant technique). A return of fluid suggests needle placement in a blind or closed space.

the upper and lower abdomen. Therefore, percussion is not a reliable test for proper insufflation. Crepitance in the abdominal fat is found when insufflation occurs above the fascial plane.

Except for the obese patient, should the gas flow into the properitoneal space, the lower abdomen will usually distend in an uneven fashion and the flow rate will decline steadily while the pressure increases rapidly. An alert surgeon will notice the uneven abdominal distention and observe the flow ball drop. Should this be observed, it is best to cease insufflation and reinsert the needle or choose an alternate insertion site.

CLOSED TECHNIQUE INSERTION OF THE TROCAR

Most laparoscopists prefer the pyramid-tipped trocar; when it is sharp, it is a delight! In fact, the sharper the trocar, the easier it is to control insertion; thus the process becomes safer. Be sure the skin incision is large enough to pass the trocar and its *sleeve* through the skin with ease. I prefer a vertical incision, which usually conforms to the stellate creases in most patients' navels (Figure 2-3.8).

Many surgeons lift the lower abdominal skin during the trocar insertion, as described for insertion of the needle through a subumbilical incision, but if, before trocar insertion, adequate distention is present, the fascia will be elevated by the intraabdominal pressure, thus placing the path of insertion in the desired location. In fact, under proper distention and pressure, one cannot lift the fascia, only the skin.

For this reason, I prefer to insert the trocar without lifting, using two hands for better control. This approach is especially helpful to surgeons with small hands. I slide the trocar and sleeve through the skin incision *parallel* to the abdominal fascia, until the edge of the trocar sleeve is under the rim of the skin incision (Figure 2-3.9). This technique con-

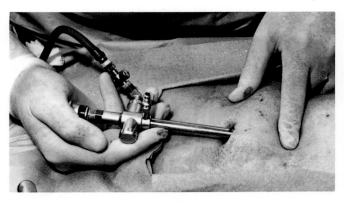

Figure 2-3.9 After the abdomen is insufflated, the trocar and sleeve are threaded through the umbilical incision in a parallel direction to the abdominal fascia (the closed technique).

firms the proper incision size and places the tip of a 10-mm trocar 1.5 to 2.0 cm below the navel. Lift the trocar handle up to a 45° angle to the fascial plane, place two fingers on the midshaft of the trocar sleeve, and firmly push the trocar and sleeve into the abdominal gas-filled space (Figure 2-3.10). Placing two fingers on the midshaft of the trocar sleeve prevents overpenetration. Never thrust the trocar forward in an abrupt manner, for one loses control of the depth of insertion; if the trocar is kept sharp, a thrusting motion is unnecessary. In teaching situations, a drop of saline placed on the insufflation port of the trocar sleeve will "blow out" of the port when the gas-filled space is entered. This alerts the student that deeper penetration is not necessary.

I never rotate or twist the parametal-tip trocar through the fascia, though many do. Twisting tears the fascia; a direct puncture cuts the fascia, leaving a triple "flap valve" to close when the trocar sleeve is removed. This flap valve

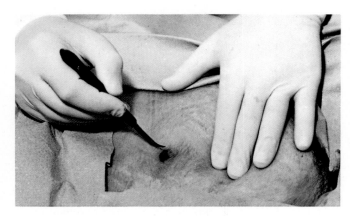

Figure 2-3.8 Using a no. 12 scalpel blade, a vertical subumbilical incision about 10 to 12 mm long is made.

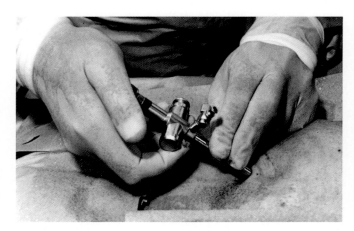

Figure 2-3.10 Inserting the trocar at a 45° angle toward the dome of the uterine fundus. Two fingers are placed on the trocar sheath to prevent deep, abrupt entry (the closed technique).

might prevent an occasional herniation of omentum through the wound.

Trocar sleeves with trumpet valves will dull the tip of a sharp trocar if the trocar is withdrawn without first depressing the valve stem; flap valve trocar sleeves tend to dull the cutting edge of parametal trocars after repeated use. Remember, proper inspection and maintenance ensures safe laparoscopy. A strong argument may be made for disposable trocars, which are of uniform sharpness.

OPEN LAPAROSCOPY

This method, developed by Harrith Hasson, MD, of Chicago, was designed to eliminate the blind entry of the insufflation needle and laparoscope trocar. Hasson recommends a vertical incision at the base of the umbilicus, 1.0 to 1.5 cm in length. Using special small Deever retractors designed for open laparoscopy, the fat is pulled laterally, exposing the fascia. After securing the fascia with two Kocher clamps, the fascia is incised vertically for 1 cm (Figure 2-3.11). Hasson punctures the peritoneum with a small hemostat and spreads the peritoneal opening with the hemostat. A suture is passed through one fascial edge and another suture through the opposite edge. The loops of suture are left long so that they may be secured to the Hasson cannula (Figure 2-3.12).

Hasson designed a blunt trocar to aid in the insertion of the trocar sleeve through the open wound (Figure 2-3.13). However, with practice, any laparoscope sleeve may be inserted without any trocar in place. A special acorn-shaped collar placed over the trocar sleeve is used to seal the junction of the abdominal skin and the trocar sleeve. This collar slides up and down the trocar sleeve and with a set screw can be secured at a desired location.

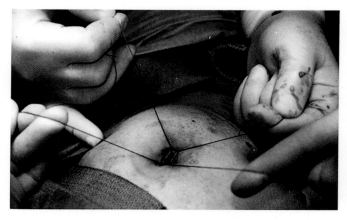

Figure 2-3.12 After the fascia and peritoneum have been incised, two sutures are placed in the fascia to secure, later, the Hasson cannula (the open technique).

Once the trocar sleeve with its acorn collar is properly wedged into the incision, the fascial sutures are tied to special hooks on the Hasson trocar sleeve or tied over the arms of the trumpet sleeve if hooks are not available (Figures 2-3.14 and 2-3.15). The insufflation of gas is then accomplished directly through the trocar sleeve via the insufflation port. Because there is less ''in-line'' resistance, it takes less time to insufflate than through the Veress needle. In experienced hands, the ''open'' technique of trocar insertion and insufflation should only take a few minutes more than the ''closed'' technique. Frequently, I use the open technique after I have insufflated the abdomen through the left upper quadrant. By doing so, it is easier to enter the peritoneum directly.

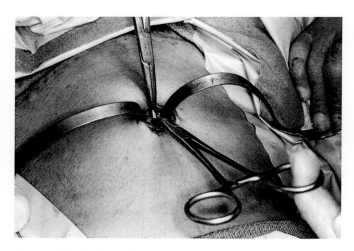

Figure 2-3.11 Using Hasson retractors, the fascia is grasped with two Kocher clamps before making a 1-cm incision (the open technique).

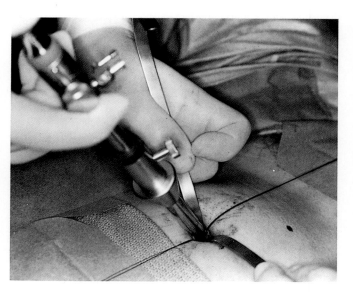

Figure 2-3.13 The blunt Hasson trocar, trocar sleeve, and acorn collar are inserted into the peritoneal cavity (the open technique).

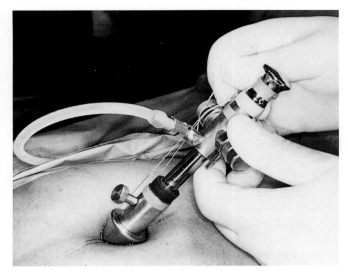

Figure 2-3.14 The acorn collar is wedged into the incision and secured in place, with the fascial sutures hooked or tied over the cannula's trumpet valve (the open technique).

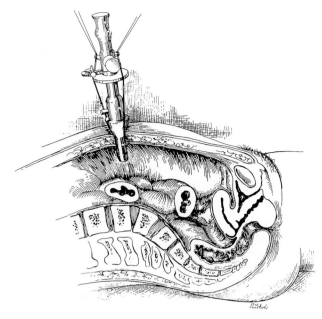

Figure 2-3.15 A cross-sectional view of the Hasson trocar, trocar sleeve and acorn collar secured to prevent leakage of gas.

SECONDARY TROCAR INSERTION

All secondary trocars should be inserted under endoscopic control. There is no proper site for secondary instrument sites; however, the suprapubic midline site is the most common. A well-drained bladder protects against accidental bladder perforation; directing the secondary trocar during insertion toward the uterus protects against accidental puncture of the vital structures that line the pelvic brim (Figure 2-3.16).

A lower quadrant site for the secondary trocar is favored by many; however, the deep epigastric vessels of the abdominal wall can be inadvertently transected, even after transillumination of the abdominal wall. Here again, aim for the uterus. On occasion, insertion of a secondary trocar into the upper abdomen may be necessary; insert the trocar slightly cephalad, toward the gutter, not the midline.

Try to pick a trocar sleeve that fits the needed instrument, because a larger trocar sleeve may lead to excessive leakage of gas. Have an assortment of trocar gaskets with different size holes, should a thin instrument be needed through a larger trocar sleeve. Many disposable trocar sleeves provide this option.

WOUND CLOSURE

When closing the wounds, fascial stitches are not necessary even with a 10-mm trocar wound; the exception is with the "open" technique. The sutures previously placed in the fascia to stabilize and seal the open trocar sleeve into the wound can be tied together for secure closure. When operating on the cancer patient, the open technique is ex-

cellent. By closing the fascia, leakage of any ascitic fluid that reaccumulates is reduced.

Most prefer a subcutaneous skin closure with absorbable sutures. Michel skin clips removed by the patient 24 hours later can be used, but on occasion the "teethmarks" remain visible. For smaller puncture wounds, 6 mm or less, Steri-Strips will suffice.

VIEWING BY LAPAROSCOPY

A systematic approach to "viewing within" should become a habit. Part of the intrigue in endoscopy is finding

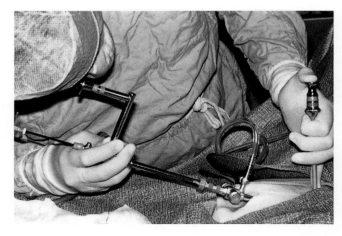

Figure 2-3.16 The secondary trocar is always inserted under direct vision. It should be pointed in the least harmful direction, as shown here. The trocar is aimed at the uterine fundus to avoid vital structures that line the pelvic brim.

the unknown or unexpected. To sterilize a patient and not inspect the upper abdomen robs the physician of an opportunity to become familiar with the upper abdomen and its anatomy as seen through the laparoscope. An enlarged spleen, a liver tumor, or the presence of diaphragmatic metastasis in an asymptomatic cancer patient may be an unusual occurrence, yet if you do not seek, you shall not find. To know the appearance of normal anatomy helps one perceive the abnormal.

Whatever inspection protocol you prefer is fine, just use one. You might explore the pelvis first and the upper abdomen last. Start with the uterus, tubes, and ovaries; the secure uterine manipulator makes this task easy. Some prefer a steep Trendelenburg position for all patients; I only use a Trendelenburg position when visualization is difficult. Inspect the anterior and posterior cul-de-sacs by using the manipulator to put the suspensory ligaments to the uterus on a stretch, thus opening hidden recesses in the pelvis.

After the pelvic structures have been surveyed, scan the right pelvic brim and continue in a clockwise fashion around the upper abdomen back down to the left pelvic brim. A word of caution: be careful not to avulse the falciform ligament with the laparoscope during the upper abdominal sweep.

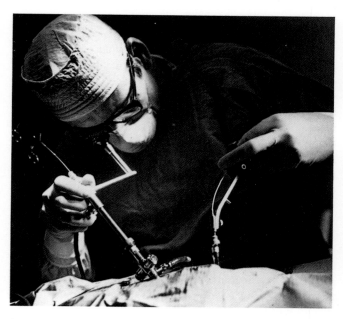

Figure 2-3.17 Using an operating laparoscope with a second puncture gives the operator two channels to grasp and manipulate tissue without a third puncture wound.

ORGAN MANIPULATION

Whether one prefers an operating laparoscope or a diagnostic laparoscope, equipment should be available for easy, atraumatic manipulation of abdominal organs. I prefer a blunt 3-mm wand or atraumatic grasping forceps. In my early years of experience, I chose the operating laparoscope but quickly learned the increased versatility of a second-puncture manipulator. Through the operating channel in the laparoscope, grasping forceps can grasp and lift structures while a blunt wand placed through a second trocar sleeve can move structures laterally or stabilize organs during inspection or operating procedures such as biopsy (Figure 2-3.17).

With experience, the surgeon can develop a feel for the mobility of internal organs such as ovaries or loops of bowel. It is fortunate that the resiliency of healthy human tissue allows the operator to move these mobile structures with ease and without trauma. Three-millimeter instruments are more flexible than 5- or 6-mm tools; thus an unexpected fixation of a vital organ can be appreciated with more sensitivity, and fixed tissue will slip out of the smaller grasping forceps if excessive traction is used.

Adhesions should be left alone unless the lysis of the adhesion will serve a purpose. Filmy adhesions can be ruptured with blunt probes or "pushed" away with grasping forceps. Adhesions attached to the abdominal wall should be severed at their abdominal wall attachment because the vascularity is minimal. Electrocoagulation is seldom necessary, but when needed it should be used with caution. Because of the current density promoted by a fine adhesion

(see Chapter 3), unipolar energy can travel rapidly down the adhesion and burn attached structures. Here, bipolar coagulation should be considered, but if the adhesion is thick, coagulation may be incomplete. Experience has shown that most cut adhesions usually stop bleeding after a brief period of time. Using scissors in the open position to "push" the adhesion off the abdominal wall is a safe technique if one can see through the adhesion. If not, a fiberoptic bundle rod passed through another trocar sleeve can transilluminate a thick adhesion and give reassurance (you can also use a small cystoscope lens as a means of transillumination). In each instance a second light source and fiberoptic card must be available. If the patient is thin, you might detach the light card from the laparoscope and transilluminate the abdominal wall over the adhesion—a helpful trick if a little eerie.

When mobile, the ovaries can be easily moved with the wand or grasper. A Palmer-Eder tong is more versatile for ovarian inspection because it can pick up the ovary, and if indicated, a generous biopsy can be obtained. The ovary can also be maneuvered into position by the fundus of the uterus. With the uterine manipulator, displace the fundus below the ovary and then push it up under the ovary, elevating it and "flipping" the lateral-inferior wall into view. The fundus can then be held as a pedestal under the ovary while an ovarian biopsy is performed.

When manipulating abdominal organs, a change in the patient's position may prove helpful. Steep Trendelenburg position will aid in pelvic organ maneuvers; the Fowler position will help in manipulation and biopsy of the upper abdominal anatomy.

IMPAIRMENTS TO VISION

Sudden or steady loss of intraabdominal gas is the most common cause of impaired vision during laparoscopy. Poor or ill-fitting gaskets are a frequent cause of gas loss. A low-volume insufflator or a closed insufflation valve (forgotten by the operator engrossed in the procedure) can render the most skilled laparoscopist powerless to proceed. This is the time when attention to detail, equipment maintenance, and having the right equipment become critical. Equipment failure runs a close second to loss of gas in causing impairment of vision. A broken light cord, a bent laparoscope, a dislodged lens, or an empty gas tank will impair the ability to see. Watch out for incompatible equipment. One company's light card attached by a conversion adaptor may cut the available light to 15% of what is available when compatible equipment is used. When an impairment to vision occurs, start from the beginning (the light source) and check each step in the pathway for a possible defect—a break in the system will be found.

TERMINATING THE PROCEDURE

As with any intraabdominal operation, at the end of the procedure be sure all is in its place. If you are confident the procedure is over, remove the instruments in preparation for deflation and then turn the laparoscope vertical. Can you see any blood dripping off the end of the laparoscope? If so, replace a 6-mm trocar sleeve in a lower quadrant position, borrow a cystoscope lens, and look at the laparoscope trocar site. If a bleeding site is seen, another trocar and sleeve can be inserted and, under direct vision, as the laparoscope trocar is removed, the bleeder can be coagulated or ligated. When multiple trocars are used, inspect with the laparoscope each intraabdominal puncture site for bleeding, after removing the trocars.

Once all is well, deflate the abdomen. If the patient is awake under local or regional block anesthesia, you might ask the patient to take a deep breath and hold it. Should gas be trapped under the diaphragm, this might help to expel it and reduce the chance of postoperative shoulder pain. You can depress the lower rib cage to create the same effect. However, the trocar sleeve should be removed before the patient or the surgeon releases this artificially increased intrapulmonary pressure, for if not, the release of the pressure will suck room air into the abdominal cavity through the open trocar sleeve, and shoulder pain may last for days.

DOCUMENTATION

Since a major part of most laparoscopic procedures is what you see, a visual record may be preferred. Several anatomic drawings are available to record findings rapidly. The American Fertility Society has an excellent evaluation sheet with drawings for patients with endometriosis. Pho-tographic slides, prints, film strips, and video recordings have all found their place in documentation. Each year some new improvement in "photoscopy" is presented at medical meetings.

Slides and Prints

Because of the light loss inherent in the light cables' connector to endoscopes, good photography requires either a matched system or a professional understanding of camera technology. Though expensive, a photographic system provided by the manufacturer of a camera, lens, and flash unit will give any surgeon marvelous pictures. For those who wish to try their hand at photography, several points and limitations should be understood.

The image seen through an endoscope is usually smaller than the frame size of the camera. The smaller the endoscope, the fewer the fiber bundles or the smaller the lens; in either case, light transfer will be reduced. To put it another way, large endoscopes have more room for fiber bundles and thus are used by the serious "photoscopist." However, since most would prefer the image to fill the frame or most of the frame, a 100-mm camera lens is usually used, which may reduce the light available to film. Some manufacturers of laparoscopes provide, for an extra charge, integral bundle laparoscopes that marry the fiberoptic cord into the laparoscope, thus eliminating the need for a cord connector. This doubles the light available to the lens system and is an excellent system for movies. These scopes require meticulous care, as the fiber bundles may break during cleaning and wrapping.

Because the endoscope light may be only available to two-thirds of the frame size, a standard, in-camera light meter that senses the available light through the lens may average the "message" over the entire frame area, and pictures will be underexposed.

Because of the wide-angle characteristics of endoscopes, the available light falls off rapidly as you move the scope back from the field for a panoramic view, thus some form of light compensation must occur to give consistent pictures of good quality. With practice, the amateur photoscopist can adjust the f-stop and obtain reasonable pictures. The optimum, however, is a system that automatically compensates for distance, image size, and available light. Such a system requires a synchronized distal flash unit and lens aperture setting, which frees the endoscopist of the guess work inherent in manual systems. To complete such a photographic package, a "databack" will record on the film selected data to identify the picture with the patient.

Thirty-five-millimeter slides may be cheaper than prints, but prints can be stored in the chart with more ease. For lecture purposes, slides can be easily made from the print. Polaroid systems are available but need to be improved.

Movies

Movies are difficult for many of the reasons described above. Movie cameras are bulky and heavy, and movie film is expensive. A good movie system requires a broad base of versatility and must be fully automatic to compensate when the laparoscope moves from light to darker areas.

Video

Video photography has progressed rapidly in the past decade. Large heavy cameras have been replaced by miniaturized cameras as small as the eyepiece of the laparoscope. Cameras that can be soaked in sterilizing solutions are attractive to operating room personnel, and each year obtainable images improve as new models are introduced. Though "tube" cameras still give the best image, "chip" cameras are competitive. Data keyboards (character generators) can imprint the video film with a vast array of data for documentation, and inexpensive copies of the operation can be stored or given to the patient on any size videotape cassette.

The experienced video photoscopist can quickly learn to operate from the monitor screen, as orthopaedic surgeons do when performing arthroscopy. Beam splitters can be used if the operator prefers to see directly through the scope.

A low light level video camera is necessary to get good pictures. It is best to field test each television camera on your equipment before making such a major investment and also to consider the interchangeability of laparoscopes and other endoscopes used within your facility. Written documentation after laparoscopy is an important feature of the procedure; photoscopy in any form is a marvelous addition.

CONTRAINDICATIONS TO LAPAROSCOPY

There are no absolute contraindications to laparoscopy; each decision should be made individually. If the patient cannot tolerate an intraabdominal pressure of 20 mm Hg then laparoscopy should not be considered. If exploratory laparotomy is not contraindicated, then neither is laparoscopy. When the blind approach of closed laparoscopy seems unwise, open laparoscopy might be considered. A patient with a large hiatal hernia may not tolerate intraabdominal insufflation. An acute bowel obstruction cannot be helped with laparoscopy. But a patient with a bleeding ectopic pregnancy, even if she is in early shock, may be managed by laparoscopy without increased morbidity.

Operative Laparoscopy, Second Edition
The Masters' Techniques in Gynecologic Surgery
Lippincott–Raven Publishers, Philadelphia © 1998.

3

Electrophysics in Endoscopy

3-1 Biophysics of Electrical Energy

Roger C. Odell

The use of electrical energy for surgical purposes dates back nearly a century. William L. Clark, MD, a general surgeon from Philadelphia, appears to have been the first to introduce into practice what in the United States is now known as "electrosurgery." The Germans and French preceded Clark in the use of electricity in surgery. Electrosurgery consists of the generation and delivery of radiofrequency current between an active electrode and a dispersive electrode to elevate tissue temperature for the purpose of cutting, fulguration, or desiccation. In contrast to electrocautery, the electric current actually passes through the tissue. Harvey W. Cushing, MD, was, with the assistance of William T. Bovie, PhD, the first surgeon to document in depth the principles of both the art and the physics of electrosurgery. These early documents detail his appreciation of Dr. Bovie's device and his enthusiasm regarding the versatility of electrosurgery. During his years of practice, he changed the course of neurosurgery as well as other surgeons' views of the potential uses of the technique. This chapter will (1) highlight the practical application of the three applications of electrosurgical energy and how to maximize their potential and (2) thoroughly review the potential pitfalls associated with the everyday use of electrosurgery. In view of today's rapid shift to minimally invasive surgical technique, a detailed discussion regarding laparoscopic use of electrosurgery will be included.

HOW ELECTRICAL ENERGY AFFECTS TISSUE TEMPERATURE

Three properties of electricity are responsible for causing a substance's temperature to rise when electricity is applied to it:

1. current (I)
2. voltage (V)
3. resistance (impedance) (R)

A direct analogy to hydraulics will be made, to define these terms. *Voltage* is electric potential or potential difference expressed in volts. The height of the water tower equates to the potential to deliver water with a great deal of force. *Current* is the practical mks unit of electric current that is equivalent to a flow of one coulomb per second or to the steady current produced by one volt applied across a resistance of one ohm. The volume of water in liters flowing through the pipe over a given period of time, is equivalent to the electric flow of current in amperes. *Resistance* is the opposition offered by a body or substance to the passage through it of a steady electric current. The diameter of the pipe from the water tower to the point of delivery is comparable to resistance or active electrode in electrosurgery. Figure 3-1.1 presents the water tower, a hydraulic energy source for the purpose of performing work. Figure 3-1.2 shows the same tower with the electrical terms current, voltage, and resistance substituted for the relevant hydraulics terms, to demonstrate the meaning and relationship of the terms. The relationship that obtains between the three terms is described in Ohm's law: $I = V/R$.

The equation $W = V \times I$ is valuable in understanding how the three modalities' waveforms cut, fulgurate, and desiccate tissue. The ratio of voltage to current of the electrosurgical waveforms is the primary factor responsible for the effects on tissue, when time and electrode size are kept equal.

$$\text{ENERGY} = \text{WATTAGE} \times \text{TIME}$$
$$E = W \times T$$

$$\text{WATTS} = \text{VOLTAGE} \times \text{CURRENT}$$
$$W = V \times I$$

Power density is a function of the size of the active electrode in contact with the tissue and the amount of energy used. In noncontact modalities (i.e., cutting and fulgurating), this is equivalent to the sparking area between the active electrode and the tissue. Only during desiccation is the exact surface area of the electrode in contact with the tissue of importance when calculating power density. During fulguration and cutting, the electrode is not in contact;

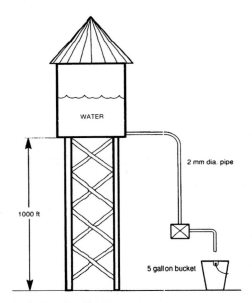

Figure 3-1.1 Hydraulic energy source.

therefore, the power density can only be approximated. In general the larger the electrode surface area, the lower the power density; the smaller the electrode surface area, the higher the power density.

The time element is the primary determinant of the depth and degree of tissue necrosis.

TEMPERATURE AND TISSUE

At or above 44°C, tissue necrosis starts. Around 70°C coagulation begins, where collagen is converted to glucose.

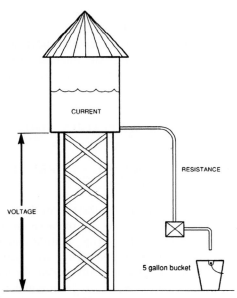

Figure 3-1.2 Analogy of electrosurgical terms inserted into the hydraulic energy source.

By 90°C tissue desiccation begins, where the tissue is dehydrated. Above 100°C vaporization occurs, where the tissue is converted into a vapor. Carbonization starts at or above 200°C; this black eschar typically can only be produced by fulguration.

EFFECTS OF ELECTROSURGERY ON TISSUE

Electrosurgical energy exerts three distinct therapeutic effects on tissue: cutting, fulguration, and dessication.

Cutting

A high-current, low-voltage (continuous) waveform, which elevates the tissue's temperature rapidly, produces vaporization or division of tissue with the least effect on coagulation (hemostasis) to the walls of the incision. Figure 3-1.3 shows a cutting waveform obtained at an electrosurgical unit (ESU) setting of 50 W. During optimal electrosurgical cutting the current travels through a steam bubble between the active electrode and the tissue. It is therefore important to recognize that electrosurgical cutting is a noncontact means of dissection. A needle or knifelike electrode floats through the tissue, and little tactile information is transmitted to the surgeon's hand (Figure 3-1.4). The continuous waveform is analogous to the constant, even, flow of the water being delivered from the valve above the bucket in Figure 3-1.1. Due to the constant flow of current and the use of the lowest possible voltage necessary to dissect, the width and depth of necrosis of the walls of the incision are minimal. Therefore, the ratio of high current to low voltage within the waveform produces less necrosis.

Effect of Varying the Cutting Waveform

With ratio modification of the cutting waveform, achieved by interrupting current and increasing the voltage, the waveform becomes noncontinuous, and a train of packets of energy consisting of higher voltage and reduced

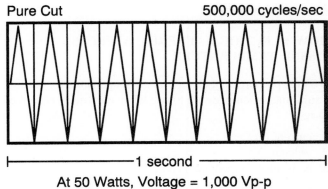

Figure 3-1.3 Pure cutting waveform.

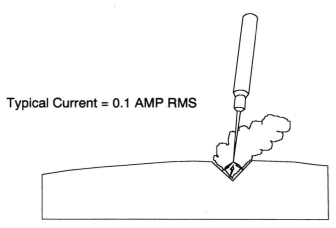

Typical Current = 0.1 AMP RMS

Figure 3-1.4 Electrosurgical cutting.

current per unit of time is delivered. Total energy remains the same, but the ratio of voltage and current is modified to increase hemostasis during dissection. Figure 3-1.5 shows three blends that may thereby be achieved. This is analogous to the garden valve in Figure 3-1.1 pulsing the water, with an increase in height to the water tower to make up for the reduction in hydraulic energy, as a result of reducing the time that the water was allowed to flow. The electrode also floats through the tissue when using the blend modes. The blend waveforms will require a longer period of time to dissect the same length of incision as compared to the cutting waveform. This is due to the interrupted delivery of current at the same power setting. With this increase in time comes an increase in thermal spread from the voltage com-

ponent of the blend waveform. This increased thermal spread improves coagulation while dissecting. When needed, these blend modes can be a valuable option, as needed, in controlling bleeding when dissecting. On the other hand, the increased width of necrosis they cause may result in a higher postoperative infection level. Blend 1 will slightly increase hemostasis, blend 2 moderately increase it, and blend 3 markedly increase it.

When dissecting tissue with a cutting or blending mode, the ESU should be activated before the electrode touches the tissue. A feathering or light stroking, similar to that employed in painting with a two-bristle paint brush for fine detail work, should be used. This will allow for the maximum power density as the electrode approaches the tissue and help start vaporization or dissection of tissue. In theory and in practice, with optimum technique and control setting, the force required to dissect tissue would be zero grams of pressure between the electrode and the tissue.

Fulguration

Fulguration is obtained with a high-voltage, low-current, noncontinuous waveform, which is designed to coagulate by spraying long electrical sparks to the surface of the tissue. Figure 3-1.6 shows a coagulation waveform set at 50 W. The most common use of fulguration is when coagulation is needed in a large area that is oozing blood, such as in a capillary or arteriole bed, where a discrete bleeder cannot be identified. It is the most effective means of arresting this form of bleeding. Cardiovascular, urologic, and general surgeons have relied on fulguration for their most demanding applications:

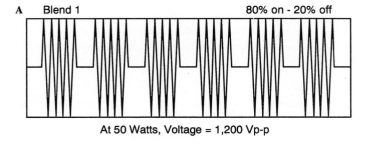

A   Blend 1   80% on - 20% off

At 50 Watts, Voltage = 1,200 Vp-p

Figure 3-1.5 A. Mode, blend 1 waveform at 50 W; **B.** Mode, blend 2 waveform at 50 W; and **C.** Mode, blend 3 waveform at 50 W.

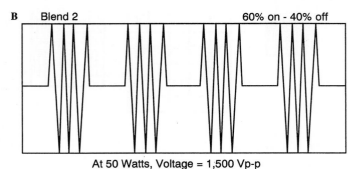

B   Blend 2   60% on - 40% off

At 50 Watts, Voltage = 1,500 Vp-p

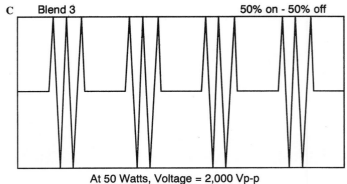

C   Blend 3   50% on - 50% off

At 50 Watts, Voltage = 2,000 Vp-p

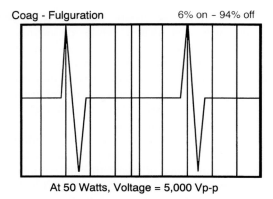

Coag - Fulguration   6% on – 94% off

At 50 Watts, Voltage = 5,000 Vp-p

Figure 3-1.6 Fulguration waveform.

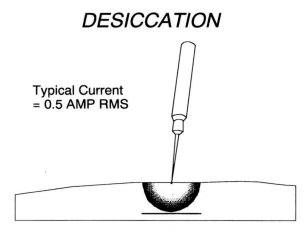

DESICCATION

Typical Current
= 0.5 AMP RMS

Figure 3-1.8 Desiccation.

hepatic resections, bleeding from a bladder tumor resection, surface bleeding on the heart. With fulguration, superficial eschar is produced; the depth of necrosis is minimal as a result of defocusing of the power density (Figure 3-1.7). By drawing the electrode away from the tissue, the power density goes down. A great deal of the energy is dissipated in the air that the current must pass through. Fulguration and electrosurgical cutting are noncontact modalities.

Fulguration can be initiated in two ways: first, by ever so slowly approaching the tissue until a spark jumps to the tissue, initiating a rain of sparks that will be maintained until the electrode is withdrawn or the tissue is carbonized to the point where the increase in resistance causes the sparks to cease, and second, by bouncing the electrode off the tissue, which will result in the same raining effect of sparks without the painstaking effort of approaching the tissue until a spark jumps.

Desiccation

Any waveform will desiccate when the electrode is in direct contact with tissue (Figure 3-1.8). Desiccation is an-

other form of coagulation. Though surgeons should, most do not make a distinction between fulguration and desiccation but refer to both as coagulation. The application of electrosurgical current by means of contact with the tissue results in all of the energy delivered by the ESU being converted into heat within the tissue. By contrast, in both cutting and fulgurating, a significant amount of the electrical energy is spent heating up the air between the electrode and the tissue. The increased energy delivered into the tissue with contact coagulation/desiccation results in deeper necrosis—as deep as it is wide, as observed on the surface where the electrode makes contact.

The most common application of desiccation is when a discrete bleeder is encountered, a hemostat is introduced to occlude the vessel, and then electrosurgical energy is applied to the body of the hemostat. In this way the current must pass through the hemostat into the tissue grasped by the jaws and back to the patient return electrode. The coaptation of vessels has been documented as producing a collagen chain reaction resulting in a fibrous bonding of the

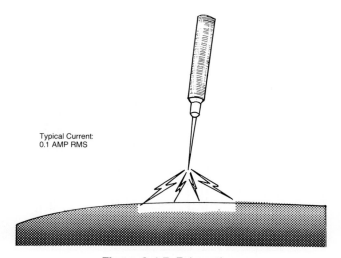

Typical Current:
0.1 AMP RMS

Figure 3-1.7 Fulguration.

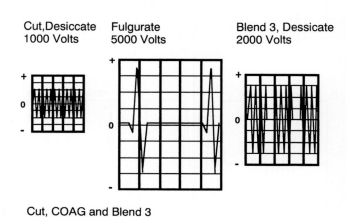

Cut,Desiccate   Fulgurate   Blend 3, Dessicate
1000 Volts   5000 Volts   2000 Volts

Cut, COAG and Blend 3
set at 50 WATTS

Figure 3-1.9 Cut, blend (desiccate) and fulgurate set at 50 W.

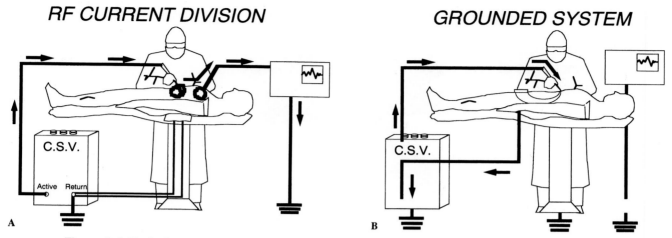

Figure 3-1.10 A. Grounded system with intended current path; **B.** Grounded system with potentially dangerous current path.

dehydrated, denatured cells of the endothelium. Because the electrode is in good electrical contact with the tissue, the voltage: current ratio is not nearly as important as it is in cutting and fulgurating. In practical application, the cut/blend waveforms are superior for this application over the fulguration waveform, when desiccation is desired. The primary reason is that the fulguration waveform will tend to spark through the coagulated tissue, resulting in voids in the bonding to the end of the vessel (Figure 3-1.9). Also, when sparks occur at the electrode in contact or near contact, the metal in the electrode will rapidly heat up, causing the tissue to adhere to the electrode when it is drawn off the target site. Bleeding will continue each time the eschar is pulled off due to this adhesion.

In bipolar desiccation, the waveform plays a far more important role. Today, for the most part, manufacturers have incorporated a continuous low-voltage, high-current waveform into the bipolar output to maximize the effect on desiccation. With older models of ESUs, manufacturers allowed the surgeon to select either a continuous cut, a blend, or a fulguration waveform when bipolar desiccation was needed. The lack of physician understanding in combination with the lack of clear explanations in the literature on the tissue effects of bipolar desiccation with these waveforms led to a number of documented associated problems. Therefore, at this time the generally accepted waveform for bipolar desiccation is a continuous low-voltage, high-current waveform. I recommend, when bipolar desiccation is critical, that a newer-model ESU with a set bipolar waveform be used. If you must use an ESU that allows you to select both cut/blend and fulguration bipolar currents, start with the pure cut (continuous) waveform for best results.

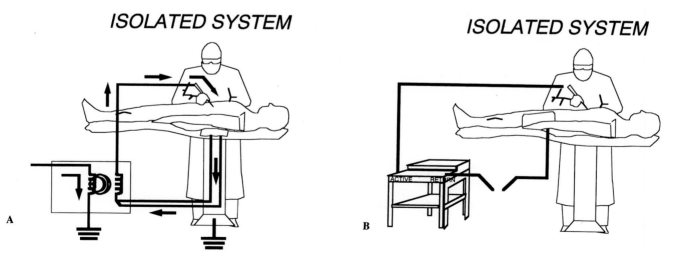

Figure 3-1.11 A. Isolated system with intended current path; **B.** current flow inhibited with cable break due to output isolated from ground.

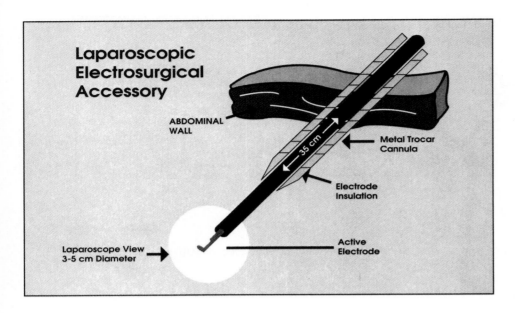

Figure 3-1.12 Electrosurgical electrode and insulation.

When performing desiccation, patience is the key to good results. Typically, the power density is much lower when desiccating; the physical size of the active electrode is therefore larger. The larger electrode or contact area to tissue will require longer activation times to attain the desired therapeutic effect. Using higher energy to speed up the desiccation process will most likely be counterproductive. Higher energy levels will increase the temperature of the tissue adjacent to the electrode(s), potentially forcing the current to spark through the necrotic region, resulting in fulguration rather than desiccation. Fulguration or sparking immediately stops the deepheating process and carbonizes only the surface of the tissue. Therefore, when sparking is observed while desiccating, stop, and reduce the power or pulse the current by keying the ESU on and off, to overcome this natural tendency of the electrosurgical energy to spark when increased voltage is applied.

IATROGENIC BURNS

Since the inception of monopolar electrosurgery, there have been three potential sites for patient burns due to the presence of electrosurgical current: one intended, two unintended. The intended site is at the active electrode where the unit is used to cut, fulgurate, or desiccate the tissue in

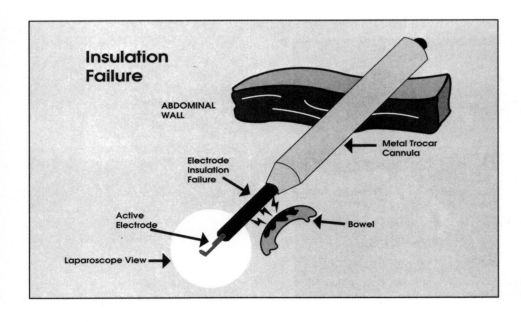

Figure 3-1.13 Defective electrode with energy diverting into the bowel.

surgery. Due to its design, the active electrode has a high power density to heat tissue rapidly. If not kept in control at all times, this electrode can burn the patient severely. Therefore, I strongly recommend that the active electrode, when not in use, be stored in an insulated holster or tray.

The first site of unintended injury is a consequence of the division of current. Current division to alternate ground points to the patient can only occur on ground-referenced ESUs (Figure 3-1.10A). The second is due to a fault condition at the site of the patient return electrode—i.e., partial detachment or a manufacturing defect that forces the current to return to the ESU via a high current density (see Figure 3-1.10B). The patient return electrode (groundplate) has a surface area of approximately 20 square inches or larger when properly applied. Therefore, very little temperature rise occurs at this site under normal conditions. Both of these potential burn sites have been overcome by improved designs within the newer ESUs; these safety circuits have been available in units sold within the past 10 years. The two major advancements in overcoming these risks are as follows.

Technical Innovations To Prevent Iatrogenic Burns

Isolated ESUs were introduced in the early seventies. The primary purpose of their introduction was to prevent alternate ground site burns due to current division. Today, the number of alternate site burns as a direct result of current division is essentially zero, with the introduction of isolated ESUs (Figure 3-1.11). A small percentage of hospitals use ground-referenced ESUs, so it would be wise to find out what type of ESU is in service at your hospital, regarding the type of output.

Contact quality monitoring circuits were introduced in the early eighties. The primary purpose of their introduction was to prevent burns at the patient return electrode site. The contact quality monitor incorporated a dual-section patient return electrode and circuit for the purpose of evaluating the total impedance of the patient return electrode during surgery. During the course of surgery, if the patient return electrode became compromised, the contact quality circuit would inhibit the electrosurgical generator's output based on this dual-section patient return electrode and circuit combination. This feature essentially eliminated the second type of unintended patient burn, those at the site of the patient return electrode.

These two technological advancements have truly reduced the incidence of patient burns during open electrosurgical procedures. These features are now found on the ESUs of major manufacturers, such as Aspen, Birtcher, and Valleylab.

LAPAROSCOPIC ELECTROSURGICAL ISSUES

Electrosurgery has been used in gynecologic laparoscopic surgery for the past 2 decades. Whether it can also be safely employed in other types of laparoscopic surgery is an increasingly important question, as interest in applying laparoscopic techniques to general, urologic, and other types of surgery continues to rise.

There are two potential pitfalls to the use of electrosurgical energy with laparoscopy, both resulting from the use of trocar cannulas to obtain access to the peritoneal cavity. Most laparoscopic accessories are approximately 35 cm long and are used with insulated active electrodes of sufficient length for the devices. Because the laparoscopic images viewed on the monitor are small—typically less than 5 cm of the distal end of the device—this insulated portion of the electrode is out of the viewing image seen on the monitor. If a breakdown of insulation occurs on the shaft of the electrode, out of view from the operator (Figures 3-1.12 and 3-1.13), a severe burn may occur to the bowel or other organs near or touching the electrode shaft at this site. These burns may not be noticed during the course of surgery and may result in severe postoperative complications. Therefore, it is important to periodically examine these electrodes.

A second hazard results from capacitive coupling of energy into other metal laparoscopic instruments or the trocar cannula. Explaining the principle of how capacitance occurs requires delving into electrical physics, which is beyond the scope of this article (Figure 3-1.14 presents the relevant equation). The bottom line is that 5% to 40% of the power level that the ESU is set to deliver can be coupled or transferred from the insulated shaft of the active electrode to the trocar cannula. This energy in itself is not dangerous, providing it is allowed to pass through a low power density pathway such as the allmetal (conductive) trocar cannula and returned to the patient return electrode. For example, the rigid urologic resectoscope is used safely even though capacitive coupling to the sheath of the working element can reach five times the energy level required for laparoscopic procedures. The problem arises when this energy is allowed to pass through a high power density pathway. For example, this can happen with the part-plastic (nonconductive) and part-metal (conductive) trocar cannulas currently on the market (Figure 3-1.15). To

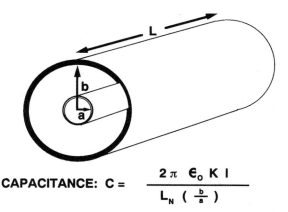

CAPACITANCE: $C = \dfrac{2\pi\, \epsilon_o\, K\, l}{L_N\left(\frac{b}{a}\right)}$

Figure 3-1.14 Formula for capacitance of cylindrical electrodes.

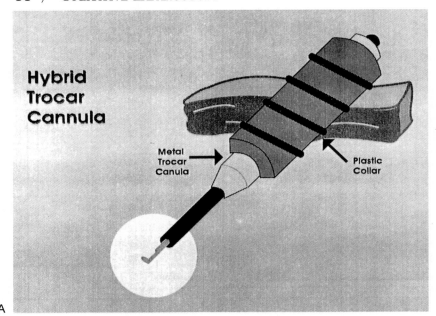

Hybrid Trocar Cannula

Metal Trocar Canula

Plastic Collar

A

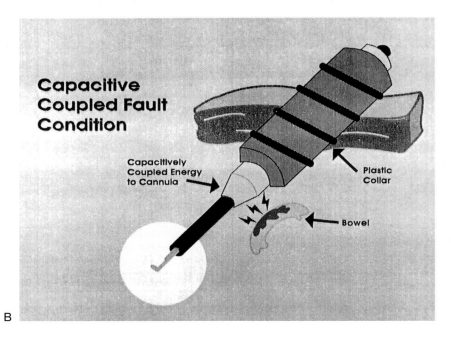

Capacitive Coupled Fault Condition

Capacitively Coupled Energy to Cannula

Plastic Collar

Bowel

B

Figure 3-1.15 **A.** Hybrid trocar cannula. **B.** Capacitative coupled fault condition.

avoid this hazard I strongly recommend the use of all-metal or all-plastic trocar cannulas. To a lesser degree, capacitive coupling can occur when crossing another laparoscopic instrument with the electrosurgical laparoscopic electrode. The energy transfer to this instrument can range from 1% to 10% of the power level set on the ESU. Caution should be exerted under this condition, especially during long activation times.

The problem of capacitive coupling was first detected in performing single-puncture laparoscopic procedures (Corson, 1974 and Engel, 1975). The laparoscope used in these procedures has a working channel to pass various instruments through. It was observed that when a 10- to 12-mm fiberglass cannula was used to pass the laparoscope,

the distal end of the metal laparoscope could deliver a portion of the power set on the ESU and burn adjacent tissue when using an active electrosurgical electrode through the operative channel. Therefore, during single-puncture operative laparoscopy where electrosurgery may be used, only all-metal trocar cannulas should be used.

The all-metal trocar cannula is also a benefit in multiple-puncture laparoscopic procedures, in the event the active electrode accidentally touches the end of the metal laparoscope during activation. The metal trocar cannula will allow this energy to pass safely into the abdominal wall via a low power density pathway. When a plastic cannula is used, the current may exit from the laparoscope to the bowel or other organs

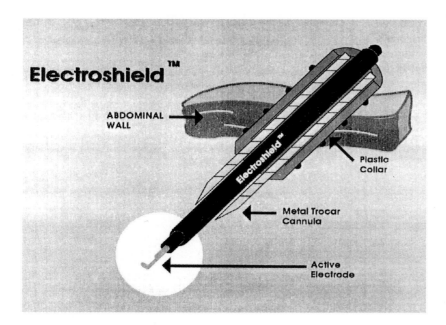

Figure 3-1.16 Electroshield.

out of view of the monitor. This is due to the plastic cannula's blocking the coupled energy from being passed safely into the abdominal wall and back to the patient return electrode.

Electroscope, Inc., of Boulder, Colorado, has recently released Electroshield, a current-monitoring system that protects against both of these primary hazards. The Electroshield system features a reusable shield that surrounds ''existing'' dissecting laparoscopic electrodes (Figure 3-1.16). The Electroshield Monitor (EM-1) dynamically detects any insulation faults or capacitive coupling (Figure 3-1.17). If an unsafe condition exists, the Electroshield system automatically deactivates the generator before a burn can occur. With this tech-

nological advancement, electrosurgical energy can be used in laparoscopy with the same efficacy as in classical open surgical procedures.

CONCLUSION

Electrosurgical energy has by far the most diverse capabilities when compared to other energy sources and is among the least expensive of them. Recent technological advancements in performance and safety have positioned this technique as one of the more useful tools in a surgeon's

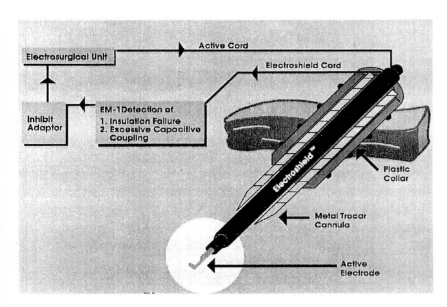

Figure 3-1.17 Electroshield EM-1 Monitor System.

armamentarium. As with any surgical tool or energy source, education and skill are required in order to use it safely. In the case of electrosurgical energy, the biophysics of electrical energy on tissue must be understood.

SUGGESTED READING

Engel T. Electrical dynamics of laparoscopic sterilization. *J Reprod Med* 1975;15:33−42.

Corson SL. Electrosurgical hazards in laparoscopy. *JAMA* 1974;227:1261.

Rioux JE. Laparoscopic tubal sterilization: sparking and its control. *La Vie Medicale au Canada Francais* 1973;2:760−6.

Sigel B, Dunn MR. Mechanism of blood vessel closure by hi frequency electrocoagulation. *Surg Gynecol Obstet* 1965;121:823−31.

Soderstrom RM. Hazards of laparoscopic sterilization. In: Sciarra JW, ed. *Gynecology and Obstetrics*. Philadelphia: Harper & Row; 1982.

Kumagi SG. Effects of electrocautery on midline laparatomy wound infection. *Am J Surg* 1991;162:620−5.

Operative Laparoscopy, Second Edition
The Masters' Techniques in Gynecologic Surgery
Lippincott–Raven Publishers, Philadelphia © 1998.

3-2   Applied Electrophysics in Laparoscopy

Richard M. Soderstrom

With the explosion of surgical procedures being developed in operative laparoscopy, many new electrodes for special procedures are being introduced at a rapid pace. Since the tissue effect of applied electrophysics depends on the size and shape of each electrode, coupled with the chosen waveform and power output, the challenge facing today's laparoscopists is to properly mix and match the electrodes and generators. For instance, because of the difference in the power density of the forceps as they grasp the tissue, a 5-mm grasping forceps will desiccate tissue much more slowly than a 3-mm forceps of similar design.

A knife electrode can be used to incise tissue; yet when coagulation is needed, one can place the flat side of the electrode on the tissue, and with a *cutting* (undamped) waveform it will desiccate and coagulate. A ball-shaped electrode will desiccate when pressed against tissue, regardless of the waveform applied. But if you hold the ball electrode away from an oozing surface and deliver a higher-voltage coagulation waveform, you can fulgurate the bleeding area without deep tissue penetration.

Fulguration can be contrasted with desiccation in several ways. First, sparking to tissue with fulguration *always* produces necrosis anywhere the sparks land. This is not surprising when you consider that each cycle of voltage produces a new spark and each spark has an extremely high current density. In desiccation, the current is no more concentrated than the area of contact between the electrode and the tissue. As a result, desiccation may or may not produce surface necrosis, depending on the current density. For an equal level of current flow, fulguration is always more efficient at producing surface necrosis. However, the depth of tissue injury is quite superficial compared to contact desiccation, because with fulguration the sparks jump from one spot to another in a random fashion; thus the energy is ''sprayed'' rather than concentrated. In general, fulguration requires only one-fifth the average current flow of desiccation.

When changing from one electrode to another, the surgeon should adjust the generator output to match the task at hand. This is especially important when needle electrodes are used after one has used a more blunt electrode. If not, the tissue touched by the high current density of the needle electrode may be severely damaged, and passive heat transfer may destroy the needle electrode.

Since speed of passage and electrode size and shape will determine the heat effect on tissue to be incised, the amount of desired thermal effect will decide what electrode to use and how fast the incision should be made. In addition, the chosen waveform may play a role. To compound the decision, the natural resistance of the tissue to be incised should be considered.

When bipolar instruments are used, a sticking phenomenon is common if a coagulation waveform is used; in general, use an undamped waveform with bipolar instruments. This is especially important when performing tubal sterilization with bipolar forceps. If one uses the coagulation or damped waveform for bipolar sterilization, the center of the tube may not be destroyed because the surface of the tube is charred too quickly, rapidly increasing tissue impedance. The same problem can happen when blood vessels surrounded by fat (i.e., mesenteric vessels) are coagulated with a bipolar instrument delivering a damped waveform. When the desiccated vessel is cut, it may bleed briskly. Using an undamped waveform, an in-line current flowmeter (Ammeter) is a valuable accessory to assure the surgeon that all of the tissue between the forceps has been coagulated before the tissue is transected.

As with laser surgery during operative laparoscopy, smoke accumulation can occur if fulguration techniques are used. For the most part, desiccation techniques create steam rather than smoke, which contains carbon particles. This problem can be reduced or eliminated by irrigating the field to be coagulated with glycine or sorbitol rather than saline or lactated Ringer's solution. Glycine, a nonelectrolytic solution, has a pH of 6.1, similar to lactated Ringer's solution. Several accessory instruments have been designed to allow the simultaneous delivery of glycine and electricity through an irrigation/aspiration cannula that contains an insulated internal electrode that can protrude beyond the tip of the cannula. At the end of the procedure, any intraabdominal glycine is aspirated. If one floods the field as electroenergy is being delivered, the energy is not dissipated within the solution, as it is with electrolyterich fluids, and in a liquid medium, smoke will not develop.

Glycine and sorbitol have another characteristic that is helpful. As one flushes the bleeding area, the individual bleeder will stream through the irrigating solution, giving the appearance of bleeding ''snakes.'' The port of bleeding can be seen with ease and quickly coagulated. These nonelectrolytic solutions are not delivered at a pressure high enough to cause intravascular infusion, which might lead to a water intoxication syndrome, as can occur with hysteroscopy or cystoscopy.

In the early 1980s, it was thought that the occasional bowel perforation following a laparoscopy, when electrodes were used, was the result of sparking or arcing to the bowel. Because the physics of fulguration will not allow an arc to be maintained in a gas-filled abdominal cavity, it is now understood that, at the worst, only a surface charring of the bowel could occur. It takes 30,000 V to spark 1 inch; therefore, the maximum spark an electrosurgical unit can produce is $\frac{1}{8}$ inch (with coagulation set at 100 W or more). To burn a hole in the bowel, the electrode must touch the bowel during the delivery of electroenergy, and remain in contact with the bowel wall for a period of time long enough to coagulate deep into the bowel wall. For this reason, it is best to disconnect the electrodes from the generator when they are not needed for the delivery of electroenergy. To prevent accidentally touching the bowel with an active electrode, one should withdraw the laparoscope from the operating field to create a wide, panoramic view before keying the generator.

At the tissue level, when the energy over time, as measured in joules, is equal between lasers and electrodes, the end result is the same. In other words, a watt is a watt is a watt.

SUGGESTED READING

Pearce JA. *Electrosurgery*. London: Chapman & Hall, 1986.
Soderstrom RM. Principles of Electrosurgery as Applied to Gynecology. In: Rock JA, Thompson JD, eds. *Te Linde's Operative Gynecology*, 8th ed. Philadelphia: Lippincott–Raven Publishers, 1996.

Operative Laparoscopy, Second Edition
The Masters' Techniques in Gynecologic Surgery
Lippincott–Raven Publishers, Philadelphia © 1998.

4

Lasers in Endoscopy

4-1   Applied Physics: Lasers in Endoscopy

Gregory T. Absten

Lasers produce waves of light energy within the electromagnetic spectrum and ultimately effect their work by producing heat. (Some laser modalities work by other than heat-generating effects, but these are specialized applications that are not included in general surgical techniques of cutting, ablation, or photocoagulation.) In order to most safely and effectively exploit these high-energy effects, the laparoscopic surgeon should be knowledgeable about the physical principles that govern the safe and expeditious use of various lasers. Even though any operative laparoscopic procedure may be effectively performed with no laser or electrosurgical assistance, the reward for those who learn to surgically harness these energy sources is extended ''reach'' through smaller endoscopic access, greater convenience and time-saving (since fewer mechanical instruments are required), and greater confidence in maintaining hemostasis and precision.

Laser devices produce their cutting, ablation, and photocoagulation effects by heat. The advantages of lasers lie in their ability to effectively create and localize this heat to produce desired surgical effects with associated hemostasis.

Lasers may be used in two basic ways. One is a general ''noncontact'' method whereby the direct absorption of light by tissue generates heat. In the other method, laser energy physically heats special fiber tips to high temperatures, which are then touched to tissue to create their effects. Before we discuss more of the specifics of these laser modalities, it will be useful to review heating and temperature concepts.

HEAT AND TEMPERATURE

Heat may be measured quantitatively as either calories or British thermal units (BTUs). *Temperature is not heat.* Temperature is a measurement of the intensity of heat, although an object at high temperature does not necessarily have more heat than an object at lower temperature. Larger or heavier objects can contain more heat, at the same temperature, than smaller objects. A 55-gallon drum of water at body temperature contains significantly more heat than a thimbleful of boiling water. This is why larger-diameter laser fibers or probes can contain more heat, and accomplish more work, than smaller-diameter devices at the same temperatures.

The transfer of heat from one object to another occurs through one or more of three basic mechanisms: conduction, convection, and radiation.

Conduction heat transfer is the flow of heat energy in matter as a result of molecular collisions. In other words, a hot object can sear tissue through direct conduction of heat. This is the mechanism of the classic cautery of tissue by hot objects. ''Cautery'' applies to simple hot objects that touch tissue. This is not the same as current-day electrosurgical units, or free-beam laser techniques.

''Contact'' laser fibers and sapphire probes (Figure 4-1.1), typically used on Nd:YAG lasers, are a type of cautery working by direct conduction of heat from an object into tissue by direct contact. These might be truly termed ''photocautery'' units since the laser supplies the energy required to heat the tip of the fiber or sapphire. This is much more effective than electrical methods and results in significantly smaller devices—less than 1.0 mm in diameter. Laser light does transmit through these fiber and sapphire devices, but the major mechanism of action is direct contact conduction heating from the crystal material to tissue.

Conduction heating can become a problem when any laser is left in contact with tissue for excessive periods of time because of low power density applications. Unwanted heat conducts from the target tissue into adjacent tissues and may cause excessive thermal injury. This is most commonly seen when using very low CO_2 laser powers for long periods of time, in order to be ''safe'' with the instrument.

Convection is the second method of heat transfer and involves larger-scale quantities of matter than conduction; an example is the heating of gases and liquids in boiling a

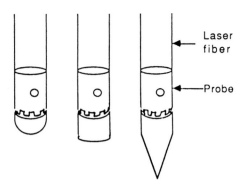

Figure 4-1.1 Sapphire Probes. Tips of various geometric shapes are used for different effects, such as vaporization or cutting. The predominant mechanism is direct heating of the sapphire tips by the laser energy. They function much like a "hot knife."

pan of water. Convection heating is not really very relevant to laser surgery.

Radiation heat transfer is very important to both electrosurgical and laser modalities. This involves the transfer of thermal energy by electromagnetic waves (light and electricity). Objects don't have to touch to transfer heat this way. Heat may even be transmitted across a vacuum by radiation since it does not depend on the presence of matter. This is the essential mechanism of laser and electrosurgical devices. Lasers (no matter what the type of light) are of higher frequency than electrosurgical units (radiofrequency electricity), but both are forms of electromagnetic radiation.

Radiation transfer means that laser beams contain no inherent heat. They transmit only radiant energy. When noncontact methods are used (i.e., no special fiber tips), heat is created only when the tissue absorbs the transmitted radiation and converts it to motion in the tissue's atoms and molecules. This is exactly the way a microwave oven works, only at lower frequencies than laser.

Heat capacity and specific heats of objects are closely related and have to do with how much heat is required to produce a certain temperature change. In other words, biologic objects of high heat capacity require much more heat to effect any given surgical effect through a temperature rise. Highly vascular tissues have a higher heat capacity than other tissues and consequently require higher laser powers to produce the same surgical effects. In particular, tissue that bleeds significantly will require higher powers to counteract the "heat sink" effect of the blood flow, unless other measures are taken to retard the flow.

LASERS

Laser is an acronym which stands for Light Amplification by the Stimulated Emission of Radiation. Radiation here does not refer to ionizing-type radiation such as x-ray. It refers to a "radiant" body, or one that "shines" light. Ion-

izing radiation is not a hazard with conventional medical laser units.

Light (photons of energy) is contained within the forces that hold together atoms and molecules. By tapping into these atomic and molecular bonds, we can release the light stored there. Regular light sources such as light bulbs release this light energy in a random, chaotic process of spontaneously emitting the light. Photons of all energies (wavelengths, or colors) are released in all directions, with no coordination between them. This results in incoherent white light (all colors combined, radiating in all directions).

Laser light consists of the same photons of light as from ordinary light sources, but they are released in an organized fashion called stimulated emission. The laser tube, with its facing mirrors at each end, serves to propagate this process and build a very intense beam of light. The light emitted is of one energy (wavelength and color) and travels in one direction through space as a tight beam. The result is a coherent beam of bright light of one color, or at least pure colors.

Lasers are devices that produce intense beams of light energy. They take electricity and convert it into light which can be further intensified to cut, vaporize, or coagulate tissue. The key mechanism of action is stimulated emission of radiation, which was described by Albert Einstein in the early 1900s. This is a special way in which atoms and molecules emit highly organized waves of light.

Through stimulated emission, atoms and molecules are energized and manipulated to produce this unique type of light. As waves of laser light, produced by stimulated emission, are emitted along the length of the laser tube (also termed the laser resonator), they reflect back and forth between the mirrors, amplifying the resulting waves of light (Figure 4-1.2). The result is a tremendously bright beam of light that exits the tube through one of the mirrors, which is only partially reflective. This is the laser beam.

Three unique qualities of laser light differentiate it from regular light: its coherence, monochromaticity, and colli-

OPTICAL RESONATOR

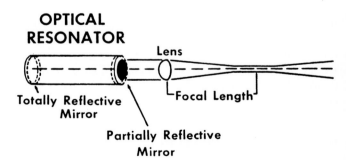

Figure 4-1.2 Laser Tube, or resonator. Laser light is amplified by reflecting back and forth between the end mirrors. One of these mirrors is only partially reflective and allows a small percentage of the light to escape as the emitted laser beam. The laser beam is focused through a lens to a small spot where it is delivered into a fiber or applied directly to tissue.

UNCOLLIMATED

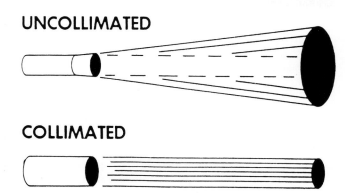

COLLIMATED

Figure 4-1.3 Unlike an uncollimated flashlight beam, a collimated laserbeam remains practically parallel. This retains the intensity of the beam over distance and allows a focusing lens to create very small spots.

Table 4-1.1 *Common laparoscopic lasers*

Laser	Color	Wavelength
Argon	Blue	488 nm
	Green	515 nm
KTP	Green	532 nm
Nd:YAG	Near infrared	1064 nm
Ho:YAG	Mid-infrared	2100 mn
CO_2	Far infrared	10,600 nm

mation. Not all of these are really important for surgery. Coherence refers to the orderliness of the wave patterns of the light. This will be very important for future diagnostic and scanning applications but is not very important in surgical uses of lasers.

Not all lasers produce only one color of light—i.e., argon, which emits light at 488 nm and 515 nm. Laser light is termed monochromatic since it produces pure colors of light. This can be important for medicine, since different tissues absorb various colors differently, but the absolute pure color is really not critical for cutting and vaporizing applications. Laser light is termed collimated because its waves travel together as a tight, parallel beam (Figure 4-1.3). This allows the beam to be finely focused to intensify its effects and is the major characteristic allowing its surgical use.

Various chemical elements emit characteristic colors of light, and the laser is named after the material used. The five primary surgical lasers (see Table 4-1.1) are the carbon dioxide (CO_2), which emits far infrared light at 10,600 nanometers (nm); the Nd:YAG (Neodymium:YAG), which emits near infrared light at 1064 nm; the Ho:YAG (Holmium:YAG), which emits mid-infrared at 2100 nm; the argon, which emits blue-green light of 488 and 515 nm; and the KTP, which produces green light similar to the argon but at 532 nm, by altering the infrared output of a Nd:YAG laser with a KTP crystal.

TISSUE EFFECTS OF LASERS

The surgical effects of the laser are due to localized heating when the light is absorbed by tissue. As tissue begins to heat, it blanches white as it coagulates, then shrivels as it desiccates, and finally turns to steam and vapor as it is vaporized above 100°C. If the light is transmitted through or reflected from tissue, then no absorption or heating will occur. This is sometimes seen in argon and KTP lasers; when used at threshold energies to ''spray coagulate'' a

bleeding peritoneal surface, the light will be absorbed by the minute oozers and cause coagulation, but will be reflected by normally light-colored peritoneal surfaces and produce no effect there. They can also transmit through the surface peritoneum to be absorbed by visible vessels underneath, as a hemostatic prelude to the laser incision in that area.

Several parameters control the delivery of laser energy to tissue. These include the power (watts), total energy delivered (watts and time), power density (the size of focused spot used to intensify the light), the color of the light, and the color and vascularity of the tissue. It is important that surgeons attend good hands-on training programs or have worked extensively with lasers in residency, to learn control of these parameters.

In some ways these energy concepts are intuitive. An analogy is the use of a magnifying glass to focus sunlight and create a burn (Figure 4-1.4). The brighter the sun (power), the more it burns. The smaller the spot created with the lens (power density), the hotter it burns. The longer the sun is focused in one place (total energy), the more extensively it burns. The wetter the target you are trying to burn (vascularity), the longer it takes to create the same effect.

The surgeon has control over a combination of three of these parameters affecting the intensity and effects of a laser: power setting, timing of application, and spot size of the

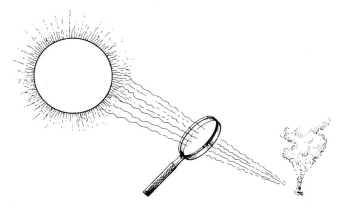

Figure 4-1.4 Focusing sunlight. The sun provides the rate of energy delivery, or power in watts. The lens intensifies the effect by concentrating the collected energy into a very small spot, increasing the power density in watts per square centimeter.

beam. The power of the laser is set at the machine by the laser specialist operating the unit. The timing of the application to achieve a given effect is controlled by the surgeon. When the laser is used in a continuous mode—i.e., the beam is delivered at a steady rate of energy—the time of application in any one spot is determined by how the surgeon moves the beam. The laser beam may also be altered to deliver energy in a timed, pulsed mode; this makes application of the beam brief, in fractions of a second usually, to provide good control of higher powers. A timed pulse gives the surgeon more control and a longer reaction time and produces less spread of heat damage, though it does go much slower than a continuous mode. The mode used is also set at the control console of the laser. (Alternatively, a good technique for laparoscopically ''pulsing'' the laser is to set the laser in a continuous mode but to pump the foot pedal to produce controlled bursts.) The spot size of the beam is directly controlled by the surgeon in the operative field and depends on the delivery device being used.

Confusion over which types of lasers are used for which procedures results from the overlap of tissue effects caused by varying these control parameters. By attaining sufficiently small spots, the ordinary color selectivity effects of the argon and KTP lasers may be overwhelmed by the resulting high power densities. Nd:YAG lasers may use sculpted fibers or sapphire tips to produce highly controlled cutting. In other words, any laser may be made to cut or vaporize tissue, though they each have their own strengths and weaknesses in various applications.

A further clarification of these energy concepts allows one to see how various laser delivery devices and fibers can achieve different surgical effects. Power is simply a measure of the rate of energy delivery in joules per second and is expressed in watts. This applies equally to lasers or electrosurgery. Of greater importance is the amount of power that can be focused into a spot. This power density, or irradiance (sometimes called spot brightness), of a laser is the number of watts per square centimeter of a spot and is the single most important factor in the effective application of a laser. The surface area of the spot (spot size controlled by the surgeon in the field) and the total power in watts (set at the laser by the operator) determine the power density, as follows:

$$\frac{(\text{Watts} \times 100) \times .86}{\text{Pi} \times r^2} = \text{W/cm}^2$$

Power density over a spot determines the rate of tissue removal within that spot. Therefore, it is not the power that determines the ''controllability'' of the beam but rather the power density. One can effectively change the size of the ''paintbrush'' (spot size) with which one is working without changing the overall rate of tissue removal (power density) within that spot, by varying the spot sizes and power. The larger the spot, the greater the power required to maintain the same power density, shown as follows:

	0.6 mm spot	2.0 mm spot
1900 W/cm²:	10 W	60 W

Laparoscopic laser delivery devices (except for contact fibers and probes) boil down to the CO_2 laser laparoscope for that laser (fibers cannot be used) and regular fibers for the argon, KTP, Ho:YAG and free-beam Nd:YAG lasers. Power density is affected primarily by spot size. Figure 4-1.5 illustrates how spot size changes with distance from the end of the laser device. The primary difference between the two systems (CO_2 versus fibers) is that fibers emit a beam that immediately begins to diverge, while a CO_2 laser laparoscope first comes to a focal point, then diverges. The range of effect with fiber systems is only an inch or two off the end of the fiber. Not much happens beyond this distance. CO_2 laser systems maintain a relatively long depth of field and may burn or vaporize tissue some distance behind the target if a suitable backstop is not selected. (Depth of field is a concept that might be familiar to amateur photographers. This is the horizontal distance, or ''depth,'' where the focal point of the lens system stays in focus. With a laser, this means that the focal point may extend virtually unchanged for an inch or two on either side of the focal point. This means that the range of effect of this device is much longer than with a fiber system.)

The advantage of fibers is that different effects can be accomplished quickly with only a slight motion of the fingers holding the fiber handpiece. A small pinch back with the fingers allows a small blood vessel to be photocoagulated, then a small pinch forward to bring the fiber end just over tissue results in a cut, both at the same power settings on the machine. The short range of effect also reduces the need for intraabdominal backstops. Many times these fibers are actually touched into tissue when cutting, but this should still not be confused with the contact type of fibers and probes, which *must* be touched to create an effect, even though part of the effect of noncontact-type fibers may actually result from heating of the end of the fiber. These fiber systems may be delivered through any conventional portal, including 3-mm sites or even smaller needle puncture sites. The argon and KTP are the primary fiberoptic lasers for laparoscopy besides contact-type modalities, which are mainly Nd:YAG lasers.

The CO_2 laser provides a great deal of versatility in the ''reach'' it provides from the end of the laparoscope, the number of angles where it can work, and the speed at which it can vaporize or cut if desired. In this sense it is probably more versatile than a fiber system, but it has a significantly longer learning curve and does not provide the hemostasis that fiber systems provide. It also requires a specialized laparoscope set and coupler to mate the laser with the scope.

CO_2 laser waveguides, which somewhat resemble a fiber for this laser, are available for laparoscopic use. Unlike

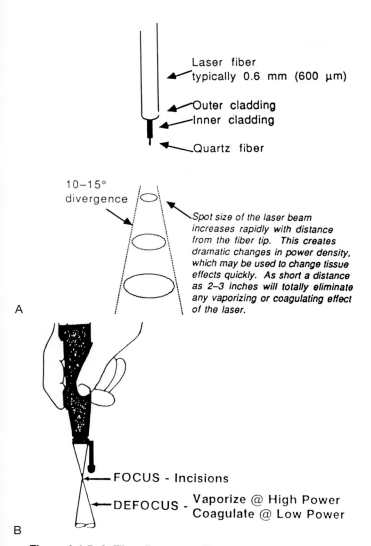

Laser fiber
typically 0.6 mm (600 μm)

Outer cladding
Inner cladding
Quartz fiber

10–15°
divergence

Spot size of the laser beam increases rapidly with distance from the fiber tip. This creates dramatic changes in power density, which may be used to change tissue effects quickly. As short a distance as 2–3 inches will totally eliminate any vaporizing or coagulating effect of the laser.

A

FOCUS - Incisions

DEFOCUS - Vaporize @ High Power
Coagulate @ Low Power

B

Figure 4-1.5 A. Fiber divergence. The spot size of the laser beam increases rapidly with distance from the fiber tip. This creates dramatic changes in power density, which may be used to change tissue effects quickly. As short a distance as 2 to 3 inches will totally eliminate any vaporizing or coagulating effects of the laser (Copyright Gregory T. Absten, 1992.) **B.** CO_2 laser-focusing handpiece. Rather than diverging like a fiber, the beam comes to a small focal point, then diverges after this point. A CO_2 laser laparoscope operates in the same fashion.

regular fibers, which are of one filament of quartz around 0.6 mm in diameter, a CO_2 laser waveguide is actually a slender hollow tube around 3 mm in diameter with an internal hollow ceramic insert or coating. The laser is focused into the proximal end of this tube and, through hundreds of internal glancing reflections, bounces down the tube until it is emitted from the end. This does destroy the focusing property of the beam, which instead diverges, somewhat like the beam emitted by a fiber. It does not diverge as rapidly as a beam from a fiber, however, and has a longer range of effect than a fiber.

Part of the original impetus for development of these CO_2 laser waveguides was the myriad alignment problems with previous laser couplers on laparoscopes. Between misaligned articulated arms on the laser and machining discrepancies in the coupler cubes and scopes, alignment of the CO_2 laser beam down the channel of the scope proved to be a constant problem. This laser has a "line of sight" delivery, and any misalignment causes the beam to bounce around on the walls of the channel, destroying its focusing abilities. This was an "in the old days" problem, and contemporary CO_2 lasers don't exhibit these problems. However, this is very manufacturer-dependent. Buy only the best.

Fibers terminating in some device such as a metal tip, sapphire probe, or even an altered shape of the fiber tip generate a significant amount of heat at this tip and are referred to as hot tip devices. They act as very intense, precise thermal knives. Energy concepts such as power density do not really apply to contact devices, since they rely on simple heat conduction. The Nd:YAG laser is the primary one used for hot tip devices, and this is a popular way to use the laser laparoscopically.

Some of the hot tip devices, such as rounded or chisel sapphire tips, do actually focus some of the laser light, so that combination effects may occur. A combination rounded tip fiber is also available, which may be backed off tissue to vaporize or coagulate as free beam or touched to tissue to cut as a hot tip. Again, the availability of various types of fibers is very manufacturer-dependent.

Sculptured fibers have increased in popularity as a laparoscopic tool. These are not as expensive as the sapphire tips but are single-use items, compared with multiple use of the sapphires. With either of these tips one must be careful not to fire the laser for extended periods (several seconds) when not in contact with tissue. This will burn up the tip, since the heat does not go into the vaporization of tissue.

Because larger objects have higher heat capacities than smaller objects, larger contact fibers or sapphires seem to cut better and are less fragile than smaller ones. This doesn't refer to the size of the very tip of the device but to the bulk behind it. For instance, a 1.2-mm sapphire, which is tapered to 0.2 mm at the tip, creates an exceptionally clean, controlled cut for applications such as salpingectomy for ectopic pregnancy.

Those that prefer the contact methods of laser point to the control they achieve by affecting only tissue that they touch. They prefer this "feel" for tissue. Those that prefer free-beam fibers point to the versatility they achieve by varying the distance from the fiber to tissue. CO_2 laser users like the precise cuts they are able to achieve, and the speed at which they can work, while, of course, maintaining surgical control.

A laser may be used with either free-beam or hot tip technique, depending on the fiber or device connected to the laser. The argon or KTP laser can be used either way, for instance. Laparoscopically, the effects of argon and KTP are indistinguishable. The KTP laser, though, because it uses Nd:YAG laser light shot through a KTP crystal to make green light, permits one to harness the capabilities of both the green KTP and near infrared Nd:YAG lasers in the same machine. The Nd:YAG laser could be used free-beam intraabdominally, but this is generally not recommended because of the potentially deep coagulation that could occur. (4 or 5 mm of deep damage is possible with the Nd:YAG laser free beam, but limiting the power to no more than about 20 W, exposure to less than 3 seconds, and a distance from tissue of no closer than about 1 cm will limit the potential damage to 1 or 2 mm.) Instead, sapphires or sculptured fibers are preferred. This limits the lateral damage to fractions of a millimeter.

For similar surgical effects, the green argon and KTP lasers don't require a special fiber tip as does the Nd:YAG, because the wavelength of light itself cuts fine at high intensities and limits more extensive damage. The Nd:YAG laser requires special tips in order to cut well and limit deep damage. There may be some very subtle differences between these three modalities, and research into this is currently underway.

The total energy within any laser beam is expressed in joules. Power multiplied by delivery time equals the number of joules. Ten watts delivered for 3 seconds is 30 J of energy. "Joules" describes the total energy delivered but does not by itself indicate how concentrated this dose of light is. This applies to electrosurgery in exactly the same way.

Fluence combines the concepts of power density (spot brightness) and dosage (joules), and is expressed in joules per square centimeter. A high fluence is like a bolus of light. It gets the job done without allowing enough time for excessive heat conduction to occur (Figure 4-1.6). Pulsing a laser is a way to achieve high fluence. This is not the same as setting the laser on a "timed" pulse such as one tenth of a second. That is simply a timer on an otherwise continuous wave beam. A true pulse delivers very high peak power bursts of light but for very short periods—usually in microseconds per burst—and may be repeated as fast as 1000 times per second. CO_2 lasers provide this feature in superpulse modes. Average powers are not high. The mode is very controllable and produces an exceptionally clean tissue effect.

A superpulse mode, where high fluences are achieved, is unquestionably the best and most precise way to use a CO_2 laser. Each pulse must contain enough energy to itself cause tissue ablation, or the beam will still result in undesirable burning or charring of tissue.

Previously, the limiting factor of superpulses on CO_2 lasers has been that only very low average powers were attainable, even with otherwise high-power lasers. The newest technological evolution of superpulse has been termed an "ultra-pulse." It is able to sustain the high power of a pulse longer than a superpulse could and deliver both higher energies in that pulse and very high average powers, at the discretion of the surgeon, and is unquestionably the best realization of the concept of superpulse.

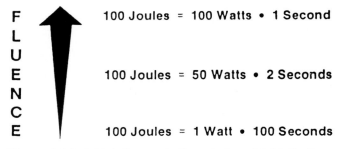

Figure 4-1.6 A high fluence is like a bolus of light. It allows the work to be accomplished without allowing much time for excessive heat conduction to occur in tissue.

A new type of pulsed system Nd:YAG laser has recently been introduced for laparoscopic use, similar to a superpulse on a CO_2 laser. This provides a much cleaner cut than would be provided by ordinary continuous-wave Nd:YAG lasers and significantly reduces concern about deep coagulation damage. Additionally, the laser incorporates an internal sensor to sense fiber tip temperatures and prevent overheating. When the tip is not in tissue, excessive powers will cause it to overheat. The laser immediately reacts by automatically throttling back the power. This is a major advantage when using contact-type fibers and an additional safety feature to prevent high laser powers from "free-beaming" in the abdomen.

CONCLUSION

Once properly mastered, lasers constitute a significantly useful tool for the laparoscopic surgeon, providing better precision and control than electrosurgery, good hemostasis, and the convenience of a tool that accomplishes several tasks. However, lasers are not a better choice than electrosurgery in all circumstances, and sometimes the ease and simplicity of electrosurgery make it the tool of choice when the advantages of lasers are not required (such as taking down a few filmy adhesions, not directly on bowel, or even dissecting the gallbladder wall from the liver).

Suggested Reading

Absten GT. *Fundamentals of Electrosurgery.* Columbus, OH: Advanced Laser Services Corporation, 1991.

Apfelberg D. *Evaluation and Installation of Surgical Laser Systems.* New York: Springer-Verlag, 1987.

Einstein A. *Relativity.* New York: Bonanza Books, 1961.

Hallmark C. *Lasers, the Light Fantastic.* Blue Ridge Summit, PA: Tab Books, 1979.

Hecht J. *Understanding Lasers.* New York: Howard W. Sams & Co./Macmillan, 1988.

Goldman L. *The Biomedical Laser: Technology and Clinical Applications.* New York: Springer-Verlag, 1981.

Laser Focus. In: *1992 Medical Laser Buyers Guide.* Littleton, MA: Penwell Publications, 1992.

Minton JP, Absten GT. Surgical lasers and how they work. *American College of Surgeons Bulletin,* 1987.

Operative Laparoscopy, Second Edition
The Masters' Techniques in Gynecologic Surgery
Lippincott–Raven Publishers, Philadelphia © 1998.

4-2 Equipment

John L. Marlow

First I must credit those masters whose endoscopic skills I was fortunate enough to observe early in my surgical career. Professor Raoul Palmer of Paris, France, Mr. Patrick Steptoe of Oldham, England, and Professor Dr. med Hans Frangenheim of Konstanz, Germany, established my basic understanding of laparoscopic surgery. My appreciation of the great value of laparoscopy was born in their operative theaters, as I looked over their shoulders. With their help, I soon realized the unique access to the inner pelvis and abdominal chamber that this instrumentation provides. Surgery remains an apprenticeship, as each generation learns from those who have gone before and in turn passes their knowledge, skills, and instruments to the next for improvement. This partnership of the past and present has brought laparoscopy to today's geometrically increasing acceptance. This chapter is dedicated to those masters who have gone before me. It will focus on laparoscopy surgery instrumentation and techniques that have proven useful in laparoscopy during the 25-plus years of my surgical experience.

THE LAPAROSCOPE

Basic to all good surgery is adequate exposure, and the laparoscope provides the best exposure possible. The ideal laparoscope optics provide a clear and sharply defined image with the widest possible viewing angle. I prefer to have several laparoscopes available on the table or in an adjacent sterile container. A large 8 to 10 mm laparoscope is useful for inspection and documentation. Angled viewing lenses allow the widest angle viewing, allowing the surgeon better access to inspect the side and back walls of structures, including the anterior abdominal wall. Forward viewing lenses give the least optical distortion and are easier for the new laparoscopic surgeon to use. Channels within the laparoscope provide additional ports to insert ancillary instruments or laser beams without the risk of inserting an additional trochar. This so-called "operative laparoscope" is useful in treating midline and cul-de-sac disease. Smaller laparoscopes may be used through secondary trochars for alternative viewing sites. Recently 1.2 mm laparoscopes which can be inserted through a Veress needle have become available. This new microendoscopy may provide new tools for use in emergency rooms and office settings. The very small incisions permitted by this technique reduce post operative recovery time. Improved optics and light-sensitive electronic imaging provide better images than have been available in the past. Hysteroscopy is frequently done with laparoscopy and can also be used as a second smaller laparoscope.

TROCARS

The correct placement of ancillary trocars will make laparoscopic surgery difficult or easy depending upon the location of pelvic pathology. Midline deep cul-de-sac adhesions or endometrial implants can be approached best through the midline operative laparoscopic channel. Adnexal disease on the other hand, is best reached through a lateral lower abdominal placement. As with laparoscopes, multiple sized trochars are used. One recent addition is a trochar that is expandable. It begins with a Veress-needle sized caliber and then can be stretched to 10-mm or larger channels. Small trochars offer less trauma while larger trochars offer easier specimen removal. Valves of the trochar are important to consider. Trumpet valve or trap door valves make specimen and instrument removal more difficult. Easy, smooth instrument exchanges and suturing through the trochar without a loss of pneumoperitoneum is desirable. The length of the trochar should correspond to the patients abdominal wall thickness. Shorter sizes increase the instruments maneuverability. Newer sealing devices come with multiple sizes which can be easily selected according to the instrument size. Fixation of the trochar to the abdominal wall or fascial anchoring is aided by spiral grooves, balloons, or expanding shafts of the trochar sleeve. The tip of the trochar is another important concern. I prefer cone-shaped trochars for lateral trochar insertions. The cone shape is less likely to cut vessels than trochars with very sharp pyramidal edges. The cost of the disposable trochars is becoming more of a consideration in selecting this instrumentation.

ANCILLARY INSTRUMENTS

To paraphrase the Marines, "All the laparoscopic surgeon needs are a few good instruments." Most laparoscopic surgeries can be done with a few good instruments, including an aspirator-irrigator system, tissue probes, injection/aspiration needles, graspers, scissors, biopsy, staple and clip applicators and coagulators. Emphasis should be on obtaining the highest quality instruments available. The composition, manufacturing, and maintenance of the instruments determine this quality. Cost considerations here also have increased the interest in reusable instruments. Sharp scissors are essential to good endoscopic surgery and are one of the most important ancillary tools. The purchase of high-quality laparoscopy instruments saves expense in the long term by avoiding delays and complications. New instruments offer single-handed rotational control. A variety of tip configurations are available including replaceable tips, shafts, and handles. Designs are increasingly made to complement the surgeons' hands. Ergonomics is becoming more important in the design. Locking and unlocking of grasping instruments can be accomplished more easily with one hand. Sharp scissors are more available with replaceable tips, at reduced cost.

INSUFFLATORS

Tympany is checked before insufflation to check for distented viscera such as the stomach. It is not difficult to find a large gas-filled stomach following muscle relaxation and hyperventilation prior to intubation. After insufflation needle placement, the flow is started at low pressure settings, usually less than 15–20 mm. During the insufflation, percussion should reveal a symmetrically enlarging tympany. The opening pressure is important to note. High or fluctuating pressure may indicate adhesions to the anterior abdominal wall. High flow rates are not used until after confirming proper trochar placement. Safety is paramount in this phase of the surgery. After an adequate pneumoperitoneum is established and the correct trochar site confirmed by intraabdominal inspection, the flow rate is set to the highest available on the insufflator. Insufflators that provide controlled high-volume gas flow are essential for laparoscopic surgery. Frequent irrigation and aspirations collapse the pneumoperitoneum and prolong the procedure without such insufflators. Visible and audible signals monitor intraabdominal pressures and flow rates during the laparoscopy. The audible monitors alert the surgical team when any safety parameter is exceeded, obviating the need to look constantly at the insufflator.

THERMAL ENERGY GENERATORS

Laser

Several lasers are available for use in laparoscopy. These include CO_2, argon, KTP, and Nd:YAG. Carbon dioxide laser was the first used through the laparoscope. Its principle benefit is the precision and control it permits. Because the tissue effect of this laser occurs at the surface, where it can be visually monitored, it can be used over very critical organs such as small bowel and ureter. At low power settings, the laser does not penetrate deeply, and because it can be visually monitored, it is my choice where removal or cutting of tissue in critical areas, such as the deep lateral pelvic walls is undertaken. Open-channel delivery through an operating laparoscope or secondary trochar is now my choice and the simplest system. This is the so called "no touch" system. Any tissue which can be visualized can be treated. One concern is that the CO_2 laser must have a backstop. This can be provided by the tissue itself, a probe, or fluid. I prefer high-power lasers 50 watts to 80 watts with computer generated options to configure the laser power density delivery to tissue. A typical power setting for thin adhesions would be 10 watts to 20 watts, delivered in 0.05 second, repeating 10 pulses per second.

The Nd:YAG laser is a fiberoptic laser that can coagulate large volumes of tissue. Its beam is delivered in higher powers than available with other fiber lasers. Delivery through a fiber has the advantage of its ability to be used through many existing instruments. The generator can be distant from the operating table and provide more open space. These lasers, i.e., can be delivered under water, while irrigating tissue. They are better for coagulation of bleeding vessels or tissue. Colored lasers, argon, and KTP, are selectively absorbed in the hemoglobin spectrum. Special eye protection is needed when using these lasers, since they can be transmitted through the lens system of the laparoscope. CO_2 laser beam would be absorbed by these lenses. Most of my laser surgery is now done with CO_2 and Nd:YAG.

Electrosurgery

Monopolar electrosurgery is still a useful tool and was the original energy source for laparoscopic surgery. I use both unipolar and bipolar electrosurgery. Safety concerns have increased the use of bipolar instruments. For most laparoscopic surgery, I use a combination of CO_2 laser and bipolar electrosurgery. For example, for dissection and destruction of lesions on the bowel and pelvic side wall, I utilize a CO_2 laser. For vascular thick omental adhesion without bowel involvement, I use bipolar electrosurgery and mechanical scissors or a cutting device in one instrument. This combination of grasping, coagulation and cutting availability in one tool has been a useful addition to the instruments. The combination of all three uses in one instrument saves significant time. Since the cutting blade is precisely in the center of the grasping jaws, only the tissue that has been coagulated is cut. Electronic monitoring of the complete coagulation to complete dessication pioneered by Dr. Kleppinger reduces the occurrence of post-transection bleeding.

SUTURES, STAPLES AND TISSUE LIGATION

Suturing through the trochar without a loss of pneumoperitoneum is now possible. I am using both intrauterine suturing and external knot-pushing techniques. Straight or ski-shaped needles simplify insertion and retrieval through ancillary trochar sleeves. Curved needle sutures can be inserted and removed through trochar site incisions after removing the rigid sleeves. Endoloops ligatures have the advantage of ease and speed of application. I prefer these for large vessel pedicles. Closed loop knot pushers have simplified external knot-tying. The braided sutures offer more resistance to pushing the knot; but are less likely to slip once in place, in my experience. Automated endoscopic suturing instruments are now available for use through the laparoscope; I await further reports of its use.

Staples reduce the operative time and are particularly useful in advanced procedures such as laparoscopy bowel surgery. The large tips of some instruments can obscure the surgeon's view of the operative site and must be used with care close to the ureter and large vessels. Absorbable staples and microstapling are two areas of new interest.

SPECIAL INSTRUMENTS

Removal of specimens during laparoscopy through small incisions have been a challenge for minimally invasive surgery. This becomes necessary for such procedures as laparoscopic myomectomy and adnexectomy. Plastic pouches speed up the removal and reduce the risk of spillage. Electronic morcellators reduce the time necessary for this removal and also eliminate the need to enlarge the incision or make an additional vaginal incision. Histological examination is possible, but loss of orientation of the specimen, (i.e., an ovary) requires additional work for the pathologist. Uterine manipulators and mobilizers provide better control of the uterus during laparoscopic surgery. Fixation of the uterine position to the desired location is more easily maintained. Injection of dye material to evaluate tubal patency and a variety of cannula tips to accommodate cervical size and configuration can be obtained.

PROBES

Probes are needed in laparoscopy to introduce irrigation fluid, manipulate pelvic organs, and to aspirate smoke and fluid. My choice of irrigating fluid is Ringer's lactate at body temperature. Since vaporization of tissue produces a plume of smoke, this must be removed for adequate visualization. The tip of the probe should be positioned near the impact site of the laser or electrosurgery. Newer lasers produce minimal carbonization and smoke production. The most used probe size is 5 mm. Aspiration of blood clots, a common need, is easier through a larger-caliber probe. Suction pressure is also a consideration. Large blood clots encountered in an ectopic pregnancy can be quickly removed, using the high vacuum pressure available in the units used for suction dilation and curettage.

TELEVISION

In an increasingly visually oriented society, almost every hospital patient has a television in her room. Likewise, today every laparoscopic surgeon must have the benefit of televised laparoscopy. Modern endoscopic operating rooms have multiple monitors, one for the primary surgeon and one or more for the assisting team. Smaller TVs, which can be positioned near the surgeon, have made this more useful. The monitors provide large, easily seen images for the surgical team, and simplify visual image documentation immediately available to surgeon and family. New camera technology has provided high definition imaging, as well as the low light sensitivities needed for smaller laparoscopic use. Fatigue during long laparoscopy cases has been reduced because the standing position is more comfortable, compared to the bent position necessary without television use. Without the strain of bending over, eye-hand coordination is also enhanced. Coordination is important for performing increasingly complex surgical procedures through the laparoscope. The use of videotapes has decreased in my practice except where it is important to document motion. Still video images are easily obtained and serve to complement the dictated operative report. These have been useful when reoperation is necessary. Although not universal, patients and family seem to appreciate a visual record of the findings and this serves to improve physician/patient communication, an important part of surgery.

I take a standard sequence of images. An overview of the pelvis, anterior, posterior, right and left pelvis, right and left mid-abdomen, and upper abdomen, are included. Closeups of any pathology before and after treatment complete the usual recording. The still images are identified in the OR with the patient's identifying label, which includes a bar code. This has simplified copying the findings for record requests.

Videotapes are cumbersome to review for specific images. This requires a VCR and TV to view, and special copying instruments to duplicate. In the near future, digital images and compact disc use will simplify this problem. Image retrieval and transmission over telephone lines for archival and other uses will make this an attractive alternative.

INSTRUMENT CARE AND REPAIR

Laparoscopic instruments require special maintenance and care. Scheduled periodic maintenance and inspection are important to keep the equipment in peak performance. Backup instruments should be available to avoid expensive operating room delays and rescheduling of cases. Instrument damage can be reduced through inservice programs and orientation for operating room personnel. Administrative assignment of coordinators and operating room personnel knowledgeable about laparoscopy equipment reduces complications from instrumentation. Surgeons also should have a good understanding of the laparoscopy instruments. This should be a part of credentialing for the surgeon and should be a renewable priviledge. New instruments and techniques which are significantly complex should be introduced as a part of the continuing education program for the hospital. Participation in this orientation and education should be documented before the surgeon is allowed to schedule cases using complex operative instruments.

NEW INSTRUMENTS

Ongoing basic research will speed the development of new laparoscopic instruments. Computer-generated virtual reality can now create instruments, test their usability and, in the near future, train laparoscopic surgeons in their use. This new technology may also be used to evaluate and maintain surgical competence, as simulators do today for airline pilots. Already we see robotics applied to laparoscopy in the form of a robot instrument that potentially could replace some surgical assistance. The unit can move laparoscope and instruments on voice-activated command to a preselected position. Multiple specialty use of laparoscopy has increased the pool of surgeons available for creative input to improve laparoscopic instrumentation. Cost of health care, including instruments, has become increasingly important. This can limit innovation. Larger economically empowered organizations are appearing in the administrative tree of health care that I hope will continue the search for improved laparoscopic instrumentation. While poor surgeons sometimes blame their tools, the best laparoscopic surgery can only be performed with the highest quality instrumentation.

SUGGESTED READING

Baggish MS. *Basic and Advanced Laser Surgery in Gynecology.* Norwalk, CT: Appleton-Century-Crofts, 1985.
Fuller TA. *Surgical Lasers, A Clinical Guide.* New York: Macmillan, 1987.
Keye WR Jr. *Laser Surgery in Gynecology and Obstetrics.* 2nd ed. Chicago: Year Book Medical Publishers, 1990.
McLaughlin DS. *Lasers in Gynecology.* Philadelphia: JB Lippincott, 1991.
Sanfilippo JS, Levine RS. *Operative Gynecologic Endoscopy.* New York: Springer-Verlag, 1989.

Operative Laparoscopy, Second Edition
The Masters' Techniques in Gynecologic Surgery
Lippincott–Raven Publishers, Philadelphia © 1998.

4-3   The CO_2 Laser

Dan C. Martin

The CO_2 laser is the most commonly used laser in gynecology. With a "what you see is what you get" effect, it is the laser of choice for techniques that require precision and predictability. The 40 to 400 μm damage to residual tissue causes little tissue distortion but is adequate for coagulation and hemostasis in most cases. The ability to project through space and cut tissue with a no-touch technique avoids problems related to mechanical tension and pressure. However, the use of the CO_2 laser requires sophisticated knowledge of beam alignment and power density. Although waveguides and fibers have been developed to make this an easier laser to use, these may interfere with the mode and limit the power density.

BASICS

Vaporization

Flash vaporization of the water component of tissue is performed with high power density. Although the water component is easily turned into vapor, the organic component itself is either sublimated into gas or thrown off as small particles. The temperature of the crater will depend on the relative amounts of water, dry matter, and carbon. Water vaporizes at 100°C while carbon sublimates at 3652°C.

Excision

Excisional techniques use a combination of laser, traction, bipolar coagulation, and scissors. The cleanest incision comes with no-touch techniques and the CO_2 laser. However, bipolar coagulation may be needed for hemostasis, and scissors can be used to spread and cut through fat layers and avoid the smoke produced by vaporization.

In beginning excision, an incision is made at the margin into healthy tissue. The lesion is placed on traction, and the laser is used to cut into healthy tissue in order to ensure complete removal of the pathologic specimen. Excision has the advantages of creating less smoke, leaving less carbon, and providing tissue for diagnosis.

LASER PHYSICS AND TISSUE INTERACTION

Basics

The CO_2 laser contains CO_2 gas in a resonator chamber. This is immediately parallel to a helium-neon (HeNe) resonator chamber that generates the aiming beam. The CO_2 laser is in the infrared spectrum while the HeNe is visible and is used for aiming. Laser energy is created by pumping electrical energy into the chamber. This electrical energy is converted into light energy. The light energy of the laser is monochromatic (a single wavelength), coherent (in phase), and collimated (parallel beams). This light energy is transmitted to the tissue site. At the tissue site, the light energy is absorbed and converted into thermal energy. A comparison of the tissue effects of CO_2 and other lasers is presented in Table 4-3.1.

When the thermal energy comes from a beam with a power density less than the threshold of vaporization, the effect is warming or desiccation (drying) (Table 4-3.2). On the other hand, higher power densities cause vaporization and are associated with less thermal coagulation (Figure 4-3.1). This is helpful in situations where a clear crater is needed. Those situations include dissections near delicate organs and areas where tissue distortion is to be avoided. However, this decreased coagulation also decreases hemostasis.

The lateral coagulation is related to the intrinsic penetration of the laser, the heat at the base of the crater, and the time of conduction of this heat from the base of the crater. Of these, the time of exposure to the heat appears to be the most important factor in the coagulation. The lower the power density, the longer the laser takes to make the crater. This increases the amount of time that the tissue is exposed to the 100°C vaporization temperature of water for the vaporization technique. If the power density is very low, desiccation and carbonization take place, and carbon itself will be sublimated at 3652°C. This technique was responsible for the 2.7-mm depth of coagulation at 20 W/cm^2 in Figure 4-3.1.

Pulsing

High power density beams decrease tissue distortion and increase speed, but may be hard to control. Control can be maintained by using a high peak power density and low average power density. This combination is developed using mechanical pulsing of the shutter or electronic pulsing of the beam. The shutter can be pulsed with the foot pedal or with a 0.05- to 0.2-second width from the panel. Mechanical pulsing is often used to control a 10- to 60-W continuous output beam. Electronic pulsing of the beam

Table 4-3.1 *General laser characteristics*

Name	Color	Wavelength	Extinction coefficient	
			Water (cm)	Tissue (mm)
CO_2	Infrared	10600 nm	0.001	0.02
Argon	Blue-green	488 to 515 nm	4000	0.5
KTP	Green	532 nm	*	*
Nd:YAG	Infrared	1064 nm	10	1.25

* Approximately equal to argon laser.

Reprinted with permission from Martin DC. Tissue effects of lasers. *Seminars in Reproductive Endocrinology* 1991;9:127–37, Thieme Medical Publishers, Inc.

produces chopped waves, superpulse waves, and ultrapulse waves with peaks of 100 to 500 W. These electronically pulsed waves have a general range of width of 50 to 600 microseconds.

Absorption, Reflection, and Transmission

Although the CO_2 laser is absorbed by water, water-containing tissue, glass, and plastic, it is reflected off of polished mirror surfaces and can be transmitted through air and zinc arsenic lenses. These zinc arsenic lenses are used for focusing the laser, since normal glass lenses would be destroyed by the laser.

SAFETY

ANSI

The American National Standards Institute (ANSI) is the combined effort of government and industry to develop safety and other standards. ANSI Z1136.3-1996 (*American National Standard for the Safe Use of Lasers in Health Care Facilities*) was updated in 1996.

Backstops

Backstops are needed with the CO_2 laser. Various combinations of water solutions, soaked sponges, etched rods, and tissue itself have been used to limit the depth of pen-

Table 4-3.2 *Power densities for CO_2 laser tissue effect*

W/cm²	Tissue effect
0 to 50	Warming
5 to 200	Superficial desiccation and contraction
400 to 4000	Slow, wide vaporization and sublimation
Greater than 1200	Rapid, narrow vaporization and sublimation

Reprinted with permission from Martin DC. Tissue effects of lasers. *Seminars in Reproductive Endocrinology* 1991;9:127–37, Thieme Medical Publishers, Inc.

etration. (Figure 4-3.2). Although rhodium front-surfaced mirrors were originally used to redirect the beam in the deep pelvis, polished metal mirrors have replaced these. However, mirror techniques are rarely used at present.

Although retroperitoneal dissection with solutions has been suggested as a technique to move endometriosis away from the ureter, there appear to be patients in whom this pushes the ureter medially rather than laterally. The use of blunt probes to push the ureter away avoids this problem. In addition, if the ureter will not push away with a blunt probe, this suggests that the ureter is infiltrated with the disease process. This has been noted with endometriosis.

Eye Protection

Although eye protection was previously suggested by ANSI, this has been avoided in endoscopic cases, where the laser is always in a contained cavity. ANSI has more recently recognized that closed systems may not require eye protection.

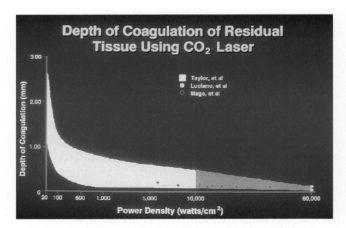

Figure 4-3.1 The depth of coagulation (tissue necrosis) decreases with increasing power density. (Reprinted with permission from Martin DC. Tissue effects of lasers. *Seminars in Reproductive Endocrinology* 1991;9:127–37, Thieme Medical Publishers, Inc.)

BACKSTOPS

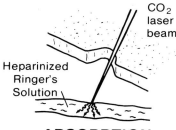

ABSORPTION

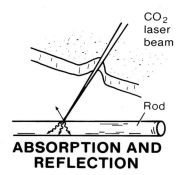

ABSORPTION AND REFLECTION

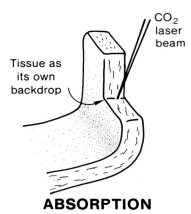

ABSORPTION

Figure 4-3.2 The CO₂ laser is generally stopped with solutions, rods, or the tissue itself. Solutions and tissue absorb the beam in its entirety. Rods both absorb and reflect the beam. Reprinted with permission from Martin DC. *Intra-abdominal Laser Surgery.* Resurge Press, 1986.

Vapor Plume

The vapor and smoke created by vaporization of tissue have produced acute episodes of bronchitis and pneumonitis in a laboratory setting. In addition, vaporization of 1 g of tissue appears to produce mutagenicity equivalent to three to six cigarettes. The possibility of disseminating immunodeficiency virus (HIV), other viral particles, and malignant tissue, causes concern.

Although many masks have been designed to decrease the inhalation of these particles, testing of these suggests that an effective face mask must be airtight and similar to the respirators used by the armed forces to avoid gas inhalation. When the simpler masks used in the operating room were tested, those efficient enough to filter out the particles also forced air around the outside edges of the mask, with little or no significant change in pulmonary protection).

High-flow evacuation systems with carbon-activated filters appear to offer the greatest protection. These must be kept as close to the target as possible.

TUBAL SURGERY

Techniques for cuff salpingostomy employ an initial incision into the lumen using a superpulse or ultrapulse laser technique to decrease the thermal damage. Once the initial incision is open, the folds are turned back and the incision is continued between the folds. With the tube completely opened, the beam is diffused by aiming it at the side of the probe and causing a mode shift of the beam. This produces a lower power density beam, which is applied to the serosal surface of the tube. This causes contraction, which everts the edge and avoids suturing. Pregnancy rates following this have been equivalent to those following microsurgery. Those pregnancy rates appear to be more related to the surgical findings than to the surgical techniques. In that these techniques are no-touch and do not require suturing, these are readily applied at laparoscopy.

Physicians who perform tubal anastomoses generally find that the laser causes more harm than good. In spite of this, term pregnancy rates of 60% to 80% have been reported. However, it is noted that Bellina used the laser for the serosa and adhesions but not for the tubal incision. Scissors were used for that incision. In spite of this, these techniques have been associated with tubal stenosis (Figure 4-3.3) and loss of the mesosalpinx (Figure 4-3.4). It still appears that sharp incision is better than laser incision for the tube.

ENDOMETRIOSIS

Small superficial lesions can be coagulated with a bipolar coagulator, whereas large or deep endometriosis should be vaporized or excised. The CO₂ laser in superpulse or ultrapulse is used to minimize tissue distortion. Vaporization is carried through the lesion until the appearance of loose connective tissue or fat is noted. This reveals a wetter appearance than the fibrosis that is associated with endometriosis.

Low power density is avoided, because this creates more carbon. This carbon interferes with recognition of the remnant tissue. At second-look laparoscopy, this may have the appearance of endometriosis.

These techniques can be used to perform extensive cul-de-sac dissections (Figure 4-3.5). However, the use of these techniques depends upon the clinical indications. Patients with infertility may be better served by limiting dissection to procedures to decrease trauma and adhesion formation,

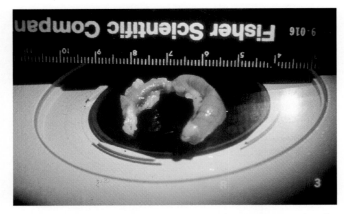

Figure 4-3.3 Stenosis occurred at the anastomotic site with resulting hydrometra when low power density was used prior to microsurgical anastomosis. (Reprinted with permission from Martin DC. Tissue effects of lasers. *Seminars in Reproductive Endocrinology* 1991;9:127–37, Thieme Medical Publishers, Inc.)

which may interfere with fertility. On the other hand, patients with pelvic pain and focal tender nodules may have an inadequate response unless the entire lesion is resected. It seems reasonable to assume that the excellent pregnancy rates for all stages of endometriosis reported by Nezhat may be achieved because he avoids extended surgery and suturing. Furthermore, life table analysis has demonstrated that laparoscopy yields the same or better pregnancy rates than laparotomy when using CO_2 laser techniques. In that these laparoscopy techniques avoid suturing, it is hard to determine which factors influence the success rates.

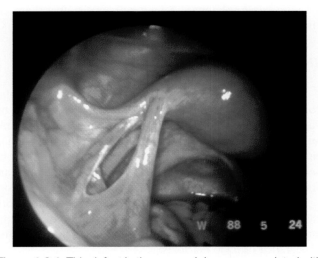

Figure 4-3.4 This defect in the mesosalpinx was associated with cornual occlusion following low power density preparation of the tube for cornual anastomosis. Note the lack of adhesions in spite of the thermal necrosis. (Reprinted with permission from Martin DC. Tissue effects of lasers. *Seminars in Reproductive Endocrinology* 1991;9:127–37, Thieme Medical Publishers, Inc.)

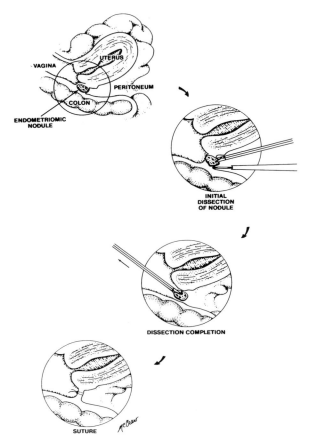

Figure 4-3.5 Deep cul-de-sac dissections have been taken from the peritoneum into the vagina using the CO_2 laser. The hemostasis provided by the CO_2 laser was adequate to maintain precise dissection throughout this level. (Reprinted with permission from Martin DC. Laparoscopic and vaginal colpotomy for the excision of infiltrating cul-de-sac endometriosis. *Journal of Reproductive Medicine* 1988;33:806–8.)

Ovarian endometriosis has been coagulated, vaporized, and stripped. Coagulation minimizes the ovarian trauma, while stripping increases histologic definition and decreases the chance of missing an ovarian cancer.

In addition to concerns regarding the amount of tissue that should be sampled or removed, ovarian closure is a major concern. Adhesions following ovarian closure appear to be more related to ischemia than to the incisional equipment. Sutures increase peritoneal adhesions and show no decrease in ovarian adhesions. The majority of surgeons who are reporting ovarian cystectomy at laparoscopy do not use suturing.

CONCLUSION

The CO_2 laser is excellent for those techniques that take advantage of the no-touch technique with the ''what you see is what you get'' tissue response. Although the use of these must be accompanied by coagulation or mechanical devices for hemostasis around larger vessels, thermal damage should be avoided in cutting across structures such as the tube, which may stenose. Increased understanding of specific use is needed to determine which techniques are optimally performed with the CO_2 laser. Although the CO_2 laser appears to have an ongoing role in surgery, its greatest role may be in encouraging the use of simpler pieces of equipment to perform procedures developed with the CO_2 laser.

SUGGESTED READING

Akale D, Streifel A, Ahrens R. A method for limiting laser plume during bronchoscopic and other angioscopic surgery. International Laser Safety Conference, 1990.

American National Standards Institute, Inc. *American National Standard for the Safe Use of Lasers in Health Care Facilities* (ANSIZ136.3-1996). Orlando: American National Standards Institute, Inc, 1996.

Boer-Meisel ME, te Velde ER, Habbema JDF, et al. Predicting the pregnancy outcome in patients treated for hydrosalpinx: a prospective study. *Fertil Steril* 1986;45:23–9.

Donnez J, Casanas-Roux F. Prognostic factors of fimbrial microsurgery. *Fertil Steril* 1986;200–4.

Kelly RW. Laser surgery of the fallopian tube. In: Keye WR, ed. *Laser Surgery in Gynecology and Obstetrics*. 2nd ed. Chicago: Year Book Medical; 1990:166–86.

Kelly RW, Roberts DK. Experience with the carbon dioxide laser in gynecologic microsurgery. *Am J Obstet Gynecol* 1983;146:585–8.

Luciano AA, Whitman G, Maier DB, et al. A comparison of thermal injury, healing patterns, and postoperative adhesion formation following CO_2 laser and electromicrosurgery. *Fertil Steril* 1987;48:1025–9.

Martin DC, Hubert GD, Levy BS. Depth of infiltration of endometriosis. *J Gynecol Surg* 1989;5:55–60.

Martin DC, Vander Zwaag R. Excisional techniques for endometriosis with the CO_2 laser laparoscope. *J Reprod Med* 1987;32:753–8.

Martin DC. Clinical use of lasers. In: Hunt RD, ed. *Atlas of Female Infertility Surgery*. 2nd ed. St. Louis: Mosby Year Book, 1992:109–16.

Martin DC. *Laparoscopic Appearance of Endometriosis*. 2nd ed. Memphis: Resurge Press, 1990.

Martin DC. Laser basics and safety. In: Hunt RD, ed. *Atlas of Female Infertility Surgery*. 2nd ed. St. Louis: Mosby Year Book, 1992:101–8.

Martin DC. Tissue effects of lasers. *Seminars in Reproductive Endocrinology* 1991;9(2):127–37.

Martin DC. Tubal microsurgery. In: Martin DC, Absten GT, Levinson CJ, Photopulos GJ, eds: *Intra-Abdominal Laser Surgery*. Memphis, TN: Resurge Press; 1986:100–4.

Nezhat C, Nezhat FR. Safe laser endoscopic excision or vaporization of peritoneal endometriosis. *Fertil Steril* 1989;52:149–51.

Operative Laparoscopy, Second Edition
The Masters' Techniques in Gynecologic Surgery
Lippincott–Raven Publishers, Philadelphia © 1998.

4-4   Laparoscopic Use of the KTP/YAG Laser

James F. Daniell

Lasers have been used laparoscopically for over 15 years. The use of the CO_2 laser at laparoscopy began independently in France, Israel, and North America. Investigators have subsequently reported use of the argon, Nd:YAG, and the KTP lasers for laparoscopic laser surgery. All four of these surgical lasers are now widely available and are used clinically for various laparoscopic procedures.

This chapter will review the laparoscopic use of both infrared and visible laser light energy from the Laserscope KTP/YAG laser.

HISTORY OF THE DEVELOPMENT OF THE KTP/YAG LASER FOR LAPAROSCOPY

In the fall of 1985, the KTP laser (Laserscope, San Jose, California) became available for clinical investigations in gynecology in North America. This laser initially had been evaluated in ophthalmology and ear-nose-throat surgery, and because of its fiberoptic delivery and its specific characteristics of vaporization, it was felt that it might be of benefit in gynecologic surgery. Initial evaluations were carried out in rabbits and laparoscopically for treatment of endometriosis and other pelvic conditions. The initial KTP laser developed produced 16 W and was water-cooled. Subsequent models allowed access to the 60-W Nd:YAG laser component, and most recently an air-cooled model has been released (Figure 4-4.1).

PHYSICS AND TISSUE INTERACTION OF THE Nd:YAG AND KTP LASERS

The KTP laser is in the visible light spectrum at a wavelength of 532 nm. Thus it does not require a helium-neon (HeNe) laser for aiming purposes, since the lime green light generated is in the visible spectrum. The Nd:YAG emits at 1064 nm and is infrared; it thus requires an HeNe laser. Both of these wavelengths can pass through flexible fiberoptic fibers for delivery to the tissue through endoscopes. They pass through clear fluids, and their primary tissue effect is coagulation. The tissue depth of penetration varies with spot size and wattage, with the KTP penetrating much less than the Nd:YAG. The KTP laser energy is generated by passing an Nd:YAG laser through a crystal of KTP. From this crystal is generated a green beam that at 532 nm is double the frequency and half the wavelength of the Nd:YAG beam. Thus the KTP laser can also be called the frequency-doubled YAG laser. Access to either laser is accomplished with a mirror system (Figure 4-4.2).

For clinical use, the energy of these two lasers can be delivered through flexible 400- or 600-um flexible fibers. Both of these lasers generate significant backscatter from tissue impact. Thus it is necessary to use safety lenses to protect the eyes and to allow adequate visual observation of the KTP laser. Tissue penetration does not exceed 2 mm with the KTP or 4 mm with the YAG laser. The primary effects are coagulation (Nd:YAG) or vaporization (KTP) when direct tissue contact with the fiber tip occurs.

ADVANTAGES AND DISADVANTAGES OF THE KTP/YAG LASER FOR LAPAROSCOPY

From working over a decade with lasers, we have found distinct advantages of fiberoptic lasers for laparoscopy. These are listed in Table 4-4.1. The main advantage of fiberoptic lasers is the tremendous ease with which the energy of these lasers can be delivered to tissue, compared to the more cumbersome coupling devices needed with the CO_2 laser. The fiber is simply delivered either through the operating channel of the laparoscope, or through an alternate probe into the abdomen and placed on or close to the impact site. No cumbersome alignment steps are needed for the application of laser energy. Since both KTP and Nd:YAG laser energy passes through clear fluids in the pelvis, the amount of smoke generated is reduced when performing operative procedures at laparoscopy, compared to the CO_2 laser. This simpler delivery system, combined with less smoke generation, means that operative procedures can usually be performed in a much shorter period of time than with the CO_2 laser. Another advantage of these lasers is the ability either to incise, vaporize, or photocoagulate rapidly merely by pulling the fiber tip back slightly, away from the tissue. We also feel that there is less potential for bleeding, because both of these lasers have greater hemostatic effects than the CO_2 laser.

These two lasers present certain disadvantages for laparoscopy. An eye safety filter must be placed over the laparoscope before firing. This filter alters the tissue color slightly and adds an extra encumbrance to the eyepiece of the laparoscope; in addition an extra cord extends out from the operating field. Using a small video insert filter that fits over the optics of the laparoscope eliminates some of these

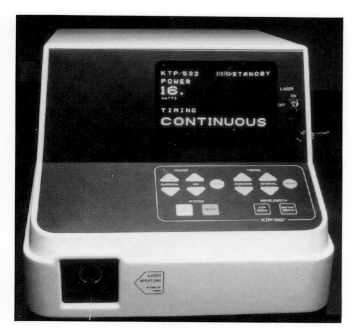

Figure 4-4.1 The front panel of the combined KTP/YAG laser can be seen in this photograph. The machine can be changed from one laser mode to another in 30 seconds and the laser energy is delivered from the same port and through the same fiber. This allows very simple intraoperative switching from one form of laser energy to the other as clinically indicated.

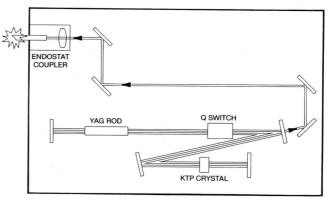

KTP/532 Laser

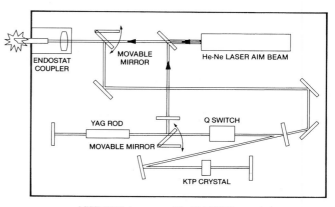

KTP/532 Laser with Nd:YAG module

Figure 4-4.2 KTP/532 laser with Nd:YAG module. These two schematic drawings demonstrate how the KTP energy can be diverted to allow direct use of the primary 50-W Nd:YAG laser present in each KTP machine. The lower panel shows the beam pathway with Nd:YAG and associated helium-neon aiming laser use, while the upper panel demonstrates the original KTP beam pathway.

problems. Another disadvantage of the KTP/YAG lasers is that they cost more than CO_2 lasers or electrosurgical systems that can be used for laparoscopic surgery.

In spite of these disadvantages of visible light laser energy, we feel that the ease and simplicity of performing certain procedures with these lasers, combined with the reduced operative time, outweigh the disadvantages for certain cases. This has led us to discard use of the CO_2 laser for laparoscopic surgery except when training physicians in its use.

DELIVERY TECHNIQUES

Since the laser energy from the KTP/YAG laser can be delivered through flexible fibers, it becomes simple to get the fiber into the peritoneal cavity for laparoscopic surgery. The method, used when a minimum amount of laser firing is necessary, is to deliver the fiber down the operating channel of a laparoscope. The system requires one extra puncture and gives the operator a good angle of attack into the pelvis by passing the fiber coaxially with the laparoscope. The disadvantage of this method is that it reduces the visible light available through the optics of the scope, because an operating scope is being used. In addition, the operator's depth perception is reduced because the fiber is passing down the axis of sight.

The alternate method of use is to deliver fibers through second puncture sites while using a standard diagnostic laparoscope. Laserscope offers small probes for delivering fibers. As an alternative, the fibers can be passed through the central channel of a 5-mm dual-channel probe, originally designed for CO_2 laser laparoscopy. In addition, a 5-mm

Table 4-4.1 *Advantages of the KTP/YAG laser for laparoscopy*

1. Simple fiberoptic delivery
2. No backstop necessary
3. Effective under fluids
4. Minimal smoke formation
5. Excellent hemostasis
6. Both vaporization and coagulation possible
7. Shortened operating time
8. Dual wavelength capability

steerable probe (Marlow Medical, Willoughby, Ohio) has been designed that allows passage of the fiber, as well as suction and irrigation. The probe tip can be moved to any degree, from 180° to 90°, with the fiber thus being directed at the necessary angle (Figure 4-4.3). This probe is specifically helpful for treating posterior ovarian surfaces. Alternatively, the probe can be used as a backstop for the fiber, or to accomplish traction on tissues in the pelvis. We have found this probe to be particularly helpful in advanced laparoscopy procedures such as salpingostomy, enterolysis, or for treatment of advanced stages of endometriosis.

Since advanced operative laparoscopy demands the placement of extra probes, it is important to select carefully the location for probe entry. We normally place our first extra trocar in the midline suprapubically, and use this with 5-mm instruments for retraction and dissection, as necessary. If inspection of the pelvis reveals a need for a third probe, we usually place it 2 to 3 inches lateral to the umbilicus at the same level and on the side opposite from the major disease. If a fourth probe is needed, we place it on the opposite side. On occasion, three probes can be placed in the midline, but this often leads to problems, such as the clashing of instruments during manipulations. Care must be taken to avoid the inferior epigastric vessels when placing lateral probes. Vascular complications can be reduced by transluminating the abdominal wall and identifying the vessels, in a briefly darkened operating room.

A plethora of ancillary instruments has been developed for laparoscopy. We feel that the minimum necessary are three 5-mm trocars with scissors, atraumatic grasping for-

Table 4-4.2 *Advantages of video use for gynecologic endoscopy*

1. Allows assistant to really help
2. Allows residents to do more
3. Permits greater involvement by the operating room team
4. Permits educational tapes to be produced
5. Increases patient enlightenment
6. Increases referrals for surgery
7. Makes possible accurate retrospective review of techniques

ceps, and electrosurgical instruments for both unipolar and bipolar use. Any gynecologist who plans to undertake extensive operative laser laparoscopy should be experienced with multiple punctures and with the use of both unipolar and bipolar cautery at laparoscopy. We now use the argon beam coagulator laparoscopic probe for many of our procedures; it produces less smoke than lasers and costs less.

The use of video can be helpful for all operative laparoscopy. There are many advantages of video; some are listed in Table 4-4.2. Since multiple punctures and extensive operative procedures require more than two hands, it is mandatory to have a coordinated, knowledgeable assistant. The assistant should be able to visualize what is occurring, to anticipate the actions necessary to obtain optimum results. Video-controlled surgery can be performed with a direct coupler, which requires the operator to work while looking directly at the video monitor, or with a beam splitter, which allows the surgeon the option of looking directly through the laparoscope or at the monitor. For us, a 90-10 beam splitter which directs 90% of the light to the video monitor and 10% through to the eye of the operator, has been adequate, giving a good diameter of view and enough light for both the monitor and recording image. Although the term "video-laseroscopy" has been coined in North America, we feel that this is a misleading term that has no real bearing on what is being performed. A more accurate description would be "laparoscopic surgery performed under video control." Some authors claim that a flat video monitor, being viewed by two eyes, permits better depth perception and finer color discrimination than is possible by using one eye to look through the laparoscope. In my opinion, no monitor or camera system will ever approach the optics of the human eye. Because of this, we still often look directly into the pelvis when we feel we are in a tight spot or are dissecting a particularly difficult area.

SPECIFIC PROCEDURES PERFORMED LAPAROSCOPICALLY

Every laparoscopic procedure that has been done with scissors, electrosurgery, and CO_2 lasers, has now been performed using the KTP/YAG laser. A partial list includes

1. treatment of polycystic ovaries
2. correction of hydrosalpinx

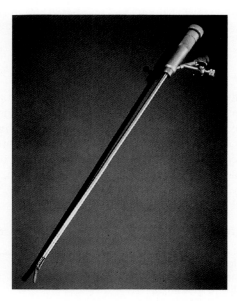

Figure 4-4.3 A steerable probe that allows simultaneous suction of smoke and irrigation. This multiple-purpose probe also can be used for traction, manipulations in the pelvis, as a backstop, or to allow bending of the fiber to target hard-to-reach areas in the pelvis.

3. conservative treatment of ectopic pregnancy
4. extensive adhesiolysis
5. treatment of stage IV endometriosis
6. myomectomy
7. uterosacral ligament transection
8. presacral neurectomy
9. pelvic lymphadenectomy
10. appendectomy
11. enterolysis
12. laparoscopic hysterectomy

Treatment of Polycystic Ovaries

Following reports of the successful use of laparoscopic ovarian electrocoagulation and ovarian biopsy to treat polycystic ovaries, we began investigating the use of laser energy to treat polycystic ovaries. First, we used the CO_2 laser, with satisfactory results. However, the volume of tissue vaporized produced a tremendous amount of smoke, requiring a fairly long operating time. In 1986, we began to investigate the KTP laser for laparoscopic treatment of polycystic ovaries. We have been able to reduce our operating time while still selectively destroying satisfactory portions of the ovarian stroma. Of 85 postoperative patients, 71% have spontaneously ovulated, with successful pregnancies in 56% (Table 4-4.3).

Our laser technique for treating polycystic ovaries involves laparoscopy with a three-puncture technique. A 5-mm grasping forceps is used to fix the ovary and the 600-um fiber is introduced through a 5-mm probe. The KTP mode at 20 W is used to vaporize the multiple sites symmetrically, over each ovary. Multiple subcapsular cysts are opened as the fiber is slowly pushed into the ovarian stroma. Small holes up to 2 cm long are thus developed into the ovary with KTP laser energy. The bilateral procedure usually can be accomplished in less than 30 minutes, and the majority of the patients are discharged within 8 hours. We feel that this is an excellent treatment for patients who desire immediate pregnancy and who have failed to respond to Clomid in maximum doses. It gives these patients a "window of opportunity" during which they might conceive without the need for expensive ovulation induction therapy or wedge resection. The effect is transient, as almost all patients failing to conceive revert back to an anovulatory state within 6 months to 1 year. In over 120 cases, we have had no complications in this procedure and recommend it to all our polycystic ovarian disease patients who fail to respond to Clomid or otherwise need a laparoscopy. For fear of excessive ovarian damage and potential ischemic ovarian failure, Nd:YAG laser energy should not be used. Switching from the CO_2 laser to the KTP laser has made this an easier, safer and quicker procedure via laparoscopy. This is of particular advantage in patients who are obese. The advantages to these patients are obvious, compared to the risks and discomfort of pelvic laparotomy, the expenses of other forms of ovulation induction, and the known risks of hyperstimulation and multiple pregnancies.

Treatment of Hydrosalpinges

In the past, the treatment of a hydrosalpinx had poor results, with the best surgeons reporting no more than 30% pregnancy rates with long-term follow-up in controlled series. Laparoscopic treatment of hydrosalpinges has been attempted since the late 1970s, with the early reports by Gomel and others. Following the reports of Bruhat on using the CO_2 laser for repair of hydrosalpinges at laparotomy, we began investigating the use of CO_2 laser energy through the laparoscope for treatment of hydrosalpinges. Our initial results were reported in 1983. We have switched to the KTP laser for this and have obtained better results by being more selective in our attempts at salpingostomy and by refining our laparoscopic techniques. When using the CO_2 laser, bleeding often occurred that required electrocoagulation of the edges of the tubes. Also, in some tubes, we could not successfully evert the fimbriae. Using the 400-um KTP fiber with four punctures, we find it easier and quicker to do laparoscopic salpingostomy.

Table 4-4.3 *Pregnancy after laparoscopic vaporization for polycystic ovarian disease[a]*

Presurgery	Patients	Postoperative results			
		No CC		CC given	
		Ovulated	Pregnant	Ovulated	Pregnant
Ovulation on CC	47	44	20	7	2
No ovulation on CC	38	20	15	17[b]	10
Total	85	60 (71%)	35	24	12

[a] Total conception = 48 (56%)—spontaneous, clomiphene citrate (CC), or human menopausal gonadotropins (hMG).

[b] One patient was anovulatory with CC and required hMG for ovulation and conception.

Source: Daniell JF, Surgical management of polycystic ovarian disease, in Collins RL (ed), *Ovulation Induction,* 1991, Springer-Verlag.

Table 4-4.4 *Results of laparoscopic neosalpingostomy with lasers[a,b]*

Type laser	Years	Total patients	Open tubes at 6 weeks HSG	Attempting pregnancy	Pregnancy results		
					IUP	Abort	Ectopic
CO_2	1982–1985	104[c]	58/71 (82%)	88	22 (25%)	11 (13%)	11 (13%)
KTP	1985–1987	36[d]	24/28 (86%)	32	10 (31%)	3 (9%)	5 (16%)
Totals		140	82/99 (83%)	120	33 (28%)	14 (12%)	16 (13%)

[a] Eighteen-month minimum follow-up.
[b] HSG, hysterosalpingogram; IUP, intrauterine pregnancy.
[c] Sixty procedures were in recurrent hydrosalpinges with at least 2 year follow-up.
[d] Only 3 procedures were recurrent hydrosalpinges.

An incision is made in the distal end of the tube and either one or two radial cuts are performed, using 15 to 20 W. After the tube is opened, the 5-mm steerable probe is placed into the tube and used both as a backstop and for traction, so that the thinnest tubal portion can be identified for the next incision. After the tube is opened, the 5-mm steerable probe is placed into the tube and used both as a backstop and for traction, so that the thinnest tubal portion can be identified for the next incision. The fiber is then held 2 cm from the lateral edges of the peritoneum of the open fimbriae, and 5 W of defocused KTP laser energy is used to contract the peritoneum. (The Nd:YAG laser should never be used on the delicate fimbria.) This causes the tubes to evert outward like the petals of a flower. This laparoscopic ''Bruhat technique'' is much easier to accomplish using a fiber than with the CO_2 laser.

Our results in patients in whom the primary treatment of tubal blockage was carried out using the KTP laser, with a minimum of 18 months' follow-up, are given in Table 4-4.4. A 31% pregnancy rate has been obtained, with an acceptable level of ectopic pregnancies in these patients. Most pregnancies in these patients do not occur until 9 to 16 months after surgery.

It is my opinion that in this age of more cost-effective in-vitro fertilization (IVF) with improved pregnancy rates, *laparotomy* for hydrosalpinges should be reserved for those patients who cannot afford or do not desire IVF, and whose fallopian tubes cannot be repaired by a laparoscopic approach. The patient advantages, from a laparoscopic approach, include reduced discomfort, minimum recuperation time, and reduction of cost and time off from work. Although further work and evaluation by other authors are needed, in the hands of experienced operative laparoscopists, it appears that laparoscopic treatment of hydrosalpinges is a reasonable alternative to laparotomy.

Laparoscopic Myomectomy

Certain uterine fibroids can be removed via laparoscopy. In patients with symptomatic leiomyomata, which are subserosal and thus amenable to laparoscopic removal, the combined KTP/YAG laser can be very helpful. The surgeon can use the KTP mode for incisions in the myometrium, and then switch to the YAG wavelength to obtain hemostasis deep in the myoma bed. Our experience with fibroids leads us to recommend use of pre-treatment for two to three months with GnRH analogues to allow correction of anemia and shrinkage of the tumors.

Treatment of Tubal Pregnancy Using Laser Energy

There have been many reports of successful treatment of ectopics using laparoscopic electrocoagulation and the CO_2 laser. However, we feel the techniques that we have used with the KTP/YAG laser have some advantages for treatment of ectopic pregnancies. In our experience, the risk of tubal bleeding is less when applying KTP laser energy through the 400-um fiber than when using the CO_2 laser. In addition, trauma to the tube appears to be less with the small laser fiber than when using the needle electrodes available for laparoscopic electrosurgery. Table 4-4.5 lists our results using KTP laser energy for laparoscopic ectopics. We agree with others that laparoscopic treatment of ectopic pregnancy is well tolerated by patients and is cost-effective.

Treatment of Endometriosis and Adhesions

Laparoscopic surgery is the ideal procedure for treatment of pelvic endometriosis of any type. It is usually multifocal and often associated with adhesions that cannot be successfully treated with drug therapy. The surgeon's ability

Table 4-4.5 *Laparoscopic treatment of ectopics January 1986 to January 1988*

Total patients	36
Ruptured tubes	2
Salpingectomy	6
Salpingostomy	30
Laparotomies done	0

Tubal patency on hysterosalpingogram: 18 of 20 tested (90%) postoperatively. Repeat ectopics: 2 of 20 attempting pregnancy (10%). Intrauterine pregnancy: 8 of 20 (40%).

to perform laparoscopic surgery combines the patient's diagnosis and therapy into one event: The laparoscopy can accomplish the diagnosis and establish the stage of the disease; then, by using a laser fiber, the experienced operator can treat the patient and accomplish successful adhesiolysis and destruction or reduction of the disease. Endometriomas can be opened, drained, and/or vaporized, and other associated pathology can be corrected, at the time of the outpatient procedure. The need for postoperative drug suppressive therapy will then depend on the amount of disease remaining and the patient's desires and symptoms. Patients who desire pregnancy can begin attempts at conceiving in the immediate next cycle, without the delays associated with drug therapy or recovery from major surgery. In addition, the likelihood of postoperative adhesions forming in the pelvis is probably less following laparoscopy, than it would be with the same techniques performed at laparotomy.

The techniques for treating endometriosis depend on the location and amount of disease present. Surface implants usually can be photocoagulated using a 600-um fiber held close to the tissue. If vaporization is desired, the tip can be touched to the tissue. An alternate method is to use accessory forceps for traction on the implants of endometriosis and then to dissect out the lesion using the tip of the laser fiber. It is important to remember that endometriosis will often tunnel subperitoneally, and active disease that is not visible may be located in the margins of visible implants. Thus we treat each implant as we do viral lesions on the perineum, using an "airbrush" technique around the visible portions of the lesion in the center.

Endometriomas need to be carefully dissected from their usual attachments to the lateral pelvic sidewalls. In our experience, it has usually been the sidewall that bleeds and not the ovary itself, so putting gentle traction on the ovary and using laser energy to vaporize the ovary free from the sidewall seems to be more effective than to dissect the ovary bluntly. Care must be taken to identify the ureter and to avoid the major vessels lateral to the ovary. Once the ovary is freed from its adherence to the sidewall, the endometrioma can be opened and the chocolate contents aspirated. Our method of handling an endometrioma depends on whether the capsule can be stripped from the ovarian stroma or not. If it is possible to tease the capsule free, it can be grasped and usually removed from the ovary with gentle traction. If the capsule remains adherent to the ovarian stroma, we use the 600 um laser fiber at 20 W to vaporize the capsule by holding the fiber close to the surface of the inside of the endometrioma and passing it over the entire surface. The endometrioma bed will usually constrict and reduce the size of the opening in the ovary. Occasionally, laparoscopic sutures or clips can be placed to close large defects. Endometriomas larger than 10 cm are probably still best handled by laparotomy, because of the large open ovarian surface areas that result from opening the cyst.

Adhesions associated with endometriomas are handled similarly to other adhesions. The advantage of the KTP/YAG laser fiber is that the energy dissipates from the tip rapidly, so that structures more than 2 cm beyond the tip will not be affected by the impact of the laser beam. This means that it is not necessary to use a backstop behind adhesions that are not close to vital structures. However, when working close to the bowel, bladder, or the fimbriae, it is necessary to use a backstop because of the potential for damage close behind the beam. The easiest instrument for providing this extra safety is the 5 mm steerable probe, which can be placed through a 5 mm second puncture and manipulated as needed, to provide both a backstop and traction behind the adhesion, while firing the laser. Gentle traction on the adhesion is usually necessary so that it can be easily vaporized. We feel the KTP laser is particularly advantageous for adhesiolysis because of the speed with which the adhesions can be lysed, with minimal risk of bleeding or smoke production.

Although some have reported the treatment of bowel endometriosis using laser energy through the laparoscope, we have minimal experience with this. Since bowel implants are usually invaginated, we feel that the risk of later bowel perforation is greater than the potential for successful destruction of the entire lesion. For this reason, we limit laparoscopic treatment of bowel endometriosis to those lesions that are exophytic or on epiploic fat, or on the tip of the appendix. We will perform an appendectomy through the laparoscope if the tip of the appendix is affected with endometriosis.

Enterolysis

Laparoscopic bowel adhesiolysis, following postsurgical or infectious processes, can also be accomplished successfully, in many cases, using KTP laser energy. We have reported our results with patients who have been referred to us for attempts at laparoscopic adhesiolysis after multiple abdominal operations. Many of these patients have had previous bowel obstructions and are at extremely high risk for potential complications at attempted laparoscopy. We counsel these patients concerning the risks of bowel injury and the possible need for immediate laparotomy and/or diverting colostomy. We do a bowel prep, and always have a general surgeon standing by to repair any bowel injuries that might occur during attempted enterolysis through the laparoscope. We will try to accomplish pneumoperitoneum in a standard fashion, usually entering at the left costal margin lateral to the upper insertion of the rectus muscle, and then introduce a 2-mm laparoscope for initial visibility. After confirming that we are in the proper peritoneal space and noting the proper site for placement of the 10-mm laparoscopic trocar, the larger laparoscope is inserted. The laser fiber placement is based on the location of any abdominal wall adhesions. Many of these patients can be helped, although some have such extensive adhesions, with bowel so adherent to the intraabdominal wall that it is impossible to cut them safely. However, patients who have significant pain from postsurgical adhesions, and who undergo successful laparoscopic lysis, report improvement in two-thirds of cases. We have not yet had any late complications and have only had one bowel perforation that required immediate laparotomy, in an initial series of over 40 patients treated with extensive laparoscopic bowel adhesiolysis.

Removal of Adnexal Structures

Our experience with laparoscopic oophorectomy, salpingectomy, or removal of periadnexal structures, has been good. In these cases, the technique is mainly nonlaser. However, if using Endoloops, we will occasionally use the KTP/YAG laser to vaporize the pedicle after the bulk of the tissue has been removed. In particular, this laser can be helpful for dissecting adhesions from the ovary and tube prior to removal.

Uterosacral Ligament Ablation

One of the more common laparoscopic operations that we perform is transection of the uterosacral ligaments (LUNA). We offer this procedure to all patients who have dysmenorrhea and who are planning laparoscopy. Doyle was the first to report successful relief from dysmenorrhea by separating the uterosacral ligaments. Data have shown laser transection via laparoscopy to be a successful therapy for dysmenorrhea, either with or without endometriosis. Initially, we used the CO_2 laser for this but encountered several cases of bleeding that required electrosurgery. As of this writing, there have been two deaths in North America as a result of bleeding from uterosacral ligaments that occurred when these were transected with CO_2 laser energy. We feel that the hemostatic properties of the KTP/YAG laser add some degree of safety when the uterosacral ligaments are being transected. Our laser technique is to identify the uterosacral ligaments, trace them out to the pelvic brim, trace the ureters, and note the area of insertion of the uterine artery to the lateral cervix. We then take a 5-mm probe and push against the posterior cervix to tent up the uterosacral ligaments. The 600-micron laser fiber is then used to transect the ligaments at right angles, just as the ligaments insert into the posterior cervix. Sometimes the ligaments will be attenuated and difficult to identify. In these cases, we may refrain from cutting if we feel it is unsafe, or if the landmarks cannot be identified. Occasionally, rectosigmoid obliteration of the cul-de-sac in cases of endometriosis will preclude the ability to cut the uterosacrals.

The majority of patients have a reduction in their menstrual pain (Table 4-4.6). In the initial postoperative period, most patients report pain, which probably reflects tissue

Table 4-4.6 *LUNA results with KTP laser (6 month follow-up)*

	Worse	Same	Improved
Endometriosis 80 patients	3 (4%)	17 (21%)	60 (75%)
Primary dysmenorrhea 20 patients	2 (10%)	6 (30%)	12 (60%)
Total 100 patients	5 (5%)	23 (23%)	72 (72%)

swelling in the healing phase. For most cases we have now converted to using the argon beam coagulator for LUNA, because it is more cost effective. We have not noted any effects on bowel or bladder functions in these patients, and no patients have reported any reduction in ability to enjoy intercourse or obtain orgasm. It is important to counsel these patients preoperatively, to make certain that they are aware that success is not guaranteed in all cases.

SAFETY

To undertake any sort of extensive operative laparoscopy without the proper safety precautions, training, equipment, and assistance, can result in unnecessary complications and their tragic sequelae. It behooves all of us who are interested in operative laser laparoscopy to be selective in the techniques we undertake to perform. This will protect us, our hospitals, and our patients.

The safe use of the KTP/YAG laser at laparoscopy includes the proper use of eye filters and protection for both the patient, the surgeon, and the assistants in the operating room. Since the laser energy of the KTP is visible, it is less likely that damage will be done to the operator's eyes. Any inadvertent firing of the laser without eye filters will be immediately recognized because of the bright green color that is seen. This improves the safety of use of the KTP component compared to the Nd:YAG, which is infrared and therefore not visible when fired. When working in a closed abdominal cavity, we do not require people in the operating room to wear safety glasses. The fiber itself is coated, which protects leakage of the energy except from the tip of the fiber.

The operator is the only person at risk when the beam is being fired intraperitoneally through the laparoscope, and his or her eyes are protected by the eye filter that is placed over the eyepiece of the laparoscope. The laser cannot be fired if the eye filter is not working properly. If an attempt is made to override the eye filter with the KTP (this can be done, for instance, by placing the eye filter on another laparoscope that might be on the table), the operator will be aware of this problem immediately because of the intense brightness that he sees when he fires the laser without the eye filter. This is *not true* with the Nd:YAG component,

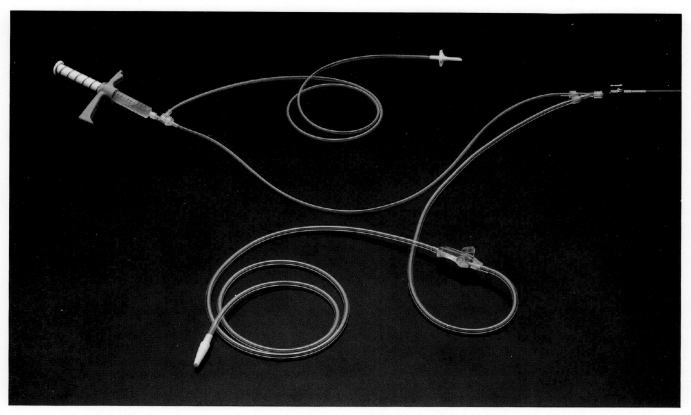

Figure 4-4.4 The disposable PumpVac system for rapid smoke or fluid suction and irrigation at operative laparoscopy. It attaches to floor suction tubing, and an intravenous bag containing irrigation solution allows aquadissection as well as simple control of smoke production. It can be operated with ease by either the surgeon or an assistant.

which is invisible, and thus requires constant awareness of unfiltered firing risks.

Because of the potential of harmful effects on those breathing the plume, we vent the smoke off through a specially designed disposable suction-irrigation system (PumpVac Plus, Marlow Medical, Willoughby, OH) that is also used to aspirate fluid and for aquadissection (Figure 4-4.4). By using in-line filters, we protect the hospital filter

system from plugging by particulate matter that might be in the plume.

Other safety precautions are those one would undertake with any sort of operative laparoscopy, such as gentle tissue handling, use of the proper instruments in the proper situations, and judicious use of both bipolar and unipolar electrosurgery. With proper attention to safety, the careful, trained, endoscopist can perform extensive operative lapa-

Table 4-4.7 *Shifting trends in gynecologic surgery*

	Old therapy	New therapy
Menorrhagia	Hysterectomy	→ Endometrial ablation
Severe endometriosis	Laparotomy	→ Laparoscopy
Ectopic gestation	Laparotomy	→ Laparoscopy
Uterine septum	Abdominal metroplasty	→ Hysteroscopic resection
Hydrosalpinx	Laparotomy	→ Laparoscopy
Cornual blockage	Cornual reanastomosis	→ Hysteroscopic probing and dilatation
Pelvic adhesions	Laparotomy	→ Laparoscopic adhesiolysis
Ovarian pathology requiring removal	Laparotomy, oophorectomy	→ Pelvoscopy à la Semm
Dysmenorrhea	Laparotomy, presacral neurectomy	→ Laparoscopic presacral neurectomy
Uterine fibroids	Laparotomy	→ Laparoscopy or hysteroscopy

Table 4-4.8 *Benefits of outpatient surgery*

1. Reduces cost to patient, insurance company, and government
2. Removes psychologic stress associated with hospitalization
3. Uses physician's (and patient's) time more effectively
4. Eliminates bed congestion
5. Lessens chance for medication error or therapeutic misadventure
6. Permits rapid return to full activity by patient

roscopic procedures with good results in the majority of cases, with minimal complications and good patient recuperation.

CONCLUSION

I strongly agree with Dr. Alan DeCherney, who said in his editorial in *Fertility and Sterility* entitled "The Leader of the Band is Tired," that the obituary for laparotomy for infertility surgery has been written but not yet published. Today, many gynecologists are becoming interested in doing more aggressive operative laparoscopic surgery. Procedures that in the past required open laparotomy can now be done with combinations of hysteroscopy and/or laparoscopy. Table 4-4.7 lists the so-called old methods of treatment for some of these disease processes, compared to the new techniques that are producing good results in the hands of experienced operators.

In this time of cost containment in medicine, it will benefit interested physicians to try to reduce costs without cutting corners or compromising patient care. Careful, selective, use of lasers and nonlaser laparoscopic techniques in gynecology can help cost containment by giving comparable results while avoiding major surgery with its increased expense, risks, morbidity, and discomfort for patients. Some of these benefits of outpatient surgery are listed in Table 4-4.8. All gynecologists should investigate the potential for using advanced operative laparoscopic laser surgery in their practices. The combined KTP/YAG laser allows the experienced operator to accomplish safely and rapidly many of these complicated laparoscopic procedures.

SUGGESTED READING

Brumsted J, Gibson C, Gibson M, et al. A comparison of laparoscopy and laparotomy for the treatment of ectopic pregnancy. *Obstet Gynecol* 1988;71:889.

Daniell JF. Surgical management of polycystic ovarian disease. In: Collins RL, ed. *Ovulation Induction* New York: Springer-Verlag;1991:145.

Daniell JF. Laparoscopic enterolysis for chronic abdominal pain. *J Gynecol Surg* 1989;5:61.

Daniell JF. Laparoscopic evaluation of the KTP/532 laser for treating endometriosis—initial report. *Fertil Steril* 1986;46:373.

Daniell JF, Brown DH. Carbon dioxide laser laparoscopy: initial experience in experimental animals and humans. *Obstet Gynecol* 1982;49:761.

Daniell JF, Kurtz BR, Lee JY. Laparoscopic oophorectomy: comparative study of ligatures, bipolar coagulation, and automatic stapling devices. *Obstet Gynecol* 1992;80:325.

Daniell JF, Kurtz BR, Nair S. Laparoscopic treatment of endometriosis with the argon beam coagulator: initial report. *Gynaec Endosc* 1993;2:13.

Daniell JF, Kurtz BR, Taylor S. Laparoscopic myomectomy using the argon beam coagulator. *J Gynecol Surg* 1994;9:207.

Gjönnaess H. Polycystic ovarian syndrome treated by ovarian electrocautery through the laparoscope. *Fertil Steril* 1984;41:20.

Keye WR, Matson GA, Dixon J. The use of the argon laser in the treatment of experimental endometriosis. *Fertil Steril* 1983;39:26.

Kurtz BR, Daniell JF. Laparoscopic terminal neosalpingostomy using the potassium-titanyl-phosphate laser. *Gynaec Endosc* 1992;1:43.

Lomano JM. Laparoscopic ablation of endometriosis with the YAG laser *Lasers Surg Med* 1983;3:179.

Operative Laparoscopy, Second Edition
The Masters' Techniques in Gynecologic Surgery
Lippincott–Raven Publishers, Philadelphia © 1998.

4-5   The Argon Laser in Gynecologic Operative Laparoscopy

Sanford S. Osher

I'm an endoscopist, and as an endoscopist I'm constantly looking for new devices and new techniques that will simplify my surgery, allowing me to perform procedures more effectively and perhaps with a little less fuss.

Over the years, as operative endoscopy has become more popular, the instrument companies have obliged us by creating a multitude of instruments, all with subtle variations, shapes, and sizes. They created not just one but a covey of different kinds of scissors with which to cut tissue, a bevy of different kinds of coagulators to coagulate tissue, and myriad different ways to vaporize tissue. As a result, operating room personnel are often overwhelmed by the number and variety of instruments on their operating room tables. This is fine for the surgical team that uses all these different tools; the subtleties of individual surgical techniques often demand this variety of instrumentation. However, some of us are trying to get away from the multitude of instruments available during our endoscopy in favor of devices that will simplify our surgery, simplify our instrument list, and allow us to perform our surgery with less effort.

Wouldn't it be nice if we had one instrument that did all things? Wouldn't it be nice if we had one instrument that I could reach for that would perform the functions of several different instruments? One instrument that would cut like a knife or scissors, vaporize like the good old-fashioned CO_2 laser, and coagulate like a Bovie? One instrument that did all things ideally at the same time or with a flick of a switch or better, say, microsurgical movement of your fingertips?

I believe that we have that instrument in the form of an argon laser fiber; it can do all things. The tissue effects include desiccation, photocoagulation, vaporization, and cutting. Remarkably, all of these things are accomplished by merely moving the fiber closer to the tissue or backing the fiber further away from the tissue. It's that simple! The argon laser energy passes through a flexible quartz fiber and then out of the end of the fiber. The laser energy diverges from the tip of the fiber at approximately a 15° angle. If you hold the tip of the fiber close to the tissue so that the fiber is perpendicular to the tissue and just off the tissue, the argon beam has had little chance to diverge and, therefore, the spot size is small, close to the diameter of the fiber from which it is emerging. Clearly, this is the distance that we would hold the fiber away from the target in order to cut the tissue. This is the hot spot! If we pull the fiber back, just off the tissue,

and allow the beam to diverge a tad more, then the spot size from the argon beam, being slightly larger, delivers less energy to the target, and vaporizes tissue. If we pull the fiber back even further, the spot size opens up, delivering still less energy to the target, and coagulation is the tissue effect. If we pull back further, superficial desiccation occurs, and further still, little effect other than warming of the tissue occurs. This simple movement of the fiber in or out to achieve different tissue effects is the magic and the wonder of argon laser surgery. Clinically, my surgery has been simplified, because I have one tool with which I merely zoom in or out to achieve a variety of tissue effects—laser surgery made easy! (See Figure 4-5.1.)

However, keep in mind that it's not the fiber itself that cuts but the laser light at the tip of the fiber; therefore, this fiber is not meant to be used in contact with the tissue. In fact, this can be injurious to the fiber and ultimately can diminish the laser's effect on tissue, as debris may collect on the tip or the tip may become slightly disfigured. The hot spot is just off the fiber tip within a few millimeters. This is where the real cutting action is; here the laser light energy is most concentrated. Depending on three variables—the power setting, the diameter of the fiber (two sizes, 300 and 600 micron(μ)), and the "freshness" of our fiber tip—the distance away from the tissue necessary to move from cutting to vaporizing and from vaporizing to coagulating varies; in general, it is a very short distance indeed. These three basic tissue effects are usually achieved within a distance of between $\frac{1}{2}$ to $1\frac{1}{2}$ cm. Again, this short "operating area" is what makes the argon laser so desirable as the endoscopic tool that does it all!

ARGON LASER HISTORY

The argon laser made its first medical appearance in the 1960s. Energy passing through an argon gas medium in a hollow laser tube with mirrors on each end generates a light spectrum of bluish-green wavelengths at 488 and 514.5 nm. The visible laser energy can then either be a free beam or can be directed down a flexible silica-quartz fiber. The bluish-green laser with its many special properties was quickly recognized as a valuable tool in several medical specialties, including ophthalmology and dermatology.

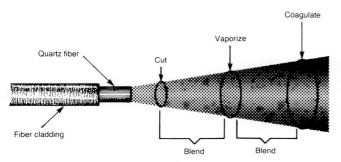

Figure 4-5.1 Laser light exits in a divergent pattern.

In the early to middle 1980s, the argon laser was investigated for gynecologic endoscopic surgery, chiefly by William "Bud" Keye, MD, and others, in an attempt to capitalize on the laser's inherent properties of selective absorption by pigmentation in general and hemoglobin and hemosiderin in particular. The early studies examined the argon laser's use in the treatment of endometriosis, but subsequently the popularity of the laser exploded as it began to be used in the management of a great variety of gynecologic conditions amenable to operative endoscopy. The only argon laser approved for gynecologic procedures is manufactured by HGM Medical Laser Systems, Inc., in Salt Lake City, Utah.

ADVANTAGES OF THE ARGON LASER

As mentioned earlier, the greatest advantage of the laser is its versatility in achieving different tissue effects by merely moving the fiber closer or farther from the tissue. Cutting, vaporizing, and coagulating can all be easily achieved with the slightest movement of the fingers holding the fiber. There are many other distinct and clinically important advantages to using this laser, but none is as appreciated as this versatility.

By comparison, with the CO_2 laser it is clinically difficult to achieve these different tissue effects, as its primary effect is cutting and vaporizing tissue, and it does little to control hemostasis. With the CO_2 laser, in order to switch from one tissue effect to another, one must manually change a power dial on the machine and/or focus or defocus a helium-neon aiming beam; not so with the argon laser, where all you have to do is move the fiber in or out. I leave the power setting on the machine on a single setting, between 6 and 8 watts, then I adjust the fiber distance from the target to control the tissue effect—simple!

By the same token, each sapphire-tipped Nd:YAG laser can't do all things or achieve all tissue effects that the argon laser can. One sapphire tip cuts, one tip vaporizes, one tip coagulates, and perhaps another tip blends effects slightly but still not as efficiently or with as little effort as zooming in or out with the argon laser. Additionally, in order to achieve different tissue effects during a case, these sapphire

tips need to be switched back and forth, screwed on and screwed off, taking up a bit of time. Tissue contact is required with the sapphire-tipped Nd:YAG lasers, and should you accidentally fire the Nd:YAG laser when the sapphire tip is out of contact with the tissue, the expensive tips may burn out or fracture, disabling them.

The bare-fiber Nd:YAG is either a blunt or sculptured, coned-down tip. The blunt-tipped Nd:YAG laser is primarily a deeply penetrating, forward scattering, coagulating laser, which can cut when in contact or near contact with tissue. The sculptured-tipped Nd:YAG laser requires contact with the tissue. Its primary task is to cut; its secondary effect is to coagulate. I don't believe either of these Nd:YAG fiber techniques provide the ease and versatility that the argon laser provides.

The argon's wavelengths are almost completely and selectively absorbed by hemoglobin and pigmented tissue, which is a nice feature as the laser favors areas where hemoglobin is or has been: oozing blood, active bleeding, hemosiderin, pigmented endometriotic implants, and, most important, blood vessels. This is a wonderful feature for the management of endometriosis and hemostasis. When sweeping across wide patches of pigmented endometriosis with the laser at the coagulating distance, the laser energy is selectively picked up and absorbed by the disease, *enhancing* the laser effect, exerting coagulating or vaporizing energy to the target. This holds true for wide areas of oozing, or raw, weeping capillary beds. All you need to do is hold the fiber at the coagulating distance and *spraypaint* the area, with immediate coagulation often occurring.

However, my favorite tissue effect is in the management of blood vessels coursing along an adhesion or the surface of an organ. I take the laser fiber and run the beam up and down the blood vessels. The laser light will pass through the transparent normal tissue and coagulate the blood vessels closed. Then the fiber can be advanced, cutting across the blood vessels already coagulated. Using one tool, I first coagulate, then move in and cut.

In other cases, once bleeding or oozing is encountered, try to stop it with the CO_2 laser—it just can't be easily done. *The argon laser shoots through water* or any clear fluid and will easily pass through irrigation fluid to zero in on a breached blood vessel or oozing bed of capillaries. Spraypainting the entire area with the argon laser at the coagulating distance, while irrigating, usually results in immediate hemostasis—wash and laser! Try that with the CO_2 laser!

Another case when lasing under water is important is in the management of endometriosis deep in a cul-de-sac, often covered with peritoneal or irrigation fluid. This area would have to be bone-dry for you to use the CO_2 laser effectively because this laser's energy is instantly absorbed by water, halting at the air/water interface. Since the argon laser shoots underwater, the same three desired tissue effects can be achieved simply by moving the fiber in or out from the endometriosis. This applies to all moist intraabdominal peritoneal surfaces, as a little moisture won't impede the laser's effect. However, when it comes to hysteroscopic surgery, the argon's ability to work under fluids is most important.

Smoke is a constant source of frustration and concern when performing CO_2 laser laparoscopy. You have to evacuate liters and liters of plume, especially when vaporizing bulky endometriosis or lysing many adhesions. This is because CO_2 explodes intracellular water into steam. Smoke is everywhere! Not so with the argon laser. It cuts and vaporizes by "melting" cellular proteinaceous material, producing much less steam and smoke. Overall, a fraction of the amount of plume is encountered when using the argon laser compared to the CO_2, giving me a nice clear view when performing laser laparoscopy.

The divergence of the argon beam makes for safe lasing for one important reason: There is little need for you to have a backstop with the argon laser in many cases. Since the spot size widens so rapidly, the energy delivered to that backstop is a fraction of that arising from the tip of the fiber. This makes backstops a few centimeters or so beyond the target fairly safe from laser burns, unlike the CO_2 laser. This will be discussed further under "Adhesions."

Finally, there is tactile feedback when you perform argon laser surgery. Holding that fiber in your hand gives you a secure feeling when performing laser surgery. We're no longer Luke Skywalkers shooting a free beam across wide expanses of space! The argon fiber gives us a chance to hold our cutting, coagulating, and vaporizing instrument in our fingertips, thus offering a degree of control that is lacking with the free beam of a CO_2 laser.

Importantly, the ability to *triangulate* by bringing the fiber down through a second puncture channel is a wonderful feature lost with most CO_2 laser surgery. CO_2 laser laparoscopy, with the laser delivered through the laparoscope, combines our operating axis with our visual axis, making depth perception impossible. When the fiber comes down any other port, that little bit of an angle makes our surgery more accurate by *triangulation,* giving us *three-dimensionality!* However, when the fiber is brought down through the operating channel of the operating laparoscope, *prepointing* and *past-pointing* is a constant problem, and I discourage this practice. Also, (*Attention, Residents*) the advantages of triangulating far outweigh the disadvantages of making a minimally morbid second puncture port.

FIBER

The argon laser energy is passed down a silica-quartz flexible fiber with diameters of either 300 or 600 μ. The 600 micron fiber is the general purpose fiber and the one I use for most of my endoscopic work. I reserve the 300-μm fiber for tuboplasty, fimbriaplasty, ectopics, and fine dissection. The smaller spot size of this fiber delivers high power densities to the tissue, making for cleaner, slicker,

finer, sharper incisions. Either of these fibers can be passed through any size port or operating channel, from a tiny hollow needle to a 3- to 5-mm hollow tube to an operative laparoscope. Beware: The fiber is sharp, and you must be careful to retract the fiber tip into its port when not lasing, to protect against inadvertent puncture of a vital structure. The fiber can be *cleaved and stripped* when debris collects on the end or when the tip begins to melt. This happens once or twice during a long case and depends upon how often the fiber tip touches the tissue. You will soon recognize when it is time to cleave and strip the fiber, because the tissue effect is diminished and your frustration level rises. Instead of turning up the power (from my usual 6 to 8 watts), I simply attend to making a new fiber tip and prepare for the full laser effect once again—after "sharpening my knife." One word of reassurance: Proper cleaving and stripping is an art form and takes time to master.

EYE SAFETY

The argon laser energy can be dangerous. Its brilliance is visible (as opposed to the dangerously invisible and painless Nd:YAG laser) and will pass through the lenses of the scope and into the eye and destroy retinal tissue. Either argon eye goggles or special argon filters attached to the endoscope must be used. A monoshutter with a colored argon filter within can be attached to the laparoscope or hysteroscope. Each time the foot pedal is pressed, a filter will drop down to protect your eyes or the camera. *Watch out!* If you take the shutter off (to take a better look through the scope, for example) and fail to put the shutter back on the scope, you'll get a brilliant, painful blast of light to your eyes that you'll likely never forget. Fortunately, there is now an interlock system built into the newer machines that will keep the laser from firing if the shutter is not on the scope.

The monoshutter filter is a bit cumbersome and will narrow the field of view when looking through the laparoscope or off a television monitor. Most surgeons quickly accommodate to this narrowed field of view, but for those who don't, there is a small filter disc that can be inserted between the laparoscope and a camera, which makes the monoshutter unnecessary. However, I find that the orange filter from this disc, or the use of eye goggles, can affect color discrimination. I much prefer the shutter, which only drops the orange filter down when the laser is being fired.

PROCEDURES

Adhesions

Thin, filmy pelvic inflammatory disease (PID)-like adhesions can be taken down in a variety of nonlaser ways. They can be snipped down with scissors easily. Bipolar forceps can be used to coagulate when there are small blood vessels within the adhesions, then scissors can be used to cut along the co-agulation line. Unipolar instruments can slice across the adhesions. Endothermy can be used to coagulate, and then scissors can be used to cut along the coagulation line as well. The Nd:YAG lasers with the sapphire tip can produce a line of coagulation, and then the sapphire tips can be switched to allow cutting along this coagulation line. Or a CO_2 laser may be used to perform adhesiolysis; however, there are usually some problems with this approach.

The CO_2 laser is wonderful for vaporizing and cutting tissue. It is not a good laser for coagulation of tissue or for providing hemostasis. If you take a typical omental or pelvic adhesion drawn up to the anterior abdominal wall, as you step back and look at that adhesion you often find some thin areas, some thick areas, and perhaps several small- to medium-size blood vessels coursing through this adhesion. On occasion, you find a sizeable arteriole or venule as well. If you take your CO_2 laser and begin to take down this adhesion, the first thing you may notice is that you create several holes in the thinner parts of the adhesion. The CO_2 laser beam then has a new backstop, mainly whatever is behind that adhesion. This is fine if whatever is behind that adhesion is something innocent—for example, a metal probe. However, if the backstop in the area behind the adhesion is the bowel or the bladder or fimbriae, then the CO_2 beam, skipping off the edge of the adhesion, will exert its undiminished effect on this new backstop. Of all injuries occurring with laser surgery, one of the most feared is hitting an undesirable backstop.

There isn't nearly the concern with backstop problems with the argon laser as there is with the CO_2. Because of the divergence of the laser beam out of the argon fiber, there is little effect much beyond several centimeters off the tip of the fiber, so that as one skips off the edge of an adhesion at the cutting distance, a tad further beyond the tip of the fiber is the vaporizing distance, the coagulating distance, and so forth. Once the backstop has reached many centimeters behind the adhesion, the power density has dropped off so dramatically that tissue warming is the only likely effect. This is a wonderful feature and adds a bit of a safety net when performing adhesiolysis. However, you must keep in mind that if I have an adhesion draped over the bowel or against the pelvic sidewall, while I'm cutting adhesions just off the tip of the fiber, I am vaporizing serosa or pelvic sidewall just beyond the adhesion. This is where instrument backstops may be employed and may even double as an instrument for traction. It is also important to keep in mind that traction and countertraction are the most basic concepts in performing adhesiolysis. An adhesion will just boil, fizzle, and crinkle, unless it's on tension while cutting with any laser.

It's nice to take advantage of the hemostatic qualities of the argon laser when performing adhesiolysis. Often, the smaller blood vessels and capillaries will not even get a chance to bleed as the argon laser cuts through the tissue. The cut edges of the blood vessels will seal immediately.

The larger blood vessels, the arterioles and venules, will bleed as you cut across the adhesion. However, I usually don't let them get a chance to bleed. When I see any blood vessels within tissue, I will back the fiber off to the coagulating distance, and I will run the fiber up and down the blood vessel until it turns white. This is the cue that the blood vessel is completely sealed over. I then move the fiber in to the cutting distance and cut across the blood vessels I just coagulated closed. If I don't back my fiber up far enough to coagulate this blood vessel closed, I may end up vaporizing through the larger vessel wall before I get a chance to seal the vessels shut by coagulation.

The ability alternately to coagulate, then cut, vascular tissue and visible blood vessels, is a remarkable feature that I use with all of my adhesiolysis. Occasionally, small bleeders are encountered during adhesiolysis, which can be managed nicely with the argon laser. I will bring my fiber through a suction irrigator probe, and once I identify the bleeding area, I will squirt some irrigation fluid over the bleeding area, wash away the blood, and identify the exact source of the oozing or bleeding. Because the argon fiber shoots under clear liquids, I simply aim the fiber at the oozing blood vessel, keeping the fiber at the coagulating distance, step on the pedal for a second or so, and the blood vessel seals immediately. This operation is so easy and useful that it saves an enormous amount of time as I cut through adhesions and coagulate blood vessels.

Of course, some blood vessels are too large to be coagulated by the argon laser. When a larger-caliber blood vessel is encountered, on occasion I will back the fiber up to the coagulating distance and run the laser up and down the tissue adjacent to the blood vessel and on either side of the blood vessel. This cooking effect will often shrink down the blood vessel to a point where I can comfortably coagulate the blood vessel itself and wink it closed and sealed. However, until you get the knack for doing this, you should stick with more traditional and reliable methods to coagulate down the larger vessels.

For thick adhesions or bowel adhesions that are glued to the ovary or uterine surface, the size and inaccuracy of the diverging beam can make adhesiolysis a bit more difficult. As you try to find a plane or create a plane, thermal injury to adjacent structures can be significant. In these cases, as with cases of tuboplasty or fimbrioplasty, I usually elect to use the smaller diameter fiber to give me a finer, more precise cut, always aiming away from the more vital organ. Still, the diverging beam can be quite damaging to surrounding tissues by either direct thermal burn or by conduction burn. Here, while lasing, I may constantly irrigate the tissues to cool surrounding tissues to avoid conduction thermal damage.

Endometriosis

Endometriosis needs to be coagulated, vaporized, and excised. Anywhere the disease occurs, where a laparoscope can find it, the argon laser can be used to treat it effectively. As mentioned, I prefer to bring the fiber through a second puncture site, triangulate, set my laser between 6 and 8 watts, and then let the fiber go to work. By merely moving the fiber forward or backward and *visually* determining the tissue effect, I can attack the endometriosis in a manner appropriate to its location.

Usually, endometriosis in the cul-de-sac along the uterosacral ligaments is in a relatively safe place to lase. I will bring in my fiber to the vaporizing distance and debulk this tissue by pure vaporization. As I inch up toward the pelvic side wall, I may move my fiber back to the coagulating distance and lase more superficially. The visual cue that will indicate the shift from vaporizing to coagulating will be less debulking and cratering, and will create less smoke. A pure coagulating effect produces no smoke. I will then alternately move my fiber from coagulating to vaporizing as I track down the endometriosis.

You must keep in mind, however, that any time you leave a laser pointed at tissue, there will be conduction of that thermal energy away from the target over a period of time. This is also the case with the argon laser, and the conduction effect may even be enhanced by the divergence of the beam. This means that you have to keep the fiber beam moving! Otherwise, you'll see much deeper thermal injury, and wider thermal injury, if you spend too much time in one place.

Several visual cues help me determine if I have removed adequate tissue. These include the appearance of smooth, unscarred symmetrical tissue fibers or occasionally even normal-appearing preperitoneal fat. I'll look for these cues in those areas where I feel comfortable lasing to deeper planes; however, in unsafe areas, i.e., over the pelvic side walls, on bowel or bladder, I have to keep my laser effect superficial indeed. In these areas, I'll back the fiber way off to the pure coagulation distance and carefully watch for peritoneal blanching and desiccation. Even at this distance, however, there is penetration into the deeper tissue, and a conduction burn is possible. I will irrigate constantly as I am lasing endometriosis superficially over vital organs. I believe that the imprecision of the argon diverging beam makes excision of endometriosis over the bowel or the bladder too dangerous, and I'll usually set aside my argon laser for a good, sharp pair of scissors.

Endometrioma

The argon laser can be helpful when entering, resecting, or coagulating the base of an endometrioma. Small, shallow, endometriomas can be easily vaporized. When the old *chocolate* material is encountered, a suction irrigator probe containing the argon fiber is used to wash out the cyst. The base of the cyst is then coagulated or vaporized to destroy the residing endometriosis. In medium- to large-size endometriomas, I use a shovel technique, employing a good

uterine elevator to lift up the ovary into the perfect position, and I try to open up the endometriomas posteriorly, for a number of reasons. This is often where the endometrioma is "pointing" and may be stuck to the ovarian fossa. The mere act of mobilizing these endometriomas may result in rupture posteriorly. Even if the endometrioma is not ruptured or "pointing," I'll still open it posteriorly. I would much rather have adhesions develop posteriorly to the ovarian fossa than medially or anterior to the tube, bowel, or uterus.

The technique is fairly simple but, on occasion, can be quite challenging. As mentioned, shoveling the ovary into position, I will bring my argon laser fiber in and first coagulate any blood vessels on the ovarian surface in the area where I'll open the endometrioma. I'll then drill a hole into the endometrioma by placing the fiber as close to the tissue as possible without touching. I'll try to open an area large enough to enter the cyst cavity with my 5-mm graspers. I then will open the prongs of my graspers inside the endometrioma and gently pull back, tenting the cyst. Coming from a different angle with my suction irrigator probe containing the laser fiber, I will lase onto the open prongs, making a long linear incision. I'll then carefully pick up the edges of the opened cyst with either 3-mm or 5-mm graspers and proceed to wash out and suction off the cyst contents. Rarely does the cut edge of the endometrioma bleed when opened with the argon laser. If it does, however, backing the fiber up to the coagulating distance and firing will quickly establish hemostasis. Once the endometrioma has been opened, I will make every effort possible to identify the thin pseudocapsule. I will then try to peel the lining of the capsule out in one or two pieces. The base of the cyst wall rarely bleeds; however, since the hilum of this cyst wall is where its blood supply is located, here bleeding is often encountered. I usually anticipate that those blood vessels are too large to coagulate entirely with the argon laser, so I'll twist the capsule several times to kink off its hilar attachment. I'll then cut off the cyst wall with the argon laser.

When the pseudocapsule of an endometrioma is completely removed, it is easy to tell the glistening white normal ovarian tissue from the hemosiderin-laden cyst wall. If I can't tease away remaining fragments of cyst wall, I will take the laser and either coagulate or vaporize at the appropriate distances. In cases where capsules cannot be identified and stripped out, I will coagulate or vaporize the entire base of the endometrioma. The darkly stained, hemosiderin-laden cyst wall rapidly absorbs the laser energy, enhancing the laser effect, so I'll lase quickly and superficially, in order not to destroy deeper normal tissue.

One final act, while using the argon laser for large endometriomas, is to do a variation of the Bruhat maneuver (designed to laser flower open a hydrosalpinx) by using the argon to desiccate the inner aspect of the opened endometrioma along its edges to invert or roll in all cut edges. This will minimize any exposure of raw ovarian tissue at the cut edges to nearby bowel, fimbriae, or uterus, perhaps reducing adhesion formation.

Ectopic Pregnancy

The argon laser is perfect for performing a linear salpingotomy on unruptured ectopic pregnancies. Once the ectopic pregnancy is properly positioned, I will bring in my 300 μ argon laser fiber and make a coagulation line, beginning proximally, over approximately one third the length of the ectopic bulge. After coagulating initially, I will then zoom into the cutting distance and make an incision directly over this coagulation line. By incising in this fashion, rarely will I encounter "cut edge bleeders." The argon laser's ability to achieve hemostasis is perfect for coagulating these cut edge bleeders before they even get a chance to bleed! However, if they do bleed after the incision, you can wash away the blood and identify the single point where the bleeding is occurring. Then while irrigating, you can spray-paint the area with the argon at the coagulating distance and seal those cut edges down immediately.

Once the ectopic is removed and the tube is irrigated, there may be troublesome bed bleeding. Bed bleeding is next to impossible to control using other techniques, but the argon is ideal for managing this difficult problem. You bring in the suction irrigator probe and wash away the blood within the lumen of the tube and zoom in with your laparoscope. Through the puddle of water, you often can identify the single area that's bleeding, "percolating" upward, filling the tube and spilling over the edges. Then simply bring the fiber in underneath the puddle of water, aim it at the direction of the bed bleeder, and step on the pedal for a split second. With the laser at the coagulating distance, you can seal these bed bleeders beautifully! For laparoscopic linear salpingotomies, the argon seems tailor-made!

Uterosacral Ligament Transection

Laparoscopic uterosacral nerve ablation, or LUNA, has become a popular procedure in recent years for the treatment of dysmenorrhea. The goal of the procedure is to transect these ligaments at their insertion into the back of the cervix, where the nerve fibers tend to converge. The uterosacral ligaments can be transected in a number of ways using laser and nonlaser technique. Using the argon laser may have several advantages for this procedure. First, I can achieve excellent hemostasis while cutting a fair amount of tissue. Second, by taking advantage of the natural forward penetration of the argon laser several millimeters beyond the surface of the target, I can coagulate deeper into the tissue, destroying more nerve fibers.

I will use my uterine elevator to tent the uterosacral ligaments to outline their course more easily. This must be done for several reasons. The two structures to fear in the area include the ureter, which commonly may drop low alongside the lateral aspect of the uterosacral ligaments, and what I call "the artery of Osher," which is really a descending branch of the cervical artery lying just lateral to the uterosacral ligaments at their insertion into the cervix. If the ligaments are scarred down with endometriosis, or are naturally thin or attenuated, you should be *extremely* careful in cutting across them.

It's best to direct the argon fiber at the uterosacral ligaments in as perpendicular a direction as possible. If the fiber is brought down through the superpubic port, a more oblique or tangential cut is likely. This is why I'll use a port higher up the abdominal wall, directing my laser 90° into the cul-de-sac. I'll then either vaporize or cut an area closest to the insertion of the uterosacral ligaments into the cervix, creating a defect approximately $\frac{3}{4}$-cm deep and $\frac{3}{4}$-cm wide. Remember, because this area is on tension, the ligament flattens out as it's being cut, never giving the appearance that you are $\frac{3}{4}$-cm deep. This can give the false illusion that you're not cutting deep enough and may encourage further cutting. This is hazardous and can lead to laparotomy, because brisk bleeding can be encountered if you cut too deeply. Also, you must be careful to avoid going too far laterally, as the diverging beam of the argon can penetrate the pelvic sidewall and injure the ureter or perhaps shrink down and coagulate those delicate, important, ureteral blood vessels. Cutting too far laterally may result in breaching "the artery of Osher," which can also result in brisk bleeding. Also, lasing posteriorly toward the sacrum offers no significant advantages, because the greatest concentration of nerve fibers is at the cervix.

One additional comment regarding this procedure, no matter how the transection is performed: Ease up on the uterine elevator following the uterosacral ligament transection in an effort to identify bleeding from the cut edges; the uterine elevator has the ligaments on so much stretch that immediate bleeding may not be identified. If, after the laparoscope and all instruments have been removed, the assistant, between the patient's legs, then eases up on the uterine elevator, bleeding or oozing from the transection site may result. Anecdotally, I've heard of postoperative bleeding from "the artery of Osher" requiring an emergent reoperation.

Fibroids

Laparoscopic myomectomies can be managed nicely with the argon laser fiber. Small, subserosal myomas can be vaporized easily, while small- to medium-sized pedunculated myomas can have their stalks coagulated initially and then cut across with the argon laser with good hemostasis. Large pedunculated myomas should probably be coagulated with either bipolar cautery or some other more powerful coagulating instrument. However, once the deeper coagulation has been accomplished, the argon laser will slice across the stalk. These fibroids can then be morcellated with the argon laser for removal.

Intramural myomas can be approached by coagulating and cutting into the myometrium. Once the intramural myoma is identified, it can be enucleated with nonlaser technique or perhaps by using the argon laser for intermittent coagulation and excision. The base of the intramural fibroid should probably be coagulated with bipolar or unipolar electrocoagulation, as the argon is unlikely to control and coagulate these large blood vessels.

Polycystic Ovary Drilling

In patients resistant to ovulation induction agents, a laparoscopic procedure has been designed where polycystic ovaries have been drilled with various devices, releasing follicular fluid and destroying internal ovarian tissue—in effect, performing a variation of the old ovarian wedge resection. Several studies have confirmed that many of these patients are ovulatory for various amounts of time postoperatively, resulting in many pregnancies. The procedure has been described with unipolar electrocoagulation, CO_2 lasers, and with Nd:YAG, KTP, and argon fiberoptic lasers.

My own experience has taught me to use fiberoptic lasers exclusively for this procedure. This is for several reasons. Anecdotally, I have heard that the widely defocused beam of a CO_2 laser, when used for drilling polycystic ovaries, has resulted in far too much superficial ovarian damage. This has resulted in massive adhesions to the ovary on second-look laparoscopy. Even when the CO_2 beam is focused, as soon as the pocket of fluid is hit, further drilling into the ovarian tissue is encumbered by the fluid itself. This not only makes for limited drilling, but also makes for a good deal of smoke!

Here, I like using the argon fiberoptic laser in a *contact mode*, which I rarely use during the rest of my endoscopic argon laser surgery. First, I will shovel the ovary up with the uterus by manipulating the intrauterine elevator. In this fashion, my assistant can rock the ovary around into any desired position without the use of extra grasping instruments. This shovel technique can flip a big, polycystic ovary onto its other side, exposing the entire lateral surface. I will then take my fiber tip and place it in a perpendicular direction onto the ovarian surface. I then step on the foot pedal, firing the laser as I push ever so gently with the laser fiber. Immediately, the fiber cuts a tiny hole directly into the ovary. I will allow my fiber to pass approximately $\frac{1}{2}$ cm into the ovarian stroma *while* I'm lasing. The follicular fluid immediately evacuates from each tiny cyst as the laser continues to fire deep within the ovary. Using this technique, there is minimal superficial ovarian tissue damage and essentially no char, while the real damage is beneath the ovarian surface to the underlying stroma. This, I believe, minimizes the chance for postoperative adhesions to the ovary and accomplishes the task of letting off the fluid while destroying a bit of ovarian tissue.

I will spend between 15 to 20 minutes on each ovary, covering the entire ovarian surface, giving the ovary a golf-ball appearance. Depending on the size of the ovary, I may make up to 100 punctures. This is the *only* procedure where I'll fire the laser, blindly, while advancing the fiber into tissue!

Hemostasis is rarely a problem; however, should I see a superficial blood vessel in the area where I am about to drill a hole, I will back the fiber up and coagulate it. I try to keep this superficial coagulation to a minimum, as I believe the more superficial damage to the ovary there is, the more likely there will be postoperative adhesions. In addition, I caution you to avoid drilling areas near the ovarian hilus. There are few follicles, yet a number of large blood vessels in this area.

Neosalpingostomy

To open up the agglutinated end of a clubbed tube or a hydrosalpinx has been shown to be an effective laparoscopic procedure. I enjoy doing this kind of surgery, and here I find that the argon laser is an exceptional tool. I will use the 300 μ fiber to perform the tubo-ovariolysis which is commonly necessary to mobilize the clubbed end. Then, once I mobilize the terminal end of the tube, I will chromotubate via an intrauterine cannula with dilute indigocarmine or methylene blue, which will often ''stiffen'' the entire tube up to the distal end. I will then identify the dimple at the end of the tube and bring in my 300 μ argon laser fiber. I will keep the laser set at my traditional 6 to 8 watts and superficially coagulate an area directly over the dimple. I will then zoom in and enter the tube by drilling a hole directly into its terminal end. At this point, all of the blue dye will spill out as I widen my entry point with the argon laser. I'll make this incision just large enough to place a 3-mm initially, then a 5-mm grasper into the intratubal lumen. By opening up the prongs of my grasper and gently pulling back, I will tent the terminal end and proceed to lase down on top of my prongs in a linear fashion. The cut edges rarely bleed, and the thermal damage is limited. I will then make radial incisions and prepare to flower back the edges of the tube.

In the past, at this point I would have turned the power of my laser down to 2 to 4 watts, backed my fiber up, and desiccated the serosa behind each new ''leaflet.'' The desiccated serosa would crinkle and contract, and ultimately the edge of the leaflet would peel back and open up like the petal of a flower. I used to do this to all leaflets, but found, by second-look laparoscopy, that reagglutination was common. Now, besides flowering the leaflets open, I routinely add a couple of micro stitches to secure the opened leaflets to the ampullary serosa. This gives me a more secure feeling that the contracture sites from the laser will not soften, releasing the leaflets and allowing reagglutination.

Any specific bleeding points, identified at the cut edges of the distal tube, can be easily coagulated by backing up the argon fiber to the coagulating distance. You may want to irrigate while coagulating to cool the adjacent delicate fimbrial tissue and endosalpinx.

Adnexectomy

In most cases where I have to perform an oophorectomy or salpingectomy, I'll use nonlaser techniques. On occasion, I will encounter some oozing on the pedicles, whether I use suture ligatures, clips, or staples. I will then use the hemostatic properties of the argon laser by spraypainting the pedicle at the coagulating distance, under irrigation to wash away the blood and coagulate the source of the bleeding. This will only work for slight oozing or bleeding and will not be effective for brisk bleeding. In cases where a suture ligature has been applied, I will be careful to do the same, using the laser at the coagulating distance but making sure that I fire the laser far from the suture material for fear of denaturing or interfering with the integrity of that suture material.

The argon laser can be helpful in carving up ovarian and tubal tissue already removed from their pedicles. An ovary can be "whittled" with the laser into several long strips for easy removal.

Open Abdominal Surgery

As much as I feel the argon laser is a wonderful tool for operative endoscopy, I don't use the argon for open cases. Old habits are hard to break, and I feel that a good old-fashioned pair of pick-ups and scissors and a microtipped electrosurgical tool can help me perform most of my adhesiolysis and excisional surgery. However, for the same reasons that I've given for using the argon endoscopically for different procedures, the argon laser can easily be used for those same procedures during laparotomy, with similar results. I suppose one of the main reasons why I don't use the argon laser at laparotomy is the need for goggles to filter the brilliant laser light. With endoscopy, I have an eye safety shutter that drops an orange filter between my eye and the scope only when I step on the pedal to fire the laser.

At laparotomy, I would need to wear goggles continuously, which would prevent me from seeing my argon-colored aiming beam. Subconsciously, this aiming beam provides critical visual cues when performing fine excisional work. With goggles, finding the critical distances needed for the three tissue effects takes a bit of guesswork each time the laser is fired.

TRAINING

It's easy to learn how to use the argon laser. However, you must take a little time to develop a feel for how the laser operates and how it's able to achieve the different tissue effects. I believe it's important for you to attend a basic laser course that will give you the background on different lasers and how they work. This basic course should allow plenty of hands-on time to help you to become familiar with the tissue effects of the different lasers. I believe that the next critical step in your learning curve is to attend some good operative endoscopy courses to learn laser technique and nonlaser technique. The best endoscopist is one who champions *all* techniques.

I feel strongly that after you attend these courses you *must* go to the table and spend time with an old seasoned laser endoscopist. This may be a nearby friend who's been doing this type of surgery for years, or you may work formally with a preceptor; many such preceptorships are available around the country. Attending a good preceptorship will make you feel comfortable and confident that you too can go home to your hospital and begin doing these procedures. This, I believe, is the most important segment on your learning curve.

SUGGESTED READING

Diamond MP, DeCherney AH, Polan ML. Laparoscopic use of the argon laser in nonendometriotic reproductive pelvic surgery. *J Reprod Med* 1986;31:1011–3.

Keye WR Jr, Hansen LW, Astin M, Poulson AM. Argon laser therapy of endometriosis: a review of 92 consecutive patients. *Fertil Steril* 1987;47:208.

Keye WR Jr, McArthur GR. The argon laser in gynecology. In: Keye WR, ed. *Lasers in Gynecology and Obstetrics*, 2nd ed. Chicago, IL: Year Book Medical Publishers, 1990.

Operative Laparoscopy, Second Edition
The Masters' Techniques in Gynecologic Surgery
Lippincott–Raven Publishers, Philadelphia © 1998.

4-6   Nd:YAG Laser Laparoscopy

Stephen L. Corson

The contact sapphire probe has transformed the YAG laser from a shotgun to a target rifle, capable of delivering energy in a discrete locus producing a predictable lesion whose shape and size can be carefully modulated according to the choice of the probe. The YAG system is compared to the CO_2 laser in Table 4-6.1; the advantages of the former are obvious and numerous. It is, in short, more user-friendly, especially because it is delivered via a flexible fiber and there is minimal smoke production within the closed space of the peritoneal cavity.

This section will cover the application technique of the YAG laser to specific gynecologic pathologies. Refer first to Figures 4-6.1 and 4-6.2 to appreciate some of the concepts of use of the sapphire contact probe in clinical situations. The figures show, respectively, energy distribution patterns and the resultant lesions produced by the probes most commonly used in gynecologic surgery.

ENDOMETRIOSIS

Lesions should be identified with a systematic laparoscopic search, mobilizing the ovaries with a grasping forceps inserted through a small trocar sleeve to inspect the lateral surfaces and ovarian fossae. A sequential order of ablation should be conducted, with posterior cul-de-sac lesions treated prior to extensive irrigation procedures that might later obscure visualization of small lesions, especially if not pigmented. A number of ancillary punctures may have to be made to accommodate irrigation probes, grasping forceps, biopsy forceps, and the YAG laser sapphire probe and handle. Bipolar coagulation forceps should be on hand if extensive dissection is anticipated and/or large amounts of tissue are to be removed.

The patient is placed in a dorsal lithotomy position, and after appropriate preparation and draping, the cervix is exposed with a speculum and grasped with a double-toothed tenaculum, so that a weighted intrauterine manipulator and cannula can be inserted into the uterus and left in place. The patient must be positioned on the table so this hangs freely. The patient is encouraged to void just before walking to the operating room from a waiting area, and we routinely try to avoid catheterization of the bladder unless it becomes full during the case.

Once a satisfactory level of anesthesia has been achieved, a Trendelenburg position of 15° is created. A small incision is made at the umbilicus, usually vertically, starting from

within the depression but on occasion horizontally, depending on topography and prior surgery. A CO_2 pneumoperitoneum is achieved with a disposable spring-loaded needle, using a syringe filled with saline, dropping fluid by gravity without a plunger, to demonstrate free entry. When sufficient distention has been reached, the needle is removed, the incision is enlarged, and the 10-mm disposable Surgi-Port trocar and sheath are inserted in a Z-track fashion, aiming toward the midline sacral hollow.

Any atypical lesion should be mechanically biopsied prior to alteration of histology by laser energy. If a lesion appearing to be an endometrioma is encountered, the surface is inspected for excrescences or other factors that might support a different diagnosis. Adhesions, if present, are lysed by sharp dissection, after which the ovary is steadied with two 5-mm toothed spring-loaded grasping forceps (one in each lower quadrant). In the interim, the laser handle has been readied, and the Surgical Laser Technologies (SLT) YAG laser has been set and calibrated to deliver 20 W of continuous power to the distal end of the probe. The laser fiber is cooled with gas (CO_2) or liquid (lactated Ringer's solution), with gas preferred for shorter cases, or when cooling fluid would tend to collect in a dependent pocket.

Using a "chisel-tip" sapphire probe, the laser is brought down, and a 5-mm diameter sheath is inserted in the midline with a 3-mm reduction adapter, to avoid loss of pneumoperitoneum. The laser probe can be inserted through the irrigator as well.

The incision is made into the cyst, or entry is made directly with a 5 mm trocar and sheath, after which a Corson irrigator aspirator (Figure 4-6.3) is inserted into the cyst cavity to remove and rinse the contents. Any spillage into the posterior cul-de-sac is removed, although usually this is quite minimal. Once this fluid returns clear, the forceps are used to enlarge the aperture in the cyst, and the telescope is inserted to view the interior, again looking for papillations or other irregularities. Most patients with adnexal masses have been prescreened with pelvic ultrasonography to help avoid confusion with patients having lesions with septation or solid components suggesting other diagnoses. When a lesion >4 cm is encountered, gonadotropin-releasing hormone agonist therapy is frequently given for 90 days preoperatively to help shrink the lesion and to reduce associated inflammatory response.

A mechanical full-thickness biopsy of the cyst wall-ovarian tunic is taken along one of the edges, using laparoscopic

Table 4-6.1 *Comparison of YAG[a] and CO₂ lasers*

	YAG	CO₂
Smoke production	Minimal	Great
Rigid arm and mirrors	No	Yes
Fiber delivery	Yes	No
Tissue contact	Yes	No
Hemostasis	Excellent	Poor
Vaporization	Fair	Excellent
Cutting ability	Adequate	Better
Need for backstop	None	Necessary
Performance at liquid interface	Yes	No

[a] With sapphire probe.

scissors; bleeding is rarely a problem. At this point, the operator has a number of options. The first and sometimes the simplest is that of laparoscopic oophorectomy. This can be achieved using a YAG laser scalpel tip with either Endoloops or electrosurgical hemostasis for large vessels, or even more easily with Multifire Endo GIA surgical staples. But when reproduction is at stake, unless the lesion has been a recurrent one or if normal ovarian tissue cannot be identified, ovarian conservation should be favored.

This may be accomplished by stripping the cyst wall away, using a forceps technique. A tedious dissection frequently ensues, and if there is an inflammatory component, this plan must be abandoned in most cases. My own preference is to destroy the cyst wall in situ, using the chisel-tip as a laser-plane (Figure 4-6.4). This ablation procedure starts at the bottom of the cyst and proceeds upward in a spiral manner with the distal side of the probe, rather than the tip, used to paint the cyst wall. Sutures are neither necessary nor desirable.

Peritoneal implants are easily vaporized with the rounded probe. Depth of penetration with this system is controlled by the (1) choice of probe, (2) wattage setting, and (3) amount of pressure at the probe-tissue contact. Thus, discrete destruction of lesions can be achieved. Since the laser energy 2 cm from the probe is minimal, one does not need a backstop as with the CO₂ laser. Small collections of irrigating fluid will not interfere with the YAG laser as with the CO₂ laser, and venting of the peritoneal space because of smoke production and accumulation is rare, unless the disease is extensive. Most important is the intrinsic hemostatic property of the YAG laser.

When endometriosis is present in bladder, bowel, or over the ureter, reduced power settings (10 to 14 W) and a light touch are recommended. After firing, the probe will remain hot for about 4 seconds, so contact with other structures should be avoided. Cooling with liquid is somewhat more efficient than with gas. Since the tissue effect is a combination of direct heat transfer from the probe plus absorption of laser energy, somewhat higher settings (about 20 W) are needed when liquid cooling is employed.

With gas cooling, about a liter of gas will be passed into the abdominal cavity for each minute that the probe is in place, but will not necessarily be fired. Thus, even with automatic shut-off of a laparoscopic insufflation device that is pressure set, overdistention is possible under these circumstances. This is far more theoretical than real, because these procedures usually require three or four punctures, and the aggregate leakage of CO₂ from the abdomen approximates the rate of flow of coolant CO₂.

Reassessment by ultrasound demonstrates a return to normal ovarian size and contour within 2 or 3 months. In patients having a secondary laparoscopic procedure, as with

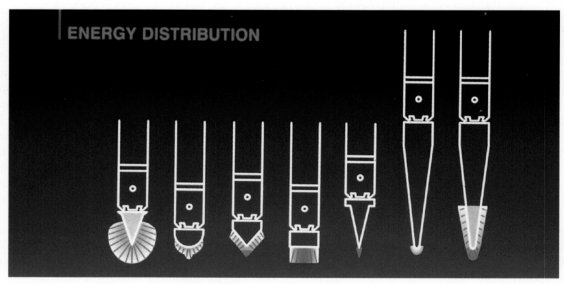

Figure 4-6.1 Energy distribution of sapphire probes commonly used in gynecologic laparoscopy. (Courtesy of Surgical Laser Technologies, Oaks, PA.)

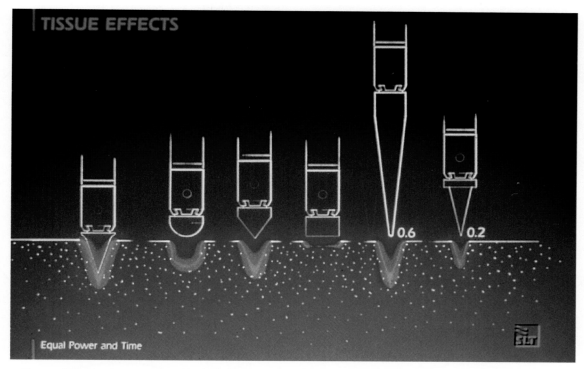

Figure 4-6.2 Lesions produced by individual probes. (Courtesy of Surgical Laser Technologies, Oaks, PA.)

gamete intrafallopian transfer (GIFT), we have observed excellent healing, usually devoid of adhesion formation.

In our study we documented that YAG laser ablation of endometriomas, as well as other pelvic implants, can be accomplished during GIFT without interference in establishing pregnancy; the fecundity rate was actually higher with this form of intervention than with GIFT alone.

In general, pregnancy rates have been satisfactory and related to American Fertility Society scores. Pain relief has been impressive, especially when the procedure has included uterosacral denervation. To summarize, I don't believe that laser surgery of any type, performed by laparoscopy or laparotomy, can produce pregnancy rates or relieve pain better than similar surgery performed by electrosur-

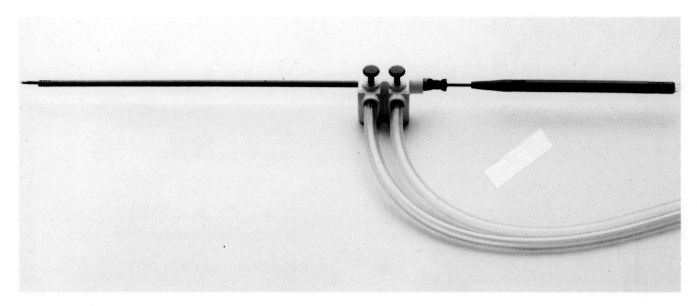

Figure 4-6.3 Corson irrigator/aspirator. (Courtesy of Cabot Medical Laboratories, Langhorne, PA.)

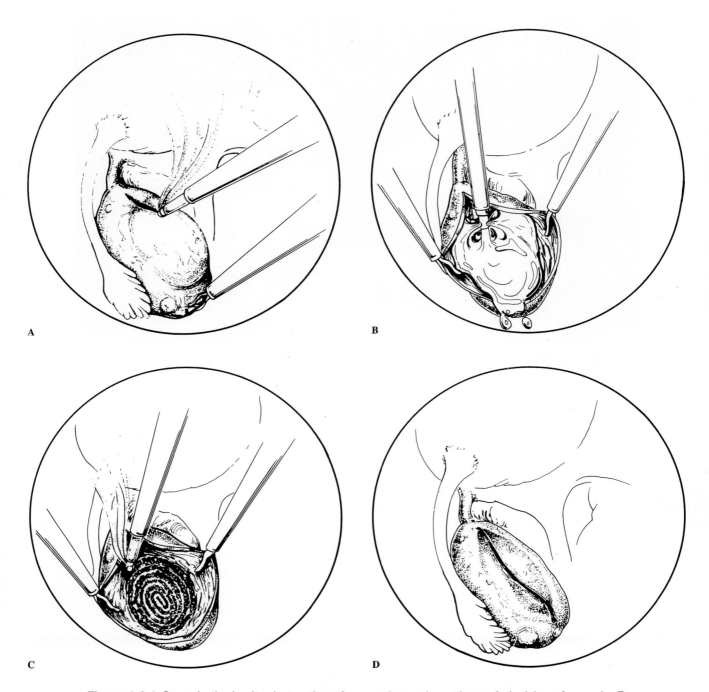

Figure 4-6.4 Steps in the in situ destruction of an ovarian endometrioma. **A.** Incision of capsule. **B.** Irrigation, then eversion of edges. **C.** Capsule destruction in an upward spiral. **D.** Edges fold in spontaneously.

gery. But I *do* believe that the use of a YAG laser-sapphire probe system allows these procedures to be done more completely and with more safety than unipolar electrosurgery because the spread of energy, and hence tissue effect, is more controllable than with unipolar surgery. Bipolar electrosurgery for endometriosis, while safe, is frequently unsatisfactory because bipolar current tends to remain super-

ficial; lesions as deep as 4 mm in the uterosacral ligaments would be incompletely treated by this modality.

UTEROSACRAL DENERVATION

Posterior compartment lesions causing persistent pelvic pain are usually those of endometriosis, although induration can be seen with the inflammation, associated with chronic salpingitis. Especially when the uterosacral ligaments are involved, partial sectioning to interrupt the sensory nerves is often salutary.

When accomplished with sharp dissection, bleeding can come from vessels within the ligament. Electrosurgery puts the ureter at some risk, and therefore the YAG laser is my preference. Usually we use either a chisel probe or a scalpel probe.

The uterus is put on anterior stretch with the intrauterine manipulator, so that the ligaments stand out. The lesion is treated horizontally near the uterine point of insertion to a depth of about 3 to 4 mm and a length of about 1 cm, dependent on thickness of the ligament.

OTHER OVARIAN CYSTS

The YAG laser sapphire scalpel can be used for ovarian cysts other than endometriomas. Cystic teratomas, for instance, can be incised, the contents aspirated and rinsed, and the wall biopsied. Then they can be enucleated or destroyed in situ. Benign neoplastic cysts can be treated in a similar fashion. Paraovarian cysts are yet another variation on that theme. Somewhat different is treatment of polycystic ovarian syndrome by laser surgery. A subgroup of patients with this diagnosis are either refractory to ovulation induction with clomiphene citrate and/or gonadotropins, or, conversely, hyperstimulate. Reduction of the bulk of subcapsular cysts will frequently bring about spontaneous ovulation or a better response to ovulation induction. Rather than resort to a laparotomy with wedge resection, via laparoscopy, 20 to 30 small holes may be drilled in each ovary to a depth of about 1 mm, to allow visual confirmation of cystic fluid drainage. A scalpel probe set at 10 to 14 W is sufficient. Remember that power density at the tip of the scalpel is great. Also, only the actual scalpel tip emits laser energy; therefore, this probe should always be used perpendicularly to tissue and not on an angle, as with a cold scalpel.

ECTOPIC PREGNANCY

When ectopic pregnancy is suspected, laparoscopy will usually settle the issue, both diagnostically and therapeutically. Now that pelvic-ultrasound has achieved better resolution, gestational sacs within the uterus can be seen quite early. It is no longer unusual to see an extrauterine gestational sac via vaginal ultrasound. This technology, plus quantitative serum β human chorionic gonadotropin (hCG) determinations, usually leads to laparoscopic diagnosis before the ectopic gestation ruptures.

Prior to surgery, a plan must be established as to the desired treatment of the tube. If the tube is to be removed, a variety of laser, electrosurgical, or mechanical approaches can be used. When conservation is planned, a discrete delivery of energy is mandatory to reduce damage to the tube. Injection into the tube with dilute vasopressin over the proposed dorsal line of incision is a helpful hemostatic maneuver. Most ectopic gestations are ampullary. Remember that the trophoblastic material often extends to the medial side of the bulge. Therefore, the incision with the laser scalpel starts medially to the distended area. Usually, intraluminal pressure will cause an intraluminal gestation to extrude intact, after which it can be extracted laparoscopically. If the implantation is extraluminal, as is often the case, a high-pressure irrigator can be used to dislodge the tissue from the implantation site. The irrigator can also be used to wash out the tubal lumen when the lumen has been entered. I never suture the edges. If hemostasis is not satisfactory, the flat-tipped probe or bipolar coagulation of discrete vessels can be employed. In the past, isthmic gestations were managed by resection (transverse) techniques. This can be done with the YAG system, but I have used the linear salpingotomy technique here also with excellent results, subsequently documented, with hysterosalpingography and by intrauterine pregnancy. Remember, monitor falling β-hCG titers to ensure that the removal of trophoblastic material was adequate and that persistent or secondary implantation has not occurred.

PELVIC ADHESIONS

Lysis of pelvic adhesions can be performed by electrosurgery, laser, or mechanical means. Excision of adhesive bands is preferable. In particular, when omentum is involved, the adhesive process often is rather vascular, and the YAG scalpel probe is the instrument of choice. Tissue vaporization and separation are more easily accomplished with the CO_2 laser, but hemostasis is minimal with that system. Moreover, under these circumstances, a backstop may be difficult to use.

MYOMECTOMY

There is increasing enthusiasm for laparoscopic myomectomy. Even when vasopressin is used, myomectomy can be associated with troublesome bleeding. Excision of the myoma with the YAG *frosted* scalpel probe is associated with significant lateral dispersion of energy, causing excellent hemostasis in vascular beds such as the liver, pancreas, and uterus. Destruction of small amounts of surrounding myometrium is not catastrophic.

If the myoma is on a stalk, the operation is merely one of severing the pedicle. If the lesion is intramural, a sagittal incision with enucleation of each half is the easiest technique. Intracorporeal laparoscopic suturing of the deep layer and often, separately, the serosa, is often necessary. The removal of large lesions can be by morcellation with laparoscopic ancillary instrumentation or simply by colpotomy. Reproductive performance following myomectomy in this fashion remains to be evaluated by sufficient patient numbers, with special attention to uterine rupture in a later pregnancy.

CONCLUSION

The use of the YAG laser contact probe system has much to offer the gynecologic laparoscopist. Tissue can be vaporized, coagulated, incised, and excised using a variety of sapphire probes. The surgeon has tactile contact with tissue, and lesions can be predictably selected by choice of probe, power setting, and tissue contact. I prefer to work in a continuous mode rather than use pulsed energy; while pulsed laser use has advantages in some CO_2 laser situations, this has not been the case with the YAG laser. Hemostasis is excellent and smoke production minimal. The surgeon has a user-friendly delivery system and the patient has the benefit of an extremely safe laser system.

SUGGESTED READING

American Fertility Society. Revised American Fertility Society classification of endometriosis, 1985. *Fertil Steril* 1985;43:351–2.

Chong AP, Pepi M, Lashgari M. Pregnancy outcome in microsurgical anastomosis using cold knife versus CO_2 laser. *J Gyn Surg* 1989;5:99.

Corson SL, Unger M, Kwa D, Batzer FR, Gocial B. Laparoscopic laser treatment of endometriosis with the Nd:YAG sapphire probe. *Am J Obstet Gynecol* 1989;160:718.

Corson SL, Woodland M, Frishman G, Batzer FR, Gocial B, Maislin G. Treatment of endometriosis with a Nd:YAG tissue-contact laser probe via laparoscopy. *Int J Fertil* 1989;34:284.

Diamond MP, Feste J, Daniell J, McLaughlin D, Martin DC. Pelvic adhesions at early second look laparoscopy following carbon dioxide laser surgical procedures. *Infertility* 1984;7:39–44.

Doyle JB. Paracervical uterine denervation by transection of cervical plexus for the relief of dysmenorrhea. *Am J Obstet Gynecol* 1955;70:1.

Filmar S, Gomel V, McComb P. The effectiveness of CO_2 laser and electromicrosurgery in adhesiolysis: a comparative study. *Fertil Steril* 1986;45:407.

Greenblatt E, Casper RF. Endocrine changes after the laparoscopic ovarian cautery in polycystic ovarian syndrome. *Am J Obstet Gynecol* 1987;156:279–285.

Luciano AA, Maier DB, Koch EI, Nulsen JC, Whitman GF. A comparative study of postoperative adhesions following laser surgery by laparoscopy versus laparotomy in the rabbit model. *Obstet Gynecol* 1989;74:220.

Luciano AA, Whitman G, Maier DB, Randolph R, Maenza R. A comparison of thermal injury, healing patterns, and postoperative adhesion formation following CO_2 electromicrosurgery. *Fertil Steril* 1987;48:1025.

Pittaway DE, Maxson WS, Daniell JF. A comparison of the CO_2 laser and electrocautery on postoperative intraperitoneal adhesion formation in rabbits. *Fertil Steril* 1983;40:366.

Tulandi T, Farag R, McInnes RA, Gelfand MM, Wright CV, Vilos GA. Reconstructive surgery of hydrosalpinx with and without the carbon dioxide laser. *Fertil Steril* 1984;42:839.

Operative Laparoscopy, Second Edition
The Masters' Techniques in Gynecologic Surgery
Lippincott–Raven Publishers, Philadelphia © 1998.

5

Infertility

5-1   Operative Laparoscopy for Tubal Disease

Victor Gomel and Christo G. Zouves

Human fertilization begins with the fusion of sperm and oocyte in the ampulla of the fallopian tube. The oviduct's functions are multiple and complex: it transports sperm in proovarian direction, picks up an oocyte which has been released from the ovary and nurtures the zygote in the ampulla before it is transported to the uterus, where it is implanted in the endometrium. Damage to the ciliated epithelium may have an adverse effect on tubal function: tubal distortion or occlusion can result either in failure of sperm to meet an egg or in tubal implantation of the zygote.

Recent technological advances permit reproductive surgeons to perform complex reconstructive procedures effectively and safely with endoscopy, but significant improvement in success rates of in vitro fertilization (IVF) forces reevaluation of the therapeutic alternatives. In addition, the higher incidence of ectopic pregnancy and the lower rate of implantation when IVF is performed could indicate an expanding role for salpingectomy in patients with hydrosalpinges.

TUBAL FACTOR INFERTILITY

Sexually transmitted pelvic infection accounts for most of the tubal damage which results in infertility and tubal ectopic pregnancies. The most common responsible organisms are Chlamydia trachomatis, Neisseria, gonorrhea, and Mycoplasma hominis. The initial attack of pelvic inflammatory disease (PID) may be anywhere from asymptomatic to life-threatening. In the latter situation, commonly, aerobic or anaerobic bacteria are also involved. More than half of the patients who present with hydrosalpinx have no clinical history of a prior pelvic infection. Incidence of PID is highest in women under the age of 24. With an ever-decreasing age of onset of first intercourse there has been an alarming increase in teenage infections. A single episode of

PID may result in infertility in up to 20 percent of affected women.

Initially, the only option available to correct tubal factor infertility was reconstructive surgery. The simplification, increasing availability, and improvement in success rates of in vitro fertilization make this an increasingly attractive alternative. The presence of additional factors such as endometriosis and/or sperm-related problems may influence the selection of IVF as the primary therapeutic approach.

INVESTIGATION

Investigation of the infertile couple must be concluded expeditiously, accurately, and economically, with as little invasion as possible, while taking into account their emotional needs. Hysterosalpingography (HSG) continues to play an important role in assessment of the uterus and especially of the fallopian tubes; to be effective, however, it must be performed accurately.

Hysterosalpingography

Hysterosalpingography should be performed after menstruation has ceased and before ovulation, and is contraindicated in patients who may be pregnant, have abnormal bleeding, or have a history of recent or recurrent PID.

The contrast medium may be either oil- or water-soluble. The latter is preferable, since it yields greater accuracy and detail about tubal architecture. Major complications are uncommon if appropriate techniques are used. Complications include pelvic inflammatory disease, perforation of the uterus, bleeding from the site of the tenaculum, or allergic reaction due to extravasation of contrast material.

HSG provides valuable information about the uterus and the fallopian tubes. With respect to the oviduct, however, HSG has an associated false positive result for proximal tubal occlusion, and has a low predictive value for periadnexal adhesions and endometriosis.

Selective Salpingography and Tubal Cannulation

Selective salpingography and tubal cannulation ideally should be performed at the time of HSG, when a cornual or proximal tubal obstruction is demonstrated. In selective salpingography, contrast medium is injected directly into the uterine tubal ostium; in tubal cannulation, a special flexible guide wire is introduced into the tube, past the site of occlusion, over which a narrow-gauge cannula is passed. The techniques may help overcome obstructions associated with tubal spasm, mucous plugs and minor synechiae. However, these techniques are unlikely to correct occlusions due to fibrosis, salpingitis isthmica nodosa, or endometriosis.

Salpingoscopy

Direct endoscopic examination of the distal ampulla may be carried out at the time of laparoscopy, using either a rigid or flexible scope. Salpingoscopy permits evaluation of the tubal epithelium allowing a rating from Grade I (normal mucosal architecture), through Grade V (tubes that are rigid and hollow with a complete loss of epithelial folds). Salpingoscopy appears to have good prognostic predictor value and may help in deciding whether to repair or remove fallopian tubes at the time of laparoscopy.

Falloposcopy

The transvaginal microendoscopic technique of exploring the fallopian tubes can be used both as a means of tubal cannulation and to assess the lumen of the tube, especially its proximal portion.

Laparoscopy

Laparoscopy permits direct evaluation of the pelvic and other abdominal viscera and observing tubal patency by chromopertubation. Whereas hysterosalpingography and laparoscopy are complementary techniques in the assessment of tubal function, HSG should always precede laparoscopy. Identifying abnormalities of the uterine cavity and the fallopian tubes prior to embarking on a laparoscopy permit operative laparoscopic procedures described below to be performed at the time of the primary laparoscopy by an appropriately trained endoscopic surgeon. This maximizes patient benefit and minimizes both the cost and the risks which go along with a second surgical procedure.

All endoscopic procedures should be performed with the aid of videolaparoscopy, with a triple- or quadruple-puncture technique. Upon entering the peritoneum, make a systematic inspection paying particular attention to the pelvis.

The patient should be in the Trendelenburg position, the bowel being displaced in a cephalad direction. Initially, examine the organs of the pelvis at a distance: first the anterior, then the posterior cul-de-sac, followed by the uterus and the tubes and ovaries on each side. Any fluid in the posterior cul-de-sac can be sent for culture, if necessary. Look carefully for endometriosis by examining the peritoneal surfaces at close quarters, and even with direct-contact laparoscopy.

Next, the extent and type of pelvic and adnexal adhesions should be catalogued and attention turned to the ovaries. The ovaries should be examined over their entire surface and should be elevated with scrutiny of the ovarian fossa and the rest of the pelvic side wall down to the uterosacral ligaments. The oviduct should be inspected, starting proximally, looking for external adhesive disease and any evidence of a proximal fusiform swelling that would suggest the presence of salpingitis isthmica nodosa or endometriosis. The distal end should be assessed for the presence of phimosis or frank occlusion, which would indicate presence of a hydrosalpinx. The fimbria should be assessed; once inspection of both sides is completed, chromopertubation should be performed. With the passage of dye, the fimbria can be evaluated further for the presence of phimosis or fine fimbrial adhesions.

SELECTION OF TREATMENT

When infertility is the result of damaged fallopian tubes, there are two modalities of treatment available: reconstructive surgery and in vitro fertilization. These treatments should be seen as being complementary rather than competitive. The choice of treatment will be influenced by both technical and nontechnical considerations. Nontechnical considerations include the age of the woman, the costs, and the wishes of the couple. The technical considerations relate to results attained in the center in which the couple is being treated, the extent of tubal damage, and associated infertility factors.

Accurate statistics for success rates of both tubal surgery and IVF in the center in which the patient is being treated should be obtained and shared with the couple, as should rates of cumulative pregnancy, ectopic pregnancy, miscarriage, and multiple pregnancy. If local expertise seems lacking, the couple should be offered the option to travel to a center of excellence.

Laparoscopy should be undertaken by a surgeon appropriately trained in endoscopy and reconstructive tubal procedures, to allow corrective surgery to be performed at the time of initial diagnostic laparoscopy.

A number of patients will be found to have extensive inoperable tubal damage at the initial HSG, with or without tubal cannulation, such as bipolar (both proximal and distal) tubal disease, marked intratubal adhesions or large hydrosalpinges with no evidence of epithelial folds. Such patients may benefit from salpingectomy, followed by in vitro fertilization, especially in the presence of an additional factor such as advanced reproductive age or compromised sperm parameters.

In Vitro Fertilization

Voluntary reporting for 1994 of centers performing in vitro fertilization in the United States indicates that each treatment cycle initiated in patients under 40 years of age carries approximately a 20% chance of resulting in a live birth. In centers of excellence, this rate is even higher. Data from France suggests that the pregnancy rate remains relatively constant in successive in vitro fertilization cycles. If we were to assume this observation to be correct and if a program has an ongoing pregnancy rate of 25% per procedure for women under 40, then a cumulative pregnancy rate for three attempts should be approximately 57%. In addition, intracytoplasmic sperm injection (ICSI) has eliminated male factor as a negative contributor to outcome, thereby improving success rates.

Hyperstimulation is a serious and sometimes life-threatening complication of controlled ovarian stimulation. However, it is now possible to eliminate this as a risk factor in most cases by coasting patients whose estradiol levels and number of follicles indicate that they are at increased risk.

With IVF, the risk of tubal ectopic pregnancy is only 2.6% of pregnancies in patients without a tubal factor, while for patients with an identified tubal factor, the risk is approximately 12%. This raises the issue of prophylactic salpingectomy, or at least, proximal tubal interruption prior to initiation of IVF in patients with an identified hydrosalpinx.

Multiple pregnancy is approximately 33% after in vitro fertilization and embryo transfer, with 6% of pregnancies being triplet or higher gestation. The Cesarean section rate increases with the incidence of multiple pregnancies and the age of the patient population. Perinatal mortality is approximately 30 per 1,000 and remains increased, even for singleton pregnancies, at about 19 per 1,000.

Reconstructive Surgery

The overall risks of reconstructive surgery, especially when performed laparoscopically, are low; these are related to anesthesia or intraoperative accidents. If successful, tubal reconstructive surgery offers multiple cycles during which conception may be attempted and also allows for repeated pregnancies. The miscarriage rate appears to be the same after reconstructive surgery as for those in the normal population. Risk of ectopic pregnancy after tubal reconstructive surgery is significant, depending on the nature and extent of the disease process.

Nontechnical considerations, which factor age, cost, and the wishes of the couple, should all be considered. Female fecundity decreases with increasing age of the egg provider.

The initial decline is noted in the early 30s, with a more significant decline starting at approximately age 37. Reversal of sterilization in patients between 40 to 42 years of age, where the minimum tubal length after anastomosis was 4 cm and the exposure at least one year, yields a pregnancy rate of 45%. The comparable figure (in centers of excellence) for in vitro fertilization after three oocyte retrievals in women between 40 and 43 years of age is 45% (18% per procedure). Younger women with proximal tubal occlusion or hydrosalpinx may consider surgery first and in vitro fertilization thereafter, if necessary, while those between 37 and 40 should be advised to consider in vitro fertilization first. The sociological and financial implications of multiple pregnancy should be considered, along with the wishes of the couple, including their values and ethical views. The physician should provide the couple with detailed and accurate information. Furthermore, the couple should be advised against active treatment when the prognosis is poor.

Selection of Treatment

The fallopian tubes may be occluded proximally and/or distally and there may be concomitant periadnexal adhesions. Tubal occlusion may be due to a disease process or prior surgical interruption. If the only apparent lesion is periadnexal adhesions, then laparoscopic salpingoovariolysis, preferably performed at the initial laparoscopy, is the treatment of choice. This modality of treatment should yield an intrauterine pregnancy rate of 51% to 62% and ectopic pregnancy rate of 5% to 8%.

Fimbrial phimosis (agglutination of the fimbriae) often coexists with periadnexal disease and can be dealt with laparoscopically. The subsequent intrauterine pregnancy rate ranges from 40% to 48% with an ectopic pregnancy rate from 5% to 6%.

Distal tubal occlusion (hydrosalpinx) is also amenable to laparoscopic surgical correction. The live birth rate after microsurgical salpingostomy ranges from 20% to 37% and the ectopic pregnancy ranges from 5% to 18%. Factors that affect outcome of salpingostomy include the diameter of the distal tube, thickness of the wall, status of the tubal epithelium, and type and extent of adhesions, if any. In cases deemed favorable, reported live birth rates may be as high as 40% to 60% but in unfavorable cases, this rate drops to less than 20%. After assessment of the tubes and pelvis by both hysterosalpingography and laparoscopy, preferably including salpingoscopy, a decision must be made regarding primary treatment modality. Salpingectomy may be carried out during the same laparoscopy, if prior consent was obtained from the patient.

True pathological proximal tubal occlusion is probably not amenable to laparoscopic correction and requires formal microsurgical tubocornual anastomosis. Laparoscopic tubotubal anastomosis after previous tubal sterilization and segmental excision, with encouraging results, have been described recently in the literature.

The development of operative laparoscopy and in vitro fertilization in the last 20 years has changed the outlook for couples with tubal factor infertility. However, the final choice, as discussed earlier, of whether to proceed with corrective tubal surgery laparoscopically or to go directly to in vitro fertilization depends on careful evaluation of both the technical and nontechnical factors outlined, and an accurate accounting of success rates with both modalities of treatment in the center in which the patient is being treated.

Endoscopic Microsurgery

Microsurgery is much more than the use of magnification. Microsurgical principles include techniques to minimize tissue injury by delicate handling of tissues, judicious intraoperative irrigation to prevent desiccation, meticulous hemostasis and avoiding introduction of foreign bodies into the peritoneal cavity. Microsurgery demands precise alignment and opposition of tissue planes with the appropriate use of fine instruments and suture materials.

The laparoscope, especially if brought close to the area of interest, can provide magnification with direct illumination. The inherent advantage of the laparoscopic approach is that the peritoneal cavity remains closed, although distended with carbon dioxide. Because of this, and the ability to carry out intraoperative irrigation, tissue desiccation can be prevented. The absence of abrasive abdominal pads and lack of exposure of the peritoneal cavity to latex gloves and talcum powder largely prevents the introduction of foreign bodies. In addition, the pressure of approximately 12 mm Hg provided by the pneumoperitoneum decreases venous oozing and allows for spontaneous hemostasis. Instruments are being developed which allow better performance of many procedures microsurgically by laparoscopic access.

SURGICAL TECHNIQUE

Access Route

The surgical techniques of procedures described in the following section are essentially the same no matter what access route is used, be it laparotomy or laparoscopy. Distal tubal disease has been treated laparoscopically for more than 20 years and appears more amenable to the laparoscopic approach. Recently isthmic-isthmic and isthmic-ampullary anastomosis, for reversal of sterilization, have been performed by laparoscopic access. It is imperative to select the access route that will yield the best outcome for the patient. Tubal anastomosis, including tubo-cornual anastomosis, may be performed using an operating microscope through a mini-laparotomy incision. We have used a special incision for this purpose since 1986; patients return to usual activity as rapidly as those who had their operation by laparoscopic access. The deserved enthusiasm for laparoscopic surgery should not blind us to the fact that some procedures are still better performed by the traditional methods of microsurgery, using instead a mini-laparotomy incision.

Intraoperative Irrigation and Pelvic Lavage

For more than 20 years we have used an irrigating solution of lactated ringers containing 1000 to 5000 units of heparin per liter. The fluid is physiologic, prevents desiccation, and can be used to verify hemostasis. Furthermore, because it largely prevents formation of blood clots, it facilitates removal of blood and debris from the peritoneal cavity.

The surgeon also can examine the operative site under water to ensure the presence of satisfactory hemostasis. At the end of an endoscopic procedure, pneumoperitoneum pressure is reduced and the region inspected with the distal end of the laparoscope under surface of the irrigation fluid. Any bleeding vessels can be clearly visualized and desiccated.

The irrigation fluid is removed and the pelvis lavaged when the procedure is completed. Some clinicians have recommended leaving either a physiological solution or Hyskon in the pelvis to reduce post-operative adhesions. We continue to use instead 200 ml of lactated ringer solution containing 500 mg of hydrocortisone succinate.

Salpingoovariolysis

The commonest cause of pelvic adhesions is pelvic inflammatory disease. These are usually not too vascular, and, in joining one structure to another, they tend to leave a space between the involved structures, which facilitates adhesiolysis. A dense, cohesive, adhesive process may result in the conglutination of tissues and the adhesed areas may be devoid of peritoneum. Adhesiolysis in this instance is not only technically difficult, but is associated with a high incidence of recurrence.

Periadnexal disease may be the only apparent lesion, but often it coexists with varying degrees of tubal disease. Even in the presence of tubal patency, adhesions distorting the physiologic relationship of the fimbriae to the ovary or encapsulating one or both of these organs will inhibit or prevent capture of the oocyte by the tube. Whether the procedure is being performed with an open abdomen or by laparoscopy, the principles are essentially very similar. Adhesions are put on the stretch and divided one layer at a time to avoid damage to the adjacent serosa. Each layer of the adhesion is put on the stretch, and once the correct plane is identified, the adhesion is transected. Care is taken to avoid direct damage to the serosal or ovarian surface. If vessels are encountered along the incision line, they may be desiccated, using the blend setting on the electrosurgical unit. Individual bleeders may be coagulated after being ex-

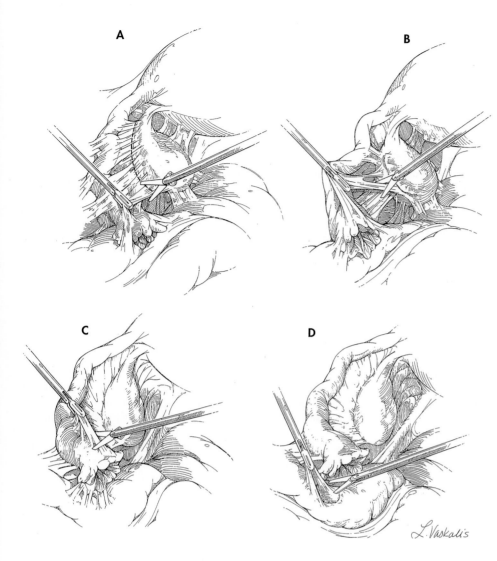

Figure 5-1.1 Salpingoovariolysis. **A.** Division of adhesions commences in a well-exposed area. **B.** Adhesions are stretched and are divided one layer at a time parallel to the organ of interest, **C.** Broad adhesions are freed at all points and removed from the peritoneal cavity. **D.** Salpingoovariolysis being completed. (Reprinted with permission from Gomel V, Taylor PJ. *Diagnostic and Operative Gynecologic Laparoscopy.* St. Louis: CV Mosby; 1995:171).

posed, by rinsing with irrigation fluid. Adhesions that are broad should be excised completely; those that are shallow may be simply transected.

During the endoscopic approach, the salpingoovariolysis is commenced, close to the tube and ovary. After putting the adhesions on the stretch, they are incised parallel to the relevant viscus, with the actual division being accomplished either electrosurgically using a microelectrode, or mechanically, with fine scissors. We prefer the latter approach. Cohesive disease is always more difficult to approach and is also fraught with the risk of inadvertent injury to one or another organ, especially the bowel. A tissue plane may be developed by entering the adhesion and spreading the jaws of the instrument, or by using hydrodissection. It is important either to avoid the use of thermal energy altogether in such instances, or to use it judiciously, because of the risks.

Adhesiolysis that is worth doing can almost always be done laparoscopically. Salpingoovariolysis, as with all fertility-promoting procedures that can be performed by lap-

aroscopic access, should be done at the time of the initial laparoscopy. This means that initial diagnostic laparoscopy should be performed after hysterosalpingography and be undertaken by a specialist able to perform the definitive treatment (Figure 5-1.1).

The Canadian Infertility Evaluation Study Group addressed the issue of treatment-dependent and treatment-independent pregnancy and showed a significant improvement, with a cumulative pregnancy rate of almost 60% after salpingoovariolysis, compared to 16% in the untreated control group. Operative laparoscopy yields the same results as those obtained by formal microsurgery. We reported a series of 92 patients who underwent salpingoovariolysis by laparoscopy; 62% achieved at least one intrauterine pregnancy and the incidence of ectopic pregnancy was 5.4%. These results have been corroborated by other centers. The reported rates of cumulative intrauterine pregnancy range from 50% to 60% with ectopic pregnancies occurring in 5% to 8% of operated cases. These results are similar to those cited in microsurgery series reports. This demonstrates that the outcome is dependent on the extent and nature of the adhesive process rather than on the mode of access.

Fimbrioplasty

Fimbrial phimosis results from the agglutination of the fimbriae. This condition often coexists with periadnexal adhesions, which are treated first. Usually there is a small distal opening which may become evident only upon distention of the tube with chromopertubation. The phimotic fimbrial end may be covered by scar tissue, which should be excised or incised to gain access to the tubal lumen. Frequently the agglutination can be corrected simply by introducing into the tube, through the small fimbrial aperture, a 3-mm forceps with the jaws closed, opening the jaws while they are within the tubal lumen, and gently withdrawing the forceps with the jaws open. This maneuver may be repeated a few times with changes in direction, in which the jaws of the forceps are open. Gentle handling of the tissues avoids undue bleeding (Figure 5-1.2).

Rarely, in the presence of fimbriae that appear normal, there may be an area of stenosis proximally, at the level of the true abdominal tubal ostium (prefimbrial phimosis). This stenosis may only become apparent upon chromopertubation. The method of treatment usually involves incision of the antimesosalpingeal border of the tube from the fimbriated end into the distal ampulla, past the area of stenosis. This is usually made electrosurgically. Alternatively, the area may be injected with a dilute solution of vasopressin and the incision made mechanically with a sharp scissors. The edges may be held back either by dessication of the serosal aspect of the flaps or everting the flaps by placing a fine suture (Figure 5-1.3).

The results of fimbrioplasty are difficult to evaluate independently, since these cases frequently have been included in the statistics of salpingostomy series. In 1983, one of us reported 40 such patients treated by laparoscopy; 48% had live births and 5% had tubal gestations. Rates of intrauterine pregnancy ranging from 26% to 61% and tubal ectopic pregnancy from 5% to 13% have been reported by other authors.

Salpingostomy (Salpingoneostomy)

Salpingostomy refers to the creation of a new stoma in a tube with complete distal occlusion (hydrosalpinx). As with most cases of tubal damage, there are usually varying degrees of pelvic and periadnexal adhesions present. This must be dealt with first and the tubo-ovarian ligament exposed to ensure that the distal end of the tube is free. If it is adherent to the ovary, the two structures must be separated. With appropriate transcervical distention, the occluded terminal end is examined, looking for the avascular areas that radiate from a central punctum. The tube usually is entered at this central point and the incision extended along an avascular line toward the ovary. This fashions a new fimbria ovarica. At this point, it becomes possible to view the tube from within and to place additional incisions between the endothelial folds along avascular areas, until a satisfactory stoma has been fashioned. Avoid cutting through vascular mucosal folds. Any bleeding points are identified under a jet of irrigating fluid and carefully dessicated. Once the stoma has been created, the flaps are everted and secured either by using fine sutures or by dessication of the serosal surface. The dessication may be performed with the CO_2 laser or electrosurgically (Figure 5-1.4).

Salpingostomy results in a birthrate ranging from 20% to 37%, with an ectopic pregnancy rate of 5% to 18%. The

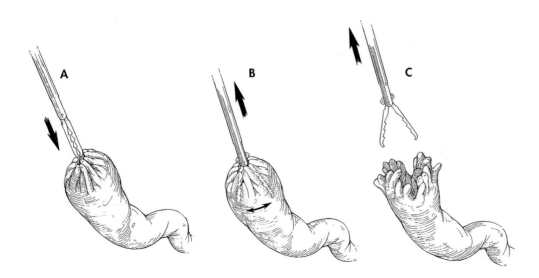

Figure 5-1.2 Fimbrioplasty; deagglutination of fimbriae. **A.** The 3-mm alligator-jawed forceps is introduced through the stenosed opening. **B.** The jaws of the forceps are opened within the tube. **C.** The forceps is gently withdrawn while the jaws are kept open. (Reprinted with permission from Gomel V, Taylor PJ. *Diagnostic and Operative Laparoscopy.* St. Louis: CV Mosby; 1995:173).

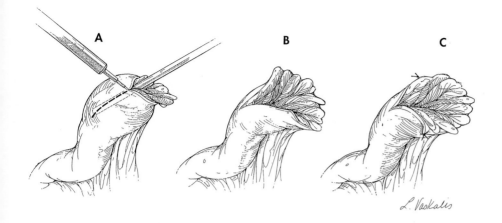

Figure 5-1.3 Fimbrioplasty: correction of prefimbrial phimosis **A.** and **B.** An incision is placed at the antimesosalpingeal border of the tube. **C.** Completed procedure with flaps everted. (Reprinted with permission from Gomel V, Taylor PJ. *Diagnostic and Operative Gynecologic Laparoscopy.* St Louis: CV Mosby; 1995:173).

major determinant of outcome is the degree of preexisting tubal damage and the extent of the periadnexal adhesive process. It appears that results achieved by laparoscopic salpingostomy are not quite as good as those achieved by the open microsurgical approach. However, there are many clear advantages to performing the salpingostomy at the time of the initial laparoscopy; these include reduced costs and avoidance of a second operative intervention.

Salpingectomy

It is unprecedented to include salpingectomy among fertility-promoting procedures. There are a number of conditions not amenable to reconstructive surgery, or where surgery is contraindicated in view of the associated poor prognosis. These include: bipolar disease, presence of extensive intratubal adhesions, and severe tubal damage (Grade V category). In such cases, IVF represents the better, if not the only, option. There is increasing evidence from the literature that patients with one or two hydrosalpinges have a lower implantation rate and a much higher incidence of tubal ectopic pregnancies when treated with IVF. Compared to tubes that are normal, where the ectopic pregnancy rate after IVF is approximately 2%, the rate may be as high as 12% to 16% where there has been at least one or more hydrosalpinges. This raises the issue of whether to perform prophylactic salpingectomy or at least proximal tubal interruption, prior to proceeding with primary or iterative in vitro fertilization attempts.

The same principles used in reconstructive tubal operations apply to salpingectomy: adhesions must be lysed and the tube must first be freed. If this is not technically possible, proximal occlusion of the tube, either with a mechanical device like a clip, or electrodessication, may be performed instead. There remains the issue of future complications associated with a retained dilated fallopian tube and the potential difficulty of access to the developing ovarian follicles for oocyte retrieval during IVF. It is preferable to remove severely damaged fallopian tubes where

possible. During the procedure care must be taken to preserve the blood supply of the ovary.

The technique we employ aims first to interrupt the two major blood supplies to the tube derived from the uterine and ovarian vessels. The proximal oviduct is desiccated at the uterotubal junction, using a unipolar or bipolar forceps. Scissors are used to divide the dessicated segment of tube. The fimbriated end of the tube is then elevated and the exposed tuboovarian ligament is then similarly dessicated and divided. Thereafter, the mesosalpinx is divided progressively, achieving dessication as necessary along the incision line. It is mandatory to dessicate the vessels that usually reach the tube at the level of the ampullary-isthmic junction. The mesosalpinx is checked then for hemostasis and the excised fallopian tube is removed through a large cannula and sent for pathological analysis. Although the procedure may be performed with the use of Endoloops or sutures, we prefer the described method because of its simplicity.

Tubotubal Anastomosis

Gynecologic microsurgery finds its ultimate application in tubotubal anastomosis, no matter where it is located and whether it is performed for occlusive disease or for reversal of a prior tubal sterilization. Tubotubal anastomosis for sterilization reversal has been performed by laparoscopic access.

The surgical technique of tubotubal anastomosis is not dissimilar to that performed by open procedure using an operating microscope. If adhesions are present, a salpingoovariolysis is performed first. The mesosalpinx under the site of anastomosis may be injected with one to two ml of dilute vasopressin solution, to reduce oozing and facilitate hemostasis. The proximal segment is distended by transcervical chromopertubation, which helps to identify the tip of occluded proximal tubal segment. The tube is then transected near the occluded end, using sharp, straight, laparoscopic scissors or a sharp micro blade. During this pro-

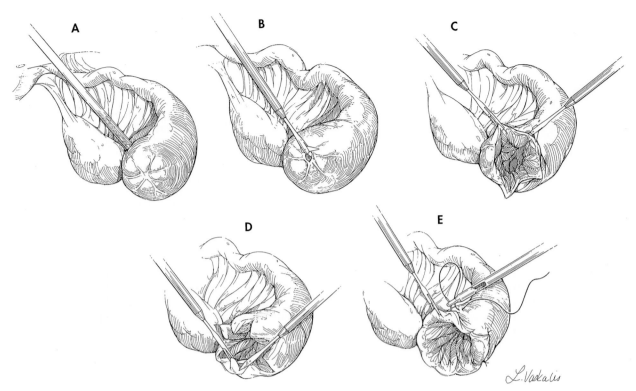

Figure 5-1.4 Salpingostomy. **A.** The occluded distal end of the tube usually has a centrally placed avascular area from which avascular scarred lines extend in a cartwheel manner. **B.** the first incision is made along an avascular line toward the ovary. **C.** Avascular lines are incised by viewing from within the tube along the circumference of the initial opening. **D.** Cutting along the avascular lines is continued until a satisfactory stoma is fashioned. **E.** The flaps can be everted by placing two or three No. 6-0 absorbable synthetic sutures. (Reprinted with permission from Gomel V, Taylor PJ. *Diagnostic and Operative Gynecologic Laparoscopy.* St. Louis: CV Mosby; 1995:174).

cess, it is essential to avoid damage to the vascular arcade in the mesosalpinx. The transected occluded end is excised from the mesosalpinx electrosurgically, using a micro-electrode. The cut surface of the tube is examined closely for normalcy and hemostasis is obtained by electrodes-sication of the more prominent bleeders and by using the microelectrode. Concurrent irrigation facilitates identifi-cation of the bleeders. Do not overuse electrodesiccation.

The distal segment is prepared similarly unless there is significant disparity in the lumina of the two segments. The distal segment may be distended by distal hydrotubation, by injecting irrigation fluid through the fimbriated end. This aids in identifying the occluded extremity of the distal stump. An opening is fashioned into the tube that is more or less equal in diameter to the proximal lumen. The tubal segments are approximated in two layers. The first joins the epithelium and the muscularis; the second, the serosa. The initial suture should be placed at the 6 o'clock position at the mesosalpingeal border. If there is undue tension in the apposition of the two segments, the mesosalpinx adjacent to the cut ends may be approximated first with a single interrupted suture. Once the 6 o'clock suture has been tied,

three or more additional sutures are placed. These can be placed using a single strand of suture and tied as multiple interrupted sutures, after dividing the loop that joins two subsequent sutures. We do not advise the use of a splint because of the risk of trauma to the endothelium and be-cause it hinders, rather then helps, the procedure. The stain-ing of the transected tubal surface with methylene blue or indigo carmine solution facilitates identification of the an-atomic layers and may be useful to the novice.

After approximation of the inner layer, chromopertuba-tion is performed to demonstrate patency as well as to es-tablish a satisfactory seal at the anastomatic site. The serosa and mesosalpinx are joined next, with interrupted sutures or two continuous sutures one apposing the anterior and the other the posterior aspect of the tube.

CONCLUSION

In spite of the tremendous progress being made in IVF/ ART, there is still a place for reconstructive tubal surgery. Laparoscopy permits the evaluation of the fallopian tubes and provides the surgical access for salpingoscopy and for reconstructive procedures, which ideally should be performed during the same setting. In more complex circumstances, one may still resort to a microsurgical procedure via a mini laparotomy.

The selection of treatment modality should be based on proper investigation, counseling of the couple, and honest disclosure with respect to the expertise and results achieved by the center in which the couple is to be treated. The wishes of the couple should also be taken into account and they should be offered access to centers of excellence, be they for surgery or ART.

SUGGESTED READING

Boer-Meisel ME, teVelde ER, Habbema JDF, et al. Predicting the pregnancy outcome in patients treated for hydrosalpinx: a prospective study. *Fertil Steril* 1986;45:23.

Bruhat MA, Mage G, Manhes H, et al. Laparoscopy procedures to promote fertility ovariolysis and salpingolysis: results of 93 selected cases. *Acta Eur Fertil* 1983;14:113.

Canis M, Mage G, Pouly JL, et al. Laparoscopic distal tuboplasty: report of 87 cases and a 4-year experience. *Fertil Steril* 1991;56:616.

Dubuisson JB, Chapron C, Morice P, et al. Laparoscopic salpingostomy: fertility results according to the tubal mucosal appearance. *Hum Reprod* 1994;9:334.

Gomel V. An odyssey through the oviduct. *Fertil Steril* 1983;39:144.

Gomel V. From microscopic surgery to laparoscopic surgery: a progress. *Fertil Steril* 1995;63:464.

Gomel V. Laparoscopic tubal surgery in infertility. *Obstet Gynecol* 1975;46:47.

Gomel V. *Microsurgery in female infertility.* Boston: Little, Brown; 1983.

Gomel V. Microsurgical reversal of sterilization: a reappraisal. *Fertil Steril* 1980;33:587.

Gomel V. Operative laparoscopy: time for acceptance. *Fertil Steril* 1989; 52:1.

Gomel V. Reconstructive surgery of the oviduct. *J Reprod Med* 1977; 18:181.

Gomel V. Salpingo-ovariolysis by laparoscopy in infertility. *Fertil Steril* 1983;34:607.

Gomel V. Salpingostomy by laparoscopy. *J Reprod Med* 1977;18:265.

Gomel V. Salpingostomy by microsurgery. *Fertil Steril* 1978;29:380.

Gomel V. Tubal anastomosis by microsurgery. *Fertil Steril* 1977;28:59.

Gomel V, Rowe TC. Microsurgical tubal reconstruction and reversal of sterilization. In: Wallach EE, Zacur HA, eds. *Reproductive medicine and surgery.* St. Louis: CV Mosby, 1995:1074.

Gomel V, Taylor PJ. In vitro fertilization versus reconstructive tubal surgery. *J Assist Reprod Genet* 1992;9:306.

Gomel V, Taylor PJ. *Diagnostic and operative gynecologic laparoscopy.* St. Louis: CV Mosby, 1995.

Kerin JF. Nonhysteroscopic falloposcopy: a proposed method for visual guidance and verification of tubal cannula placement for endotuboplasty, gamete and embryo transfer procedure. *Fertil Steril* 1992; 57:1133.

Marana R, Muscatello P, Muzii L, et al. Perlaparoscopic salpingoscopy in the evaluation of the tubal factor in infertile women. *Int J Fertil* 1990;35:211.

Munro MG, Gomel V. Fertility-promoting laparoscopically-directed procedures. *Reprod Med Rev* 1994;3:29.

Musset R. *An atlas of hysterosalpingography.* Quebec: Les Presses de l'Universite Laval, 1979.

Reich H, McGlynn F, Parents C, et al. Laparoscopic Tubal anastomosis. *J Am Assoc Gynecologic Laparoscopists* 1993;1:16.

Rowe TC, Gomel V, McComb P. Investigations of tuboperitoneal causes of female infertility. In: Insler V, Lunenfeld B, eds. *Infertility, male and female.* Edinburgh: Churchill Livingstone, 1993:253.

Sart T. Assisted reproductive technology in the United States and Canada: 1994 results generated from the American Society for Reproductive Medicine/Society for Assisted Reproductive Technology Registry. *Fertil Steril* 1996;66:697–705.

Sedbon E, Bouquet de la Joliniere J, Boudouris O, et al. Tubal desterilization through exclusive laparoscopy. *Hum Reprod* 1989;4:158.

Tan SL, Royston P, Campbell S, et al. Cumulative conception and live birth rates after in-vitro fertilization. *Lancet* 1992;339:1390.

Thurmond AS. Selective salpingography and fallopian tube recanalization. *AJR Am J Roentgenol* 1991;156:33.

Trimbos-Kemper TCM. Reversal of sterilization of women over 40 years of age: a multicenter survey in the Netherlands. *Fertil Steril* 1990; 53:575.

Tulandi T, Collins JA, Burrows E, et al. Treatment-dependent and treatment-independent pregnancy among women with periadnexal adhesions. *Am J Obste Gynecol* 1990;162:354.

Urman B, Gomel V, McComb P, et al. Midtubal occlusion: etiology, management, and outcome. *Fertil Steril* 1992;59:747.

Urman B, Zouves C, Gomel V. Fertility outcome following tubal pregnancy. *Acta Eur Fertil* 1991;22:205.

Yoon TK, Sung HR, Cha SH, Lee CN, and Lee KY. Fertility outcome after microsurgical tubal anastomosis. *Fertil Steril* 1997;67:18–22.

Zouves C, Erenus M, Gomel V. Tubal ectopic pregnancy after in vitro fertilization and embryo transfer: a role for proximal occlusion or salpingectomy after failed distal tubal surgery? *Fertil Steril* 1991;56:691.

Zouves C, Gomel V. Gamete intrafallopian transfer (GIFT): procedure-dependent and procedure-independent pregnancy. *Infertility* 1990; 13:163.

Operative Laparoscopy, Second Edition
The Masters' Techniques in Gynecologic Surgery
Lippincott–Raven Publishers, Philadelphia © 1998.

5-2   Ectopic Pregnancy: Linear Salpingostomy

Michael P. Diamond and Kenneth A. Ginsburg

The options for clinical management of tubal ectopic pregnancies have greatly expanded over the past decade. In a woman with an ectopic pregnancy who wishes to conceive in the future, the standard surgical options of salpingectomy or salpingo-oophorectomy are often replaced by salpingostomy. Furthermore, these procedures are now frequently performed at laparoscopy as opposed to laparotomy, thereby reducing the morbidity and expense associated with these procedures. The ability to perform a linear salpingostomy requires timely diagnosis of the eccyesis using serial β-subunit determinations of human chorionic gonadotropin (hCG) in combination with pelvic ultrasound scanning. Ultrasound scanning is optionally performed by the transvaginal route, at times additionally employing Doppler to assess placental/adnexal flow. These newer ultrasound modalities have increased the ability to identify an intrauterine pregnancy and adnexal masses that may represent the ectopic gestation earlier and with confidence. A full description of techniques of β-subunit monitoring and ultrasound for diagnosis of ectopic pregnancies is beyond the scope of this chapter, and specific guidelines are difficult to offer because management is highly dependent on the complete clinical presentation of the patient, and on the sensitivity, specificity, and accuracy of βhCG titers and ultrasound scans in your own institution. At our hospital, we recommend βhCG testing beginning with a missed menses in the patient at high risk for ectopic pregnancy. Titers are then repeated at approximately 2- to 4-day intervals. Vaginal ultrasound can identify intrauterine sacs with βhCG titers as low as 1200 to 1500 mIU/mL in some patients; most patients should have sacs visible by transvaginal ultrasound when the βhCG titer is $\geq$ 3000 mIU/L. For abdominal scanning, intrauterine sacs should be identified once the titer has reached a βhCG of 6500 mIU/mL. In these cases, the absence of a visible intrauterine gestational sac when βhCG titers are above these discriminating levels is highly suggestive of an extrauterine gestation. For additional reading on these diagnostic techniques, the reader is referred to two recent publications. (Diamond, et al. and Meyer, et al.)

The technique of linear salpingostomy for the treatment of ectopic pregnancy can be performed either at laparotomy or laparoscopy. In this chapter, while the laparoscopic technique will be described, these principles can be applied to performance of the procedure at laparotomy as well. The performance of laparoscopy for a definitive diagnosis of

ectopic pregnancy is based on clinical history, physical exam, and laboratory and diagnostic imaging findings. Timing of diagnostic laparoscopy is important since there are potential perils if one waits too long to make this diagnosis, or if one attempts to make this diagnosis too early in pregnancy. Prolonged observation has resulted in rupture of a pregnancy, with hemorrhage and death. However, when diagnostic laparoscopy is performed too early, it may be difficult or impossible to identify the eccyesis. Figuratively, the physician is between a "rock and a hard place." The decision to perform laparoscopy is dictated, in part, by the experience of the endoscopist and the availability of appropriate equipment and personnel. For example, for all but the most experienced endoscopist, a hemodynamically unstable patient with a ruptured ectopic pregnancy is best treated by a laparotomy.

For the hemodynamically stable patient suspected of having an ectopic pregnancy, diagnostic laparoscopy is performed to confirm the diagnosis; operative laparoscopic intervention for surgical treatment is often appropriate. For diagnostic laparoscopy, the bladder is drained and an umbilical incision for placement of the laparoscope is used, with a suprapubic second puncture site for introduction of a probe to manipulate the pelvic organs. The second puncture site is placed two to three finger widths above the symphysis pubis in the midline, and the trocar advanced under direct vision through the anterior peritoneum at a site noted to be free of adhesions. The incision is placed in such a position that, if a laparotomy is indicated, it can be made through this suprapubic incision. The second puncture site must be placed cephalad enough to allow manipulation of an instrument behind the uterus.

Upon introduction of the laparoscope, the status of the bladder and other viscera are ascertained. This is of particular importance in a patient who has had a prior laparotomy, during which the bladder may have been advanced along the anterior abdominal wall or when intrapelvic adhesions, which predispose to ectopic pregnancy, would distort the anatomy or limit bowel mobility.

The entire pelvis is then examined carefully to assess both the fallopian tubes and other pelvic structures. Standard criteria for laparoscopic linear salpingostomy to treat ectopic pregnancy include: (1) eccyesis in the ampullary segment of the fallopian tube, (2) the tube is no more than 3 cm in greatest diameter, and (3) the tube is freely mobile or can be easily mobilized in the hemodynamically stable patient. These recommendations may be modified based on the clinical situation and the experience of the endoscopic surgeon.

While ampullary ectopic pregnancies are usually treated by linear salpingostomy, some debate exists about whether isthmic ectopic pregnancies should be treated in this fashion. While postoperatively ampullary ectopic pregnancies are rarely complicated by either fistula formation or tubal obstruction, these complications have been reported commonly when isthmic ectopic pregnancies are treated by linear salpingostomy. Therefore, some advocate segmental resection for isthmic ectopics. After segmental resection, however, the potential exists for developing a repeat ectopic pregnancy in the distal segment of the residual tube. In some situations, primary resection and anastomosis have been advocated; however, the potential for a successful anastomosis at this time is reduced because of the edema and increased vascularity, along with the presence of operating room personnel who may be inexperienced in microsurgical techniques if it must be done as an emergency procedure in the nights or on weekends. Thus, if linear salpingostomy is performed on an isthmic ectopic pregnancy and a fistula or obstruction does not form, the patient can continue to try to conceive, eliminating a second operative procedure. If fistula formation or an obstruction does occur after linear salpingostomy, then resection and anastomosis can be performed at a later time. To summarize, with both ampullary and isthmic ectopics—when a linear salpingostomy is possible, the patient has little to lose by the attempt, despite the greater likelihood that an additional operative procedure may be needed to correct the fistula or obstruction that results from an isthmic salpingostomy.

On occasion, linear salpingostomy has been completed using only a two-puncture technique. Frequently, however, we require two or sometimes three assessory punctures. Some surgeons will routinely place two lower punctures, one each to the left and right of the midline; however, as noted, we usually place a second puncture in the midline and a third one to the side of the ectopic gestation. With this third puncture, the tube is grasped with a self-retaining atraumatic grasper distal to the site of the planned salpingostomy incision. This places the tube on stretch so that it can be manipulated with ease during the operative procedure. A dilute vasopressin solution (1 ampule of 20 units in 100 mL normal saline) is injected into the antimesenteric border of the tube overlying the ectopic gestation. This is done by placing a spinal needle through the anterior abdominal wall, aimed directly at the ectopic pregnancy. Place the spinal needle after palpating the anterior abdominal wall, while viewing through the laparoscope for proper location near the fallopian tube. If a large pneumoperitoneum is present, reaching the ectopic gestation with a thin needle may sometimes be difficult; release of some of the distending gas is helpful. Some surgeons also inject the mesosalpinx or cauterize vessels within the mesosalpinx. An alterna-

tive to the use of a spinal needle is a laparoscopic instrument with a fine needle for injection.

After the injection of vasopressin, an incision is made along the antimesenteric border of the ectopic (Figure 5-2.1). This is performed either with the CO_2 laser, the argon laser, electrosurgery, sharp knife, or scissors. The choice depends on instrument availability, along with physician preference and experience. We are unaware of any benefit of one incision modality over the other. Carry the incision down deep enough to expose the clot surrounding the ectopic gestation, covering approximately two-thirds of the length of the ectopic gestation. At this point, the ectopic gestation and the surrounding clot often extrude from the incision. When this happens, grasp the tissue and remove it through one of the second puncture probes. If this does not occur, an atraumatic grasping instrument can be placed into the incision that has been created and the tissue gently removed, or an irrigator can be placed into the incision. Irrigation, under pressure, may dislodge the eccyesis (Figure 5-2.2). Alternately, pressure applied to the outside of the tube often will dislodge the products of conception and clot. Remove all tissue that comes out of the incision from the patient's pelvis; there are multiple reports in the literature of trophoblastic tissue re-implanting on normal peritoneum elsewhere in the pelvis.

Attempt to remove all tissue that comes away easily. Judge this by gently grasping tissue that remains at the base and irrigate within the salpingostomy incision. Any tissue that is grasped but does not come easily is left behind. Be-

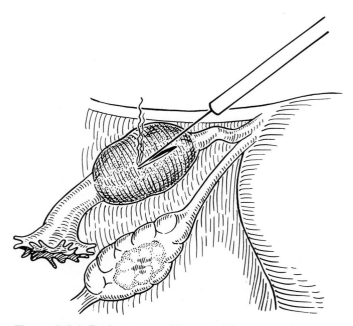

Figure 5-2.1 Performance of linear salpingostomy in an ampullary ectopic pregnancy. Procedure being performed with the use of CO_2 laser beam on a tube where the site is easily accessible. (Reprinted with permission from *Clinical Obstetrics and Gynecology* 1987;30:206, JB Lippincott.)

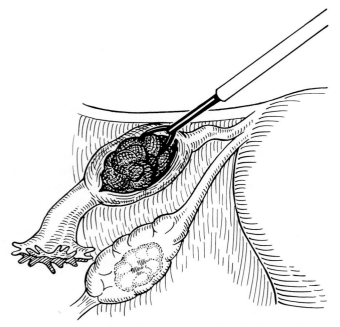

Figure 5-2.2 Products of conception being removed with the use of grasping forceps from the mesosalpinx after creation of the linear salpingostomy. (Reprinted with permission from *Clinical Obstetrics and Gynecology* 1987;30:206, JB Lippincott.)

cause of the risk of a persistent ectopic pregnancy, grasp the tube gently both proximally and distally to the site of the incision and gently palpitate to search for remaining placental tissue. If found, grasp the tissue from the existing incision or extend the incision so as to allow easy removal of any remaining trophoblastic tissue.

At completion, the site of the salpingostomy is copiously irrigated to ensure hemostasis. If oozing is noted and bleeding points inside the tube can be identified, these can be coagulated using precise bipolar instrumentation. Oozing from the incision often comes from the proximal or distal angle of the incision, and these sites can be point-coagulated. If extensive bleeding occurs, the area can be extensively coagulated in a fashion similar to what would be done for a tubal ligation and, in extreme cases, partial salpingectomy may be indicated. This can be performed using either laser, electrocoagulation, Endoloops, linear cutter or endoscopic staples. By definition, the salpingostomy incision is not sutured closed, but rather left to heal by secondary intention. (Figure 5-2.3). Salpingostomy, in which the incision is sutured closed, has been associated with higher rates of postoperative adhesion formation and/or obstruction. At the completion of the procedure, the entire pelvis should be irrigated and hemostasis confirmed. It is helpful at this point to deflate the pneumoperation slightly, thereby demonstrating any irregular bleeding that requires attention. We have not routinely utilized anti-adhesion intraperitoneal adjutants in these patients. Skin closure and recovery room

care of these patients are no different from that of other patients undergoing intra-abdominal surgery.

All patients treated in this conservative fashion must be followed postoperatively by serial β-subunit titers since persistent ectopic pregnancy has been described after salpingostomy. While observation must always be individualized based on the complete clinical picture, this is usually performed at weekly intervals until the β-subunit level falls below the sensitivity of the assay. In general, as long as the titer continues to fall, and the patient's clinical condition permits, the titer is followed without intervention even if the rate of fall is slow. While uncommon, it may take two to three months for the β-subunit titer to fall to negativity. If clinically warranted, further evaluation of the subjects with ultrasound or other modalities is sometimes needed. In a recent report, eleven (11) persistent ectopic pregnancies were identified after salpingostomy because of patient symptoms or rising titers. (Seifer, et al.) Ten of these were treated by repeat operative procedures, while one was treated by methotrexate. In this same report, it was demonstrated that, in approximately 25% of persistent ectopic pregnancies, the trophoblastic tissue was not discovered in the pathology specimens—a rate equal to those patients whose ectopics were treated successfully by conservative laparoscopic procedures.

Linear salpingostomy is followed by achievement of pregnancy in approximately 40% of subjects. This frequency is the same as in patients treated by salpingectomy. Of equal importance, the rate of recurrent ectopic pregnancy is not increased by performance of linear salpingostomy. In patients who do have recurrent ectopic pregnancies, the likelihood of development in the ipsilateral and contralateral fallopian tubes is equally divided.

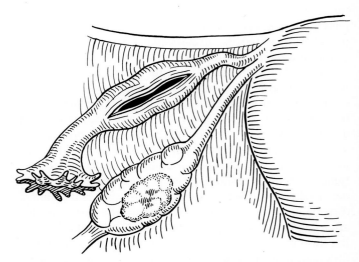

Figure 5-2.3 Appearance of the tube after completion of removal of the products of conception. The incision is allowed to heal without primary closure. (Reprinted with permission from *Clinical Obstetrics and Gynecology* 1987;30:206, JB Lippincott.)

Recently, several centers have advocated treatment of ectopic pregnancies by chemotherapy—some without a laparoscopic diagnosis of an ectopic gestation. Some of these centers are evaluating observant time and expectant management of ectopic gestations. The appropriate role of chemotherapy and expected management as opposed to surgical management of ectopic pregnancy is now being reevaluated, and attempts are underway to define which patients are best served by various treatment alternatives. These studies may be particularly relevant if we can diagnose ectopic gestations with certainty without performing a diagnostic operative procedure.

While there are obvious advantages to performing linear salpingostomy by laparoscopy (cost, decreased morbidity, etc.), at times this will not be possible and laparoscopic salpingostomy or laparotomy will be warranted. While it is reasonable to attempt laparoscopic salpingostomy, prolonged operating time can be harmful. If it appears that the procedure will be protracted by the laparoscopic approach, convert the procedure to another technique or method. The specific circumstances under which surgeons should change their goal from laparoscopic linear salpingostomy to salpingectomy or laparotomy will be highly dependent on the clinical situation, and will need to be individualized in every case.

SUGGESTED READING

Diamond MP, Lavy G, DeCherney AH. Diagnosis and management of ectopic pregnancy. In: Seibel M, ed. *Infertility: A Comprehensive Text.* East Norwalk, CT: Appleton-Century-Crofts; 1989:447–55.

DeCherney AH, Diamond MP. Laparoscopic salpingostomy for ectopic pregnancy. *Obstet Gynecol* 1987;70:948–50.

Meyer WR, DeCherney AH, Diamond MP. Tubal ectopic pregnancy: contemporary diagnosis and reproductive potential. *J Gynecol Surg* 1989;5:343–52.

Seifer DB, Gutmann JN, Doyle MB, Jones EE, Diamond MP, DeCherney AH. Persistent ectopic pregnancy following laparoscopic linear salpingostomy. *Obstet Gynecol* 1990;76:1121–5.

Operative Laparoscopy, Second Edition
The Masters' Techniques in Gynecologic Surgery
Lippincott–Raven Publishers, Philadelphia © 1998.

5-3   Endometriosis

Dan C. Martin

The method of treatment of endometriosis is determined by the goals of treatment. Endometriosis may be diagnosed as a probable cause of or associated with pain, tenderness, infertility, pelvic nodularity, ovarian cysts, or other pelvic mass. Endometriosis may be a coincidental finding at the time of sterilization, appendectomy, cholecystectomy, or other abdominal endoscopy that includes an examination of the pelvis and abdomen.

When the indication for surgery is pain, tenderness, or mass, complete resection is frequently needed for histologic confirmation or for complete destruction of the lesions. However, when endometriosis is associated with infertility, surgery to remove endometriosis may cause adhesions. Extended surgery, tissue manipulation, and suturing may interfere with fertility more than the endometriosis itself. In addition, the exact role and relationship of infertility to endometriosis therapy is poorly defined. Many studies in the past have relied on the endstage appearance of superficial puckered black lesions, which are the most endocrinologically inactive. Conclusions regarding the treatment of puckered black lesions may not be the same as conclusions regarding the treatment of superficial red or blistered lesions.

Of the available equipment there is no one unit that will be optimally effective in all circumstances. Combining various equipment components appears to offer a better approach than trying to concentrate on any one. Coagulation (desiccation), vaporization and/or excision (Figure 5-3.1) of endometriosis has been performed with combinations of scissors, bipolar coagulators, thermal coagulators, unipolar electrosurgical knives, lasers, loops, sutures, and clips.

In addition to the goals of surgery, the number of previous surgeries also influences the approach. Although superficial coagulation of endometriosis appears to be a useful and beneficial approach at the time of first laparoscopy, vaporization or excisional techniques may be more reasonable at second and later surgeries. In addition, persistent pain following laparoscopic treatment can be associated with deep bowel or retroperitoneal involvement that is not noted at laparoscopy.

RECOGNITION AND CONFIRMATION

One of the most difficult areas of education has been in relearning how to recognize endometriosis. Like many other surgeons, I was trained to look for puckered black or dark lesions. However, experience and the literature showed that superficial darker lesions are older and less metabolically active. My experience and publications on this are based on using excisional techniques at second-look laparoscopy, looking for changes related to previous laser surgery. This study showed that carbon was associated with the development of foreign body giant cell reaction in a fashion similar to suture. There were no premalignant or other transformations noted. However, many areas that did not appear to be endometriosis were shown to be endometriosis by the pathologist. Due to this, excisional techniques were used on all lesions of any description and published in a series of articles, with the conclusion that any appearance can be endometriosis but there was no appearance that was always endometriosis. Furthermore, subtle, white and ''atypical'' lesions have been endometriosis, endosalpingiosis, calcification, or cancer.

When I began these studies in 1982, I had only a concept of typical lesions. As a concept of subtle lesions developed, the percent of patients with endometriosis rose from 47% in 1986 to 71% in 1988. More recently, endometriosis has been reported in 72% of all patients and 83% when patients had negative *Chlamydia* titers. At present, lesions that were considered to be subtle in 1986 are the most common, as demonstrated in Table 5-3.1.

In addition, the percent of patients with specimens sent and with specimens confirmed increased, as shown in Table 5-3.2. Since that time, the percent of patients and specimens confirmed has remained at 97% to 99%. Perhaps more important is that when the confirmation of 55 physicians was examined, 31% of patients had endometriosis found by pathologists that had not been noted on the operative note or discharge summaries. This study showed that 14% to 59% of patients presented with appearances that were not documented as endometriosis at the time of surgery.

INFERTILITY

The most common approach at the first laparoscopy is removal or coagulation in areas where this can be performed with controlled trauma to adjacent tissue and in areas away from vital organs. Coagulators include bipolar, thermal, and laser, while vaporization can be performed with high power density laser or electrosurgery. Excision utilizes various combinations of scissors, coagulators, loops, clips, and lasers. The equipment used is generally

Surgical Technique

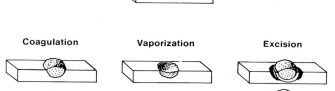

Figure 5-3.1 Surgical techniques include coagulation, vaporization, and excision. Coagulation leaves the lesion intact. Vaporization turns the lesion into a vapor or cloud of smoke. Excision produces a specimen for histologic confirmation. (Modified from Martin DC. *Intra-Abdominal Laser Surgery.* Resurge Press, 1986. Used with permission.)

Table 5-3.1 *Endometriosis and forms of endometriosis as a percent of all laparoscopies*

Year	1986	1987	1988
Endometriosis	47%	63%	71%
"Typical"	43%	53%	60%
"Subtle"	15%	58%	65%

Note: "Typical" are those lesions I used for diagnosis of endometriosis prior to 1986. "Subtle" were those not felt to be endometriosis prior to 1986.
Source: Martin DC, Hubert GD, Vander Zwaag R, et al. Laparoscopic appearances of peritoneal endometriosis. *Fertility and Sterility* 1989;51:63–7, American Fertility Society.

determined by the equipment available and by past surgical experience. Although there may be specific equipment that is most useful in certain situations, there is no one instrument that provides all that is needed in patient care.

When these techniques have been used in patients with infertility, the success rates for laparoscopic techniques have been equal to or greater than those of laparotomy techniques. Furthermore, when these techniques are used, the success rates have been independent of stage and more dependent upon other factors such as years of infertility and coexistent male factor.

However, long cases are associated with more tissue distortion. This tissue distortion can create an appearance similar to endometriosis, and it can hide endometriosis. Furthermore, extensive procedures increase tissue trauma and ischemia, and may predispose toward pelvic adhesions. This increase in adhesions following tissue manipulation has been observed clinically in situations where a first laparoscopy was used to correct endometriosis and a second was used to correct the adhesions. New adhesions are uncommon following laparoscopy, but have been reported in 10% to 25% of cases. Adhesions are more common following laparotomy.

PAIN AND TENDERNESS

In the treatment of pain and tenderness, techniques are more definitive than those used for infertility. Pelvic nodules associated with focal tenderness do not commonly respond to superficial coagulation and require deep vaporization or excision. Coagulation has been so unreliable for these lesions that it has been abandoned; either deep vaporization or excision is used. If deep vaporization is used, the technique requires that vaporization be carried down to healthy tissue. Healthy tissue can be recognized by the ap-

pearance of loose connective tissue, fat, or a water-containing layer. Fibrotic, infiltrating endometriosis has a whitish, scarred, appearance that is relatively dry except for occasional loculated areas of brown or clear fluid. Although vaporization may be adequate for these lesions, excision creates less smoke, speeds up the operation, and produces a tissue specimen for confirmation. Confirmation can be helpful, as lesions that were clinically thought to be endometriosis have been other pathology, including ectopic pregnancies, psammoma bodies associated with positive *Chlamydia* titers, splenosis, reaction to oil-based hysterosalpingogram dye, carbon from previous laser surgery, old suture material, and cancer.

The degree of resection at the first operation will depend upon informed consent after discussion with the patient. Certain patients will want as much done through the laparoscope as can be done but with the intent of avoiding laparotomy. Others will want all tissue cared for at the first operation, even if this means laparotomy. In the first group of patients, the plan is to remove as much endometriosis as reasonable through the laparoscope and then stop. This is followed by observation or postoperative medical suppression. If there is adequate pain relief, further surgery is avoided or delayed. If this does not produce adequate pain relief, longterm medical suppression and/or further surgery is used. This technique is particularly advantageous when endometriosis is around the ureter, bowel, or major blood vessels. For the second group of patients, bowel preparation and permission for elective laparotomy are completed routinely. In addition, self-blood banking is considered.

Table 5-3.2 *Changes in tissue sampling and confirmations*

Year	1982	1984	1986
Patients	97	91	119
Specimens	13	65	119
Specimens positive	8	59	116
Percentage of specimens positive	62%	91%	97%
Percentage of patients confirmed	8%	65%	97%

Source: Martin DC and Vander Zwaag R. Excisional techniques for endometriosis with the CO_2 laser laparoscope. *Journal of Reproductive Medicine* 1987;32:753–8, Journal of Reproductive Medicine Inc.

Publications suggest that the first approach may be the most useful in younger patients in whom recurrence is likely. The second approach would be more useful in older patients with more deeply infiltrating lesions, who do not have as much evidence of active formation.

Laparotomy in patients with persistent pelvic pain can reveal bowel lesions not seen at laparoscopy. I have cared for patients with as many as 20 small nodules and 6 large nodules that had been missed at laparoscopy. The patient with the 6 large nodules had had three previous laparoscopies that had not noted the infiltrating sigmoid colon lesions. In addition, my first three patients with endometriosis of the sigmoid mesentery had this level of involvement missed at laparoscopy.

SPECIFIC TECHNIQUES

Frequently, coagulation is all that is needed on peritoneal lesions with infiltration up to 2 mm. Bipolar and thermal coagulators can coagulate any lesion that can be held between the jaws. With large lesions, remember that the thermal coagulator is active only on one side of the jaw. It may be useful to turn the thermal jaws over for such lesions. Coagulation with lasers is a combination of the effects of penetration of the laser light, conversion of this light into thermal energy, and secondary thermal conduction. Although the argon laser penetrates to 0.3 to 0.8 mm, the heat coagulates tissue to about 2 mm. YAG fibers can penetrate as deep as 4 mm.

With deeper and larger lesions, vaporization or excision becomes increasingly important. Either technique is taken to the level of healthy tissue. Excision produces tissue margins that are easier to identify than those produced by vaporization. Excision generally starts by cutting through the healthy margins and then extending the incision beneath the lesion. Lasers, electrosurgery, and scissors are used for the excision. Bipolar and thermal coagulators as well as clips and loops can be used for hemostasis, when bleeding occurs during the course of the incision. A deeper incision has been taken into the vagina to remove full-thickness penetration in this area.

Lesions infiltrating deeper than 5 mm in the mid cul-de-sac and in the anterior peritoneum have an increased chance of being into the bowel or bladder muscularis. Although the author and others have performed full-thickness excision of bowel endometriomas at laparoscopy, this is still an approach that requires close coordination and planning. This may require consultation with a general surgeon and/or the operating room committee.

Tissue specimens less than 10 mm in size are removed through the trocar sheath. Larger specimens are cut into strips or morcellated, then removed by minilaparotomy or colpotomy. Tissue removal bags may limit fragmentation and seeding into the incision. Medical equipment companies are now producing lines of trocars from 15 to 30 mm in size that will increase the size of the specimen that can be removed by dilating and expanding the trocar site.

A previous study has documented that 94% of the lesions of 4 to 9 mm, but only 22% of the lesions that were 10 mm or greater, were removed at laparoscopy. The majority of those lesions that were 10 or more mm in depth required full-thickness resection of the muscularis of the bowel. In addition, an attempt to partially resect deep bowel lesions resulted in inadequate pain relief in all five of the patients in whom this was attempted. Although full-thickness resection is being used at laparoscopy in select circumstances by a small group of surgeons, laparotomy and bowel resection are commonly used in my patients.

Ovarian Lesions

Endometriosis on the ovary is treated according to size in a fashion similar to peritoneal lesions. Biopsies are taken of small lesions, and then the base is coagulated or vaporized (Figure 5-3.2). Healthy ovarian tissue has a whitish appearance, and vaporization is taken approximately 2 mm past this appearance to ensure that deep irregular infiltration is not present. This technique is used on lesions of up to 10 mm in size on the ovary. However, large ovarian endometriomas are easier to strip.

The stripping technique uses an incision followed by drainage and irrigation of the internal cavity (Figure 5-3.3). The edge of the endometrioma is then grasped. A relaxing incision is used when needed to facilitate grasping. The stripping techniques have been described by Semm. If the

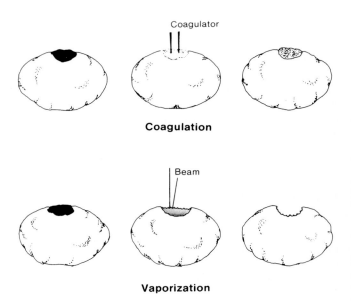

Coagulation

Vaporization

Figure 5-3.2 Although bipolar coagulation is useful for surface lesions of endometriosis, deeper lesions require vaporization. (Reprinted with permission from Martin DC. *Intra-Abdominal Surgery*. Resurge Press, 1986.)

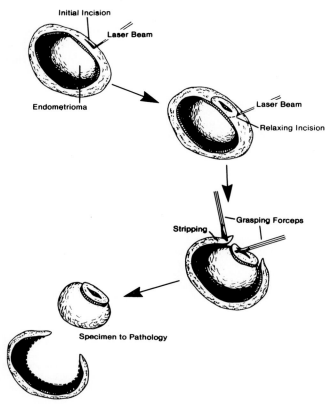

Figure 5-3.3 An ovarian endometrioma is resected by techniques patterned after those of Semm (1987). The cyst is drained, and this is followed by a relaxing incision into healthy ovary. The purpose of the relaxing incision is to make the edge easier to grasp. After the cyst wall is removed, it is sent to pathology for examination. (Modified from Martin DC. *Intra-Abdominal Laser Surgery.* Resurge Press, 1986. Used with permission.)

deep margin of a large endometrioma is adherent to the hilar vessels, the stripping is abandoned and coagulation used. Trying to strip adherent ovarian tissue off the hilar vessels can cause hemorrhage from these vessels.

The amount of lavage solution used to clean the area is controlled to limit its spread into the upper abdomen. The cul-de-sac has a capacity of less than 80 mL (Figure 5-3.4).

Once the endometrioma has been removed or coagulated, the edges are pushed together, and sutures are avoided. These techniques have produced excellent results in several series.

If a cystic ovary with the possibility of stage IA ovarian cancer is to be removed, spill is avoided. This can be performed by use of a minilaparotomy or colpotomy for intact removal or by bagging the specimen. When bagging the specimen, the ovary is separated from the sidewall before being placed in the bag. The neck of the bag is pulled through the incision and the cyst decompressed extraabdominally.

Ureter Involvement

When endometriosis is over the ureter, the technique is similar to that used at laparotomy. An incision is made into the healthy peritoneum above and away from the ureter. Grasping forceps are used to pull the lesion medial. The ureter is pushed off the peritoneum under direct visualization, using a blunt probe. If the ureter cannot be visualized or pushed off the peritoneum, the procedure is continued only if there is adequate preparation for a laparotomy and ureteral repair.

As long as the ureter pushes away easily, the peritoneum is pulled medial and resected with the ureter lateral and out of the dissection field. These techniques appear relevant in patients with pelvic pain, but may be counterproductive in infertility. Although subperitoneal injection of water solutions has been said to separate the ureter from the peritoneum, there is some concern that this injection may push the ureter toward the peritoneum in certain patients.

Bladder Involvement

Small lesions over the bladder are handled similarly to peritoneal lesions. These have not infiltrated the bladder muscularis and can be lifted up with recognition of healthy loose connective tissue. However, deeper lesions can invade the bladder muscularis, so be prepared for this possibility before attempting to dissect these through the laparoscope.

Bowel Involvement

Bowel lesions are resected and the bowel repaired at laparoscopy in a small group of patients. Small surface le-

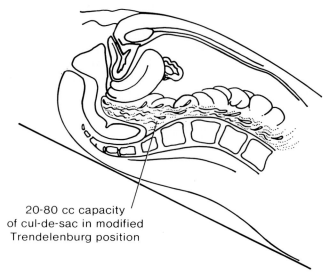

Figure 5-3.4 The capacity of the cul-de-sac is no more than 80 mL. If upper abdominal contamination is to be avoided, positioning of the patient in a flat or heads-up position may be desired. (Modified from Martin DC. *Intra-Abdominal Laser Surgery.* Resurge Press, 1986. Used with permission.)

sions or the superficial component of deep lesions can be biopsied, coagulated or vaporized superficially. This is in the hope that limited destruction of these bowel lesions may help avoid further surgery. This hope must be balanced against the chance of inadvertent bowel perforation.

DISEASE OF COPING

All the symptoms of patients with endometriosis may not be related to endometriosis and/or may not resolve following excision. Patients may continue to have pelvic pain, pelvic discomfort, dyspareunia, marital discord, infertility, and miscarriages. These frustrations require counseling and/or support. Physicians, counselors, and self-help groups such as the Endometriosis Association and Resolve, Inc., are useful for these patients.

LAPAROTOMY

Although laparotomy is frequently avoided in the treatment of endometriosis, it has a place when palpation, examination of retroperitoneal spaces, examination of bowel, and delicate tissue handling are needed. Laparotomy is also useful in patients with persistent pelvic pain following laparoscopic treatment. On the other hand, laparoscopy provides better exposure and visualization for the majority of endometriotic lesions.

CONCLUSION

Laparoscopy is sufficient for the treatment of endometriosis in many patients. Small surface lesions can be handled with basic techniques, using biopsy forceps, thermal coagulation, or bipolar electrosurgery. Deeper lesions require a combination of scissors, electrosurgery or lasers, accompanied by hemostatic techniques when needed. Suturing hemostatic techniques is generally avoided as this may increase the chance of adhesions.

Ongoing development of laparoscopic techniques for such procedures as bowel resection and anastomosis, nephrectomy, lymph node dissection, and cholecystectomy, is responsible for producing equipment and techniques that may be useful in pelvic surgery for endometriosis.

SUGGESTED READING

Ascher SM, Agrawal R, Bis KG, et al. Endometriosis: Appearance and detection with conventional and contrast-enhanced fat-suppressed spin-echo techniques. *JMRI* 1995;5:251–7.

Evers JLH. Endometriosis does not exist; all women have endometriosis. *Human Reproduction* 1994;9:2206–9.

Kempers RD, Dockerty MB, Hunt AB, Symmonds RE. Significant postmenopausal endometriosis. *Surg Gynecol Obstet* 1960;111:348–56.

Koninckx PR, Martin DC. Deep endometriosis: a consequence of infiltration or retraction or possibly adenomyosis externa? *Fertil Steril* 1992; 58:924–8.

Koninckx PR, Oosterlynck D, D'Hooghe T, Meuleman C. Deeply infiltrating endometriosis is a disease whereas mild endometriosis could be considered a non-disease. *Ann NY Acad Sci* 1994;734:333–41.

Martin DC, Hubert GD, Vander Zwaag R, El-Zeky FA. Laparoscopic appearances of peritoneal endometriosis. *Fertil Steril* 1989;51:63–67.

Martin DC, Berry JD. Histology of chocolate cysts. *J Gynecol Surg* 1990;6:43–6.

Martin DC. Pain and infertility—a rationale for different treatment approaches. *Brit J Obstet Gynecol* 1995;102, Supplement 12:2–3.

Moen MH. Is a long period without childbirth a risk factor for developing endometriosis? *Hum Reprod* 1991;6:1404–7.

Moen MH, Muus KM. Endometriosis in pregnant and non-pregnant women at tubal sterilization. *Hum Reprod* 1991;6:699–702.

Moore JG, Binstock MA, Growdon WA. The clinical implications of retroperitoneal endometriosis. *Am J Obstet Gynecol* 1988;158:1291–8.

Nesbitt RE, Rizk PT. Uterosacral ligament syndrome. *Obstet Gynecol* 1971;37:730–3.

Nezhat C, Nezhat FR. Safe laser endoscopic excision or vaporization of peritoneal endometriosis. *Fertil Steril* 1989;52:149–51.

Perper MM, Nezhat F, Goldstein H, Nezhat CH, Nezhat C. Dysmenorrhea is related to the number of implants in endometriosis patients. *Fertil Steril* 1995;63:500–3.

Redwine DB. Age-related evolution in color appearance of endometriosis. *Fertil Steril* 1987;48:1062–3.

Redwine DB. Conservative laparoscopic excision of endometriosis by sharp dissection: life table analysis of reoperation and persistent or recurrent disease. *Fertil Steril* 1991;56:628–34.

Reich H, McGlynn F, Salvat J. Laparoscopic treatment of cul-de-sac obliteration secondary to retrocervical deep fibrotic endometriosis. *J Reprod Med* 1991;36:516–22.

Ripps BA, Martin DC. Correlation of focal pelvic tenderness with implant dimension and stage of endometriosis. *J Reprod Med* 1992;37:620–4.

Vercellini P, Vendola N, Presti M, Bolis G. Multifocal endometriosis: a case report. *J Reprod Med* 1993;38:815–19.

Operative Laparoscopy, Second Edition
The Masters' Techniques in Gynecologic Surgery
Lippincott–Raven Publishers, Philadelphia © 1998.

5-4   Laparoscopic Electroexcision of Endometriosis

David B. Redwine

Since no medicine eradicates endometriosis, surgery is often used by clinicians treating patients with pain or infertility related to the disease. While laser vaporization or electro-coagulation have the potential of destroying superficial endometriosis, invasive disease often escapes complete treatment, since the surgeon may not judge accurately the depth of destruction required, or may be hesitant to burn near vital pelvic structures. Additionally, electrocoagulation has not been described sufficiently in the literature to allow clinicians consistently, safely, or completely to treat the many manifestations of endometriosis in human females. Vaporization and electrocoagulation techniques do not return a pathology report, so the surgeon's opinion is the sole determinant of what is being treated and how completely it was destroyed. The inconsistencies in treatment can lead to a high rate of persistent disease. The modern view of endometriosis is that it is a chronic, highly recurrent, disease which has no effective treatment. This modern view is completely opposite to the view of the disease held by experts half a century ago, when Meigs stated in confident, unequivocal, terms that ". . . recurrence is not frequent, and cure of the lesion by conservative surgery is usual."

Has the disease changed that much? Or has the profession adopted unproven, ineffective treatment techniques? How was endometriosis treated in women who wanted to bear children before laparoscopes, lasers, electrocoagulation, or expensive medical therapy? The ancient surgeon had only one option: the abdomen was opened, and the disease was cut out of the body. While removal of disease from the body may seem to modern gynecologists like a primitive mode of treatment of endometriosis, it is apparent that other surgical specialists frequently remove disease from the body of their patients, so this method of treatment should not be rejected out of hand.

Mature techniques exist which allow laparoscopic electroexcision of endometriosis from anywhere in the pelvis. Resection of the uterosacral ligaments for invasive disease, ureterolysis for retroperitoneal fibrosis, ovarian cystectomy or oophorectomy for ovarian disease, full thickness anterior resections of the sigmoid colon and rectum, segmental resection of the sigmoid colon with anastomosis, and retroperitoneal dissection, all are existing components of the laparoscopic surgical armamentarium.

INSTRUMENTS AND TECHNIQUES

The instruments needed for basic or advanced electroexcision of endometriosis are very simple and inexpensive (Table 5-4.1). The simplicity of these items places the surgical premium where it belongs—in the skill of the surgeon to identify and separate diseased tissue from healthy tissue. Identification of endometriosis is as important as is its complete removal. Aspiring endometriosis surgeons should be familiar with the visual appearances of the disease.

The patient is placed in the low lithotomy position with an intrauterine manipulator in place. The left arm is tucked along her side, the bladder is catheterized, and a return electrode is applied to the anterior thigh. After prepping and draping the patient, I stand on the patient's left, and make a midline incision from the inferior depth of the umbilicus up to the crescenteric reflection of skin at the inferior margin of the umbilicus. This not only hides the incision well, but places the incision closer to the peritoneum, which tents up to the base of the umbilicus. The skin lateral and inferior to the umbilicus is grasped by the surgeon's left hand and the assistant's right. I then palpate the pubic symphysis with the little finger of my left hand, while elevating the abdominal wall. With the patient's body largely hidden by drapes, this serves as a useful final confirmation of landmarks before blind insertion of a reusable 10-mm trocar sheath, which is directed toward the bottom of the pelvis to intersect a coronal plane midway between the umbilicus and the pubis. The reusable trocar is less sharp than a disposable trocar, which makes it safer to use.

Although most of my patients have had previous surgery, I make only two concessions to a previous vertical midline laparotomy incision: (1) if the incision travels above the umbilicus, I will make my umbilical incision on the side opposite the laparotomy incision; (2) rather than an open technique for insertion of the trocar and sheath, I frequently insert the 10-mm trocar and sheath just through the fascia, then insert the laparoscope and use *intra-sheath dissection* with the 3-mm operating scissors passed down through the laparoscope to incise the peritoneum exactly as one would do at laparotomy. Once the laparoscope is in, the inferior epigastric vessels are identified as they travel cephalad from the vicinity of the internal inguinal ring. Two 5.5-mm trocars and sheaths are inserted lateral to these vessels. I place the suction-irrigator in the right lower quadrant and a 5-mm grasper in the left lower quadrant.

The 3-mm scissors are passed down the operating channel of the laparoscope, and I work by looking directly

Table 5-4.1 *Equipment needed for excision of endometriosis (triple-puncture technique)*

BASIC: PERITONEAL EXCISION, OVARIAN CYSTECTOMY, URETEROLYSIS, ANGIOLYSIS, RESECTION OF UTEROSACRAL LIGAMENTS, HEMOSTASIS

10-mm Operating laparoscope with 3-mm channel
3-mm Hook scissors
5-mm Graspers
Suction-irrigator
Light source, insufflator
Bipolar coagulator
ValleyLab Force 4 electrosurgical generator

ADVANCED: HEMOSTASIS, LAPAROSCOPIC BOWEL RESECTION
Endoloops
Internal suturing technique

through the scope, which gives me the highest possible optical resolution as well as a magnified view down the axis of surgery. This also avoids the "helpful interference" of an assistant. I draw the eyepiece of the laparoscope into the nasal bridge of my right eye by continually pulling the scissors toward my head. You can duplicate the feel of this by putting the point of a pencil in the thenar web of the back of your right hand, then putting the pencil's eraser against the right side of your nose just below your eyebrow. This allows a stable 3-point operating platform to be constructed, the points consisting of the right hand, the bridge of the nose, and the umbilicus. This allows extremely precise control of the tip of the scissors, as well as of the depth of the laparoscope within the abdomen. Ninety watts of pure cutting current (also known as 'unmodulated' current), or 50 watts of coagulation current (also known as 'modulated' current), are passed through the scissors, which serve as the active electrode. Although both waveforms can be used either for cutting or coagulation, I find that cutting current is most useful for making initial peritoneal incisions, while the higher voltage potential of coagulation current is useful for severing retroperitoneal fat or parenchymal structures such as the uterosacral ligaments. Electroexcision depends on extremely high current densities, achieved by touching only the tip of the electrically activated scissors to tissue, which is kept on traction. It is important to activate the scissors before touching the tissue, to avoid "pillowing" of tissue around the tip of the scissors; this would lower the current density and slow surgery down. Only rarely will the activated scissors be used to "gnaw" through tissue, since this results in messy coagulation rather than a quick, clean cut. It is important to realize that electroexcision of endometriosis depends approximately 75% on blunt dissection to prepare the tissue, and 25% electrosurgery, to sever the last tendrils of attachment once the surgeon sees that vital structures are sufficiently separated. Short bursts of electrosurgery and a constantly moving active electrode will prevent lateral thermal spread to vital structures. Experienced electrosurgeons use high power cutting current directly on the bowel, bladder or ureter with safety when those structures are involved by disease.

Hemostasis

Avoiding injury to vessels is my primary method of hemostasis. When this has been unsuccessful, 50 watts of coagulation current, in short bursts, can be used to stop most bleeding. It is important to try to see the individual vessel. These will usually be rather small and may retract slightly into surrounding tissue, so near-contact laparoscopy and irrigation are used to see it better. When the vessel has been visualized, it can be grasped gently with the scissors and coagulated. This keeps the thermal effect as shallow as possible. Remember that the pneumoperitoneum acts as a tamponade in all directions, and venous bleeding may stop due to this tamponade, only to resume when the gas is released from the abdomen. The larger the vein, the lower the blood pressure within it and the more likely the increased intra-abdominal pressure will stop it from bleeding during the procedure. This physical fact can lead to serious problems with blood loss after the abdomen is closed. Cutting current can also be helpful in controlling bleeding in parenchymal tissue such as the uterus, although the power setting must be reduced from 90 watts to about 50 watts to result in a slower, deeper, more widespread coagulation effect. Bipolar coagulation will be necessary for larger vessels which do not respond to monopolar coagulation.

Excision of Endometriosis

Since endometriosis is a disease primarily of the peritoneal surface, with greater or lesser degrees of invasion, excision of the abnormal peritoneum is the basic method of treatment. A surgeon just beginning to use this technique can simply use the graspers to pick up the peritoneum at various spots around the pelvis. The transparent nature of normal peritoneum will allow retroperitoneal structures to be seen, and the movement of the peritoneum over these vital structures will suggest natural planes of dissection that can be used to remove endometriosis. The normal peritoneum adjacent to a lesion is tented up with the graspers, then the electrically activated 3-mm scissors with 90 watts of cutting current are used to touch the resulting peritoneal pleat, resulting in instant vaporization of a small hole. The closed jaws of the scissors are then inserted into this hole, and the scissors bluntly dissect the peritoneum from the underlying areolar fatty tissue, while the graspers hold the cut edge next to the lesion. The scissors are then withdrawn and used to incise the peritoneum around the lesion as the graspers lift and begin to peel the peritoneum away from the underlying tissue. The fatty tissue which adheres to the peritoneum has vessels within it, and by using the scissors

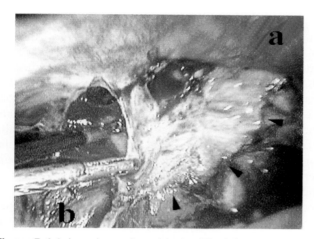

Figure 5-4.1 Invasive endometriosis of the left uterosacral ligament is being resected. A peritoneal incision has been created medial to the ligament (*arrows*). While the lateral edge is being elevated by graspers, the scissors are undermining the involved peritoneum laterally. The ligament is still attached to the posterior uterus (**a**). The lateral incision and blunt dissection has kept the ureter (**b**) well out of harm's way.

in a blunt dissecting mode, this tissue can usually be stripped away from the overlying peritoneum. Cutting current is then used to complete the line of incision around the lesion, which is eventually removed. Troublesome small vessels will often be found in the lower right or left of the cul-de-sac adjacent to the sigmoid colon. These can hide in the peritoneal pleat which is first cut with the scissors, and this is why it is important to elevate and incise just the peritoneum when possible. If the lesion is invasive, this will be immediately obvious, and the scissors will be used to probe and dissect the softer, normal, tissue beneath the lesion. With invasive lesions, the ureter or large pelvic vessels may be encountered, and with practice these can be dissected out of harm's way.

Invasive disease of the uterosacral ligaments will frequently require resection of a portion of the ligament for complete removal. Using 90 watts of cutting current, first make peritoneal incisions around the posterior, lateral and medial edge of involvement (Figure 5-4.1). The lateral incision is the key to avoiding injury to the ureter and large vessels, allowing the peritoneum to separate. Blunt dissection laterally will allow the ureter and vessels of the broad ligament to be kept out of harm's way. Fifty watts of coagulation current can then be used to shave the ligament off the pelvic floor, taking care to palpate any fibrosis or nodularity with the scissors as you go so you can be sure to remove all invasive disease. Once the diseased ligament has been shaved up to its insertion into the posterior cervix, 50 watts of coagulation current can be used to transect the ligament adjacent to the cervix (Figure 5-4.2). Patients do not have a sensation of uterine prolapse following resection of the uterosacral ligaments.

Superficial endometriosis of the ovaries can be removed by cortical resection. Pure cutting current at 90 watts can be used to cut a square around small lesions, or to incise around the perimeter of larger lesions. The lesions can then be undermined with the scissors and dissected out of the ovary. Endometrioma cysts will invariably rupture during dissection, and the cyst can be opened, irrigated, and further drained. Then the open edge of the cyst can be grasped with the graspers and the scissors can cut the normal ovarian cortical tissue parallel to the open edge of the cyst. This opens a plane of dissection between the fibrotic cyst wall and the overlying normal ovarian cortex. The cyst wall can then be grasped and pulled one way while the side of the scissors is used to push the ovarian cortex the other way (Figure 5-4.3). In this fashion, the cyst wall can be stripped completely out of the ovary. Monopolar or bipolar coagulation can be used to control bleeding near the base of the cyst.

Bowel Endometriosis

The colon has 4 layers: serosa, outer muscularis, inner muscularis, and mucosa. Endometriosis of the bowel almost never penetrates all the way through the mucosa, but is usually localized on the serosa and in the layers of muscularis. For this reason, preoperative barium or sigmoidoscopy studies will usually be negative, even in patients requiring segmental resections at laparotomy. However, this lack of full-thickness penetration of the bowel also allows an advantage to the laparoscopist, since it is possible in most cases to remove colonic lesions by partial thickness resection without penetration into the bowel lumen. Very superficial lesions are removed in a manner similar to resection of peritoneum, and these do not require suture. The frequency distribution of sites of intestinal

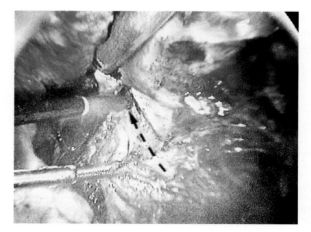

Figure 5-4.2 The 3 mm-monopolar scissors with 50 W of "coagulation" (modulated) current transects the parenchymal tissue of the insertion of the left uterosacral ligament (*dashed arrow*).

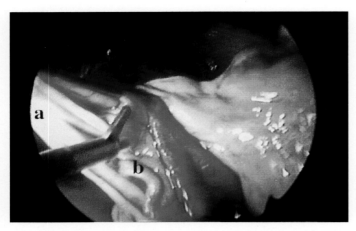

Figure 5-4.3 A large endometrioma cyst of the right ovary is being removed. The cyst wall (**a**) is being pulled medially, while the scissors are used bluntly to push normal ovarian tissue (**b**) away.

endometriosis in the author's practice is shown in Table 5-4.2. The ileum is so thin that perforation of the bowel during dissection is likely. Nodularity of the cul-de-sac or rectal wall is a cardinal sign of endometriosis of the lower bowel. If the lower bowel is not involved by endometriosis, the rest of the bowel is usually free of disease, so rectal nodularity is a sentinel sign of the possible presence of disease higher in the bowel. Patients with endometriosis frequently have non-specific intestinal symptoms such as diarrhea, constipation, and bloating. The cardinal symptom of rectal involvement is a description of rectal pain, whether with bowel movements, passing flatus, or sitting. Rectal bleeding is usually absent. A bowel prep of 4 liters of Go-Lytely (Braintree Laboratories, Inc., Braintree, MA) can be given the afternoon before surgery, based on the presence of symptoms or physical exam, to be followed by intraoperative Unasyn (Roerig Division, Pfizer, Inc., New York, NY) (3 g). At laparoscopy, palpation of the bowel is at least as important as visualization. A ring forceps passing up and down the rectum will give evidence of a mass effect in the wall of the bowel by the presence

of the "snap" sign: as the ring forceps is withdrawn slowly, a nodule in the bowel wall will snap off the end of the forceps, while normal bowel wall will glide smoothly. Palpation of the bowel wall with the graspers also is useful, since a bowel nodule will slip out of the grasper jaws. The rectosigmoid must be evaluated from the cul-de-sac to the pelvic brim. The appendix, cecum, and terminal ileum must also be examined. Based on the size and location of the lesion and the experience of the surgeon, laparoscopic bowel wall resection may be in order. The normal bowel adjacent to the nodule is grasped and the scissors cut directly into the serosa next to the nodule. Since the serosa is quite thin, this initial incision will usually enter the first layer of muscularis. The cut edge is grasped, and the line of incision can be made in the serosa around part of the nodule. The scissors are then used to undermine the nodule. The layers of muscularis usually will peel apart, and the nodule can be lifted off. When the nodule has been undermined completely, the dissection exits out through the muscularis and serosa. Some nodules will have invasion and fine, granular fibrosis down to the submucosa, and these will require mucosal skinning with dissection immediately adjacent to the mucosa under magnification with the laparoscope. Large areas of mucosa can be denuded through the laparoscope, (Figure 5-4.4). During mucosal skinning, nodules with significant submucosal fibrosis will result in entry into the bowel lumen (Figure 5-4.5). In this case, complete the dissection by cutting the mucosa around the bottom of the nodule, then cutting back out through the muscularis and

Table 5-4.2 *Sites of disease among 450 patients with intestinal endometriosis*

Intestinal site	Number of patients	% of patients with intestinal endometriosis
Sigmoid	300	66.7
Rectal nodule	200	44.4
Ileum	68	15.1
Cecum	28	6.2
Appendix[a]	42	9.3

[a] Some patients had previous appendectomy.

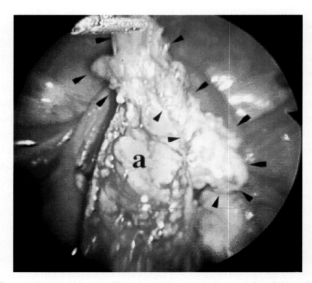

Figure 5-4.4 A large, fibrotic endometriotic nodule of the mid-sigmoid (*arrows*) has been dissected off the mucosa (**a**) by blunt dissection. This technique is called mucosal skinning. The seromuscular layer is then closed with interrupted 3-0 silk suture. Antibiotic therapy is optional if the bowel lumen is not entered.

serosa after the nodule has been passed. The bowel can be closed transversely with 3-0 chromic in the mucosa, and with interrupted 3-0 silk for the seromuscularis. The suture is cut to a length of about 4 inches before insertion into the abdomen, to make suturing easier. Be sure to start the seromuscular suture layer at each lateral angle of the defect in the bowel wall and work toward the central anterior bowel wall.

Laparoscopically-assisted transvaginal segmental resection of the sigmoid colon for endometriosis has been performed on 11 patients with very large intestinal nodules. The affected segment of bowel is isolated from its mesentery with monopolar techniques and then prolapsed through a colpotomy incision to the vaginal introitus (Figure 5-4.6) where the segment is resected. Transvaginal hand-sewn anastomosis is accomplished and the bowel is returned to the pelvis. An intracorporeal stapled technique has also been described, as well as a transanal pull-through approach accomplished with a circular stapler. Laparoscopic segmental bowel resection usually follows a challenging pelvic dissection and should be attempted only by skilled laparoscopists.

THE FUTURE

As reports on the long-term efficacy of laparoscopic treatment of endometriosis reach the literature, laparoscopic techniques inevitably will assume an increasingly dominant role in treating the disease. It is already known from the laparotomy era that recurrence after conservative excision is uncommon, and this has been found to be the case with

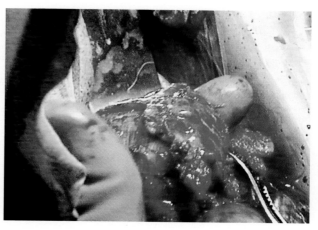

Figure 5-4.6 Laparoscopically assisted transvaginal segmental bowel resection can be performed in selected patients. The affected bowel segment is isolated from its mesentery, then prolapsed through a colpotomy incision to the introitus where segmental resection and hand-sutured anastomosis are accomplished.

laparoscopic excision. Society, patients, and scientific journals will demand long-term outcome analysis and biopsy validation of the efficacy of surgical procedures. For these reasons, laparoscopic excisional techniques will emerge as a frequent choice of treatment for most cases of endometriosis, whether by sharp dissection, laser or electrosurgical methods.

Endometriosis surgery is not for every gynecologist, however. The fibrosis and retroperitoneal or visceral invasion accompanying severe disease can be daunting. Gynecologic oncologists often would not operate on malignancy with a similar presentation, since such a case would likely be considered inoperable. Yet severe endometriosis is far more prevalent than advanced cancer. Endless patience, meticulous attention to detail, and excellent hand-eye coordination are required, as well as the knowledge that it is up to the surgeon to remove the disease completely. The learning curve may be long and steep, whether the surgery is done at laparotomy or laparoscopy, and can be made longer by a busy obstetrical practice. Although simple cases of minimal or mild disease may be within the capability of some general gynecologists, more complex cases should be referred until experience is gained.

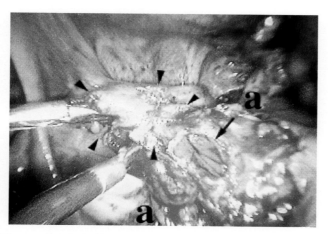

Figure 5-4.5 A fibrotic nodule of endometriosis (*arrowheads*) was associated with intense submucosal fibrosis, resulting in entry into the prepared bowel (*arrow*) during mucosal skinning. After removal of the nodule, the mucosa is closed with running 3-0 chromic. The seromuscularis is closed with interrupted 3-0 silk suture, with the first sutures placed at each angle (**a**) of the defect and working toward the center of the bowel wall.

SUGGESTED READING

Meigs JV. Endometriosis. Etiologic role of marriage age and parity; conservative treatment. *Obstet Gynecol* 1953;2:46–53.
Nezhat F, Nezhat C, Pennington E, Ambroze W. Laparoscopic segmental resection for infiltrating endometriosis of the rectosigmoid colon: A preliminary report. *Surg Laparoscop Endoscop* 1992;2:212–6.
Redwine DB. Laparoscopic excision of endometriosis with 3-mm scissors: comparison of operating times between sharp excision and electroexcision. *J Am Assoc Gynecol Laparosc* 1993;1:24–30.

Redwine DB. Treatment of endometriosis. In: Tulandi T, ed., *Atlas of Laparoscopic Technique for Gynecologists,* London: WB Saunders, 1994.

Redwine DB. Bowel Resection for Endometriosis. In: Tulandi T, ed., *Atlas of Laparoscopic Technique for Gynecologists,* London: WB Saunders, 1994.

Redwine DB. Treatment of Endometriosis of the Cul-de-sac. In: Nezhat, Buttram, Berger, Nezhat, eds., *Modern Surgical Management of Endometriosis.* New York: Springer-Verlag, 1995:105–15.

Redwine DB, Koning M, Sharpe DR. Laparoscopically assisted transvaginal segmental bowel resection for endometriosis. *Fertil Steril* 1996;65:193–7.

Redwine DB. Conservative laparoscopic excision of endometriosis by sharp dissection: life table analysis of reoperation and persistent or recurrent disease. *Fertil Steril* 1991;56:628–34.

Redwine DB, Koning M, Sharpe DR. Laparoscopically assisted transvaginal segmental bowel resection for endometriosis. *Fertil Steril* 1996;65:193–7.

Redwine DB, Sharpe DR. Laparoscopic segmental resection of the sigmoid colon. *J Laparoendosc Surg* 1991;1:217–20.

Sharpe DR, Redwine DB. Laparoscopic segmental resection of the sigmoid and rectosigmoid colon for endometriosis. *Surg Laparosc Endosc* 1992;2:120–4.

Wheeler JM, Malinak LR: Recurrent endometriosis. *Contr Gynecol Obstet* 1987;16:13.

Operative Laparoscopy, Second Edition
The Masters' Techniques in Gynecologic Surgery
Lippincott–Raven Publishers, Philadelphia © 1998.

5-5 Pelvic Abscesses

Richard M. Soderstrom

Although the development of powerful broad-spectrum antibiotics has reduced the occurrence of pelvic abscess formation, incision and drainage are usually necessary if it does occur. The success of in vitro fertilization has precluded the need for total abdominal hysterectomy with bilateral salpingo-oophorectomy, at times the only alternative available to patients several decades ago. Today, the incision, drainage, and irrigation of pelvic abscesses, large and small, is possible via operative laparoscopy. In such cases, I prefer the open laparoscopy technique, after I have insufflated through a Veress needle placed in the left upper quadrant of the abdomen. If the peritoneum is free of the underlying bowel, it will balloon up through the fascial incision, giving one a sense of security as the peritoneum is cut.

In most circumstances the adhesions surrounding the abscess can be teased away with ease. Gentle traction on adherent loops is important to prevent inadvertent perforation of the bowel wall, which may be edematous and fragile. Once the abscess is exposed, I will insert a disposable 10-mm trocar and sleeve through the abdominal wall and into the abscess wall. Once the wall has been punctured, the protective sleeve will spring forward and lock in place. After removing the trocar, large-bore suction tubing can be threaded into the trocar sleeve down to the purulent fluid,

to aspirate it. When the pus is removed, copious irrigation can be performed through the trocar sleeve, which is still housed in the abscess cavity. Using a circular motion, the irrigator/aspirator cannula can explore the abscess cavity for possible loculations.

Once the irrigation fluid returns clear, I remove the large trocar sleeve and insert my gloved finger through the trocar stab wound. On occasion, I will extend the fascial incision to accommodate my finger, but not so much as to allow leakage of intraabdominal gas. Under endoscopic view, I will place my finger into the abscess cavity and palpate the cavity, searching for occult loculations. If necessary, I digitally break up the loculations, remove my finger, and replace the large trocar sleeve through the abdominal wall. I repeat an irrigation/aspiration process many times, exchanging small amounts of irrigating fluid, but using enough to wash down the surrounding pelvic structures. The purulent material is sent to the laboratory for aerobic and anaerobic cultures, and a Jackson-Pratt drain is threaded through the trocar sleeve into the open abscess cavity. I do not use intraabdominal antibiotics.

As with laparotomy, the drain is removed 24 to 48 hours later. The length of hospital stay is usually brief, and the patient's recovery period is substantially shorter than following laparotomy.

Operative Laparoscopy, Second Edition
The Masters' Techniques in Gynecologic Surgery
Lippincott–Raven Publishers, Philadelphia © 1998.

6

Management of the Pelvic Mass by Operative Laparoscopy

William H. Parker and Jonathan S. Berek

The operative approach to the pelvic mass has routinely been via laparotomy. This provides for early detection, resection, and proper staging, should ovarian cancer be found. However, most adnexal masses in premenopausal and postmenopausal women are benign. In women operated on for the presence of a pelvic mass, various studies have reported finding malignancy in 7% to 13% of premenopausal and 8% to 45% of postmenopausal patients.

Dermoid cysts and endometriomas have also been managed via laparotomy, to allow complete resection and thus decrease recurrence. Laparotomy was also felt to allow removal of dermoid cysts with minimum spill, thus decreasing the potential for chemical peritonitis. Recent studies have shown good results for operative laparoscopic management of dermoid cysts, with low risk of recurrence and only rare evidence of mild adhesion formation seen at second look laparoscopy. Likewise, management of endometriomas by operative laparoscopy has been associated with low risk of recurrence and good fertility rates.

The role of operative laparoscopy in postmenopausal women has been more controversial. However, with careful preoperative screening, as described below, we have managed 61 postmenopausal patients with adnexal masses, via operative laparoscopic surgery. All the women had benign masses, and only three required laparotomy. Operative laparoscopy has also been shown to have a role in the management of paraovarian cysts, paratubal cysts and adnexal torsion.

Therefore, with proper preoperative evaluation, women who are likely to have benign masses may be candidates for operative laparoscopy.

PREOPERATIVE EVALUATION

The patient's age, the clinical exam, and ultrasound findings provide important information that help to determine the operative approach. Postmenopausal women should also have a serum CA-125 value determined.

Clinical Examination

Adnexal masses that are fixed, irregular, and firm are suggestive of malignancy. An adnexal mass found in the presence of ascites or an upper abdominal mass is highly suspicious for cancer. A recent study found that clinical examination was more accurate in predicting malignancy than either sonography or tumor markers. Therefore, masses that are suspicious for malignancy based on clinical exam should be approached via laparotomy.

Sonography

Sonographic examination of the pelvis is a reliable and consistent method for evaluation of a pelvic mass. Therefore, a sonogram should be performed to determine the size and consistency of the mass. Transvaginal sonography is able to achieve greater resolution and clarity of image, and thus is prefered over transabdominal exams. Sonographic findings of irregular borders, papillations, solid areas, thick septa, ascites, or matted bowel raise concern regarding the possibility of malignancy.

BENIGN ULTRASOUND CHARACTERISTICS

1. Regular borders
2. No papillations
3. No solid parts
4. No thick septa (>2 mm)
5. No ascites or matted bowel

With the use of specific ultrasound criteria, Herrman accurately predicted benign masses in 177 of 185 (96%) patients studied. In addition, all 48 purely cystic masses <10 cm were benign and 8 out of 10 stage I ovarian cancers were predicted accurately. Granberg, in a large study of 94 postmenopausal and 86 menstruating women, found that the number of papillations detected sonographically correlated to the likelihood of malignancy. Ninety-two percent of tumors without papillations were benign, whereas all 37 tumors with more than 5 papillations were malignant. If the sonogram shows suspicious characteristics, operative laparoscopic removal is not appropriate and laparotomy should be performed without delay.

Dermoids, endometriomas, hemorrhagic cysts, cystadenomas, and persistant functional cysts, will often have a characteristic sonographic appearance. Along with the clinical picture and other laboratory data, the ultrasound may help select patients who can be approached by operative laparoscopy. Functional cysts are usually unilocular and have regular, thin, borders on sonogram. In premenopausal women, the majority of purely cystic masses > 7 cm will resolve spontaneously. Therefore, these cysts may be followed for eight weeks. Recent studies show that the use of oral contraceptives does not help to suppress these cysts, and that most will regress spontaneously.

Hemorrhagic cysts contain internal echoes that can vary in intensity from low to high level and can be either focal or diffuse. These cysts characteristically change over time and often regress spontaneously. Cysts that appear to be functional or hemorrhagic on sonography, but persist for more than eight weeks may also be removed by operative laparoscopy to rule out neoplasia. Dermoids have a variable appearance on ultrasound. They may appear as a cystic mass that contains an echogenic mural focus, echogenic material in a nondependant area, or highly echogenic areas suggesting bone or teeth. Endometriomas usually have regular but slightly thickened borders. They often will contain low level and diffuse internal echoes, although fresh hemorrhage may appear more highly echogenic.

Investigators have proposed that measurement of blood flow within a tumor by color Doppler sonography may help distinguish benign from malignant masses. Malignant tumors are associated with the formation of thin walled vessels and arteriovenous shunts that have high diastolic blood flow. Hata et al found that, in 36 patients with benign masses and 27 patients found to have malignant masses, transvaginal Doppler sonography had a sensitivity of 92%, but a specificity of only 52%. In that study, the authors concluded that transvaginal Doppler sonography did not provide more useful information than either transvaginal sonography or CA-125 values. Kurjak found, in an analysis of Doppler sonography in 254 women with adnexal masses, that vessels with a low resistance index near the center of a mass or within papillations or septations, were highly correlated with malignancy. This analysis explains discrepancies in prior studies that evaluated a variety of vessel locations, using inconsistent resistance cut-off values. A consistent approach to the use of Doppler sonography will provide more helpful information for the preoperative evaluation of the adnexal mass, but at present it should be considered investigational.

CA-125

CA-125, a tumor-associated antigen, has been studied to determine its value in preoperative differentiation of benign and malignant pelvic masses. Vasilev found that 128 of 132 (97%) patients with pelvic masses who had a CA-125 of <35 U/ml had benign masses. Eighty percent of patients over 50 with elevated CA-125 levels had malignant masses. However, in patients less than 50 years old who had an elevated CA-125 value, 34 of 40 patients (85%) had a benign mass. Endometriosis, leiomyomata, adenomyosis, dermoid cysts, and acute or chronic salpingitis may all be associated with elevated levels. Due to this high false positive rate, the use of CA-125 values unnecessarily excludes many premenopausal women who would benefit from operative laparoscopy. Therefore, we do not perform this test for premenopausal patients with an adnexal mass. In the same study, 80% of patients over age 50 who had a CA-125 level of >35 U/ml had a malignant mass. For this reason, we find the CA-125 value helpful in the preoperative evaluation of the postmenopausal patient. However, a review article found that only 50% of patients with stage I ovarian cancers had elevated CA-125 values of >35 U/ml. This test will miss many early cancers and is, therefore, too insensitive to be used alone for selecting appropriate patients for laparoscopic management.

A number of other tumor markers have been studied in an effort to increase both sensitivity and specificity in the preoperative determination of ovarian tumors. One study that measured serum sialyl-Tn, sialyl-Lewis Xi, CA-19.9, CA-125, CEA, and tissue polypeptide antigen in 65 women with early stage ovarian cancer, and 317 women with benign pelvic masses, found that even with the combination of all six of these markers, 20% of the patients with stage I or II ovarian cancer had false negative results. The authors concluded that a combination of clinical examination, imaging and serum assays would be necessary to detect malignant masses at an early stage.

Combination of Ultrasonography and CA-125 Values

Finkler combined the use of clinical impression, CA-125 values, and sonographic findings for the preoperative evaluation of ovarian masses. In 74 premenopausal women, sonography alone had a negative predictive value of 86%, which was not improved by the addition of CA-125 values.

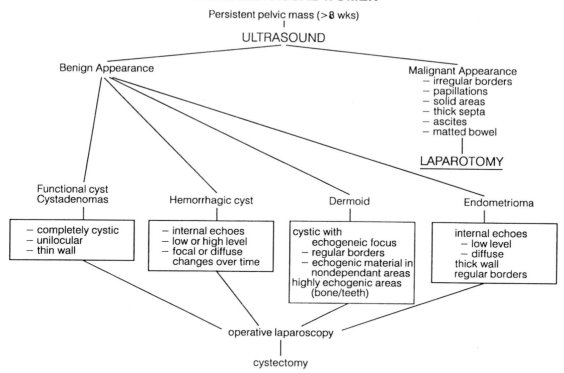

Figure 6-1 Management of premenopausal women with adnexal mass.

Therefore, in premenopausal women we use only clinical and sonographic criteria to select patients for laparoscopic management (Figure 6-1). However, for postmenopausal patients in the same study, sonography had a negative predictive value of 71% but, when combined with CA-125 values, all 10 postmenopausal patients predicted to have benign masses were predicted accurately. Using similar criteria, Jacobs found that in nine postmenopausal patients predicted to have benign masses, seven had benign processes and two had a normal pelvis. Using a selection process that included benign sonographic findings, a benign pelvic examination and CA-125 values <35 U/ml, we have thus far evaluated 61 postmenopausal patients with adnexal masses and have accurately predicted benign masses in all patients. Therefore, in postmenopausal patients, the combination of benign clinical exam and sonogram, and normal CA-125 value, appears to be a reasonable process to select patients for management via operative laparoscopy (Figure 6-2).

TUMOR SPILL

Laparoscopic removal of a pelvic mass has been avoided because of the fear of rupturing a malignant mass during removal, and decreasing the patient's survival chances by ''spilling'' cancer cells into the peritoneal cavity. This concern, however, resulted from early studies of tumor rupture that did not analyze other variables, such as tumor grade, the presence of adhesions, or ascites. In addition, the patients evaluated were not properly staged, as they did not have peritoneal washings, omental biopsies, or evaluation of retroperitoneal lymph nodes. However, Dembo and colleagues studied the rate of relapse in 519 stage I epithelial ovarian cancer patients by logistical regression, multivariate analysis. These patients were managed by appropriate staging laparotomy at the time of diagnosis. Dembo and colleagues found that the only factors that influenced the rate of relapse were the tumor grade, the presence of dense adhesions, or the presence of large volume ascites. The rate of relapse and prognosis was not influenced by intraoperative rupture of the tumor. While this study lacked complete staging information, the large size of the sample generated data that was statistically significant. Another strength of Dembo's study was a design that used data from one hospital to create a hypothesis, which was then validated on patients from another institution.

Sjovall et al. reported the 10-year survival rates for 394 women with stage I and stage IIa ovarian cancers. In the 147 women who had the tumors removed with the capsule intact, 78% survived 10 years. For the 47 women who had intraoperative puncture of the tumors and the 98 women who had intraoperative rupture of the tumors, the 10-year

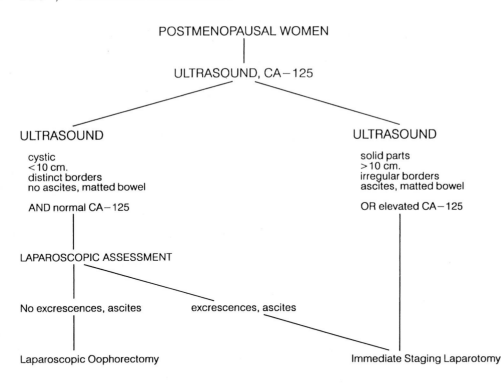

Figure 6-2 Management of postmenopausal women with adnexal mass.

survival was 87% and 84% respectively. Seventy-seven percent of women with intact tumors were treated postoperatively, compared to 90% of those with punctured or ruptured tumors. No patient with a well differentiated tumor died, regardless of rupture or use of postoperative treatment. The authors concluded that neither intraoperative puncture nor rupture of the tumor had any impact on survival.

A recent study by Sainz de la Cuesta et al. suggested that intraoperative rupture of stage I ovarian cancers did worsen the patients' prognoses. Only 1 of 36 women with stage Ia tumors had recurrences compared to 4 of 29 women with stage Ic-rupture. However, all women with grade I tumors survived without recurrence and the number of remaining patients was too small to reach statistical significance. Therefore, the conclusions of the study were stated more broadly than the result justified. It is apparent that a prospective study of sufficient numbers in similarly evaluated patients will be needed to make definitive conclusions about the risk of tumor spill. However, the evidence at present suggests that tumor rupture at the time of laparoscopic surgery should not decrease the patient's survival.

Reported Studies

A number of studies now provide evidence that operative laparoscopic management of a pelvic mass can be appropriately accomplished in most patients. Mecke et al. managed 678 of 809 (84%) adnexal masses by operative laparoscopy in 773 patients >45 years old. They found 11

(1.4%) ovarian cancers; all 9 patients considered operable were subjected to laparotomy. Only two masses (0.2%) were found to be stage I ovarian cancers. Canis et al found that after careful preoperative and intraoperative evaluation, only 7 of 819 (.9%) masses were found to be malignant and 12 were borderline tumors. In addition, all the borderline and malignant tumors were considered suspicious at laparoscopy and were managed by immediate conversion to laparotomy. Findings in the other patients managed by operative laparoscopy included 149 functional cysts, 190 endometriomas, 192 serous cysts, 129 teratomas, 67 mucinous cysts and 73 paraovarian cysts. Therefore, it appears that the risk of finding an unsuspected ovarian cancer in selected patients is very low.

Endometriomas have been managed routinely via laparotomy in order to improve fertility. Prior reports have indicated that pregnancy rates in women following resection of endometriomas approach 40%. Marrs, however, reported 10 of 23 patients (43%) achieved pregnancy after laparoscopic management of their endometriomas. In that study, surgical time averaged 52 minutes, mean postoperative recovery time was 5 hours, and there were no complications. Dermoid cysts have been managed routinely by laparotomy to decrease the risk of cyst rupture and the possibility of chemical peritonitis. Canis reported that of 129 patients who had laparoscopic excision of a dermoid cyst, 2 had chemical peritonitis following the procedure. A retrospective analysis of dermoid cysts managed by laparotomy, compared to those managed by laparoscopy, found that while intraoperative rupture of the dermoid was greater for the patients subjected to laparoscopic surgery, no patient in either group had evidence of chemical peritonitis following the procedure.

Canis found that eight of 757 patients (1.1%) had complications of the laparoscopic procedure, including: one laceration of the stomach by a trocar, one sigmoid laceration, two ovarian abscesses, one unexplained peritonitis, two cases of chemical peritonitis following spillage of dermoid cyst contents, and one patient with endometriosis of a trocar site, found 18 months after laparoscopic removal of an endometrioma. Although no randomized studies have been performed, these results compare favorably with the morbidity described following laparotomy for an adnexal mass.

The role of operative laparoscopy in postmenopausal women has been even more controversial. We have just published a multicentered study of postmenopausal patients with adnexal masses. The patients were carefully selected with sonography and CA-125 values before laparoscopic adnexectomy. All 61 women were found to have benign masses and only three patients (5%) required laparotomy. The size of the cysts on sonograms ranged from 3–10 cm, with a mean of 5.4 cm. Operative time averaged 63 minutes, average postoperative hospital stay was 12 hours, and average before return to normal activity was 5 days.

Laparoscopic Management of the Adnexal Mass During Pregnancy

An adnexal mass has been reported to occur during pregnancy in 1/160 to 1/1300 women. With the frequent use of early obstetrical sonography, the present rate of discovery may be higher. Current management of these masses involves observation of cysts not suspicious for malignancy until the second trimester, which allows for spontaneous resolution of non-neoplastic masses. One study of adnexal masses detected sonographically during pregnancy found that all 15 masses >5 cm resolved spontaneously and 19 of 39 (49%) simple cysts < 5 cm also resolved spontaneously. Persistent tumors are often removed in order to rule out malignancy, avoid torsion or rupture during pregnancy, and prevent the mass from obstructing delivery. Also, one study demonstrated that elective removal of an adnexal mass during pregnancy was less morbid than removal of a symptomatic mass in an emergency setting. Of fifteen women who had an emergency laparotomy, 8 (53%) had a spontaneous abortion and 3 (20%) delivered before 37 weeks' gestation. For 39 women undergoing elective surgery for an adnexal mass, 2 (5%) had a spontaneous abortion and none delivered before 37 weeks. In order to avoid the potential risks of a surgical emergency, the authors recommend elective removal of any adnexal mass <6 cm that persists for 16 weeks, regardless of its sonographic appearance.

Management of an adnexal mass during pregnancy via operative laparoscopy has been approached with caution because of the high level of technical ability needed to perform laparoscopic surgery in a limited operative field, and because of concern that the surgical technique might endanger the fetus. The effect of a carbon-dioxide pneumoperitoneum on the fetus during laparoscopic surgery are not well understood. However, recent animal studies suggest there are no deleterious effects. Also, laparoscopic removal of an ovarian cyst is more likely to result in cyst rupture than if it is removed via laparotomy. Furthermore, the possibility of chemical peritonitis following rupture of a benign cystic teratoma has raised concern regarding the laparoscopic approach.

The shorter hospital stay and faster recovery associated with laparoscopic surgery may be of benefit to the pregnant patient; however, experience with laparoscopic surgery in pregnant women is limited.

In order to ensure the safety of the fetus, careful operative technique is recommended during the laparoscopic management of an adnexal mass during pregnancy. Surgery should be performed early in the second trimester, when the risk of inducing a spontaneous abortion is reported to be low, and the uterus is small enough to allow adequate operative exposure. Open laparoscopy, or initial placement of the Veress needle and trocar in the left upper quadrant, may be considered to protect the gravid uterus from injury. Exposure of the operative field may be more difficult because of the size and position of the gravid uterus and because an intrauterine elevating device cannot be used. Ovarian cystectomy is recommended in these women in their reproductive years, in order to preserve ovarian tissue. Careful inspection of the peritoneal cavity, copious irrigation, and removal of all spilled cyst contents, should be performed to prevent peritoneal irritation.

We recently reported that 12 women had laparoscopic removal of a benign cystic teratoma during pregnancy. Patient ages ranged from 21 to 36, with a mean of 29. Gestational ages at the time of surgery ranged from 9 to 17 weeks, with a mean of 14 weeks. Cyst size ranged from 5 to 13 cm, with a mean of 8.5 cm. Intraoperative rupture of the cyst occured in 7 of 8 (88%) women with cystectomy and in 3 of 4 (75%) women who had an oophorectomy. A laparoscopic sac was used to remove the cyst from the abdomen in 6 cases. Estimated blood loss ranged from 5 to 100 ml, with a mean of 52 ml. Operating times ranged from 60 to 130 minutes, with a mean of 87 minutes. Postoperative hospital stay ranged from 8 to 72 hours, with a mean of 44 hours. No patient had evidence of chemical peritonitis and no intraoperative or postoperative maternal or fetal complications occurred. Subsequent to surgery, two women underwent elective termination of the pregnancy for fetal anomalies. Ten women delivered at term without incident. Our preliminary experience suggests that laparoscopic removal of these masses is feasible and safe, and that further study of this approach is warranted.

General Considerations for Surgery

All patients scheduled for operative laparoscopy should also consent to a possible laparotomy, and the surgeon should be prepared to proceed with staging laparotomy without delay, if malignancy is found.

SURGICAL CONSIDERATIONS

1. Consented for laparoscopy and laparotomy
2. General endotracheal anesthesia
3. Foley catheter
4. Intraoperative assessment of abdomen and pelvis
5. Pelvic washings
6. Biopsy and immediate frozen section of suspicious areas
7. Immediate staging laparotomy for obvious cancer, ascites or positive frozen section

The proper intraoperative management of the patient with an adnexal mass who is approached by operative laparoscopy is important. Under general endotracheal anesthesia, surgery is performed in the low-lithotomy position. Foley catheters are used in all patients to avoid bladder injury and prevent overdistention during prolonged cases. Under direct vision from within the peritoneal cavity, the inferior epigastric vessels are identified lateral to the obliterated umbilical vessels. Taking care to avoid the epigastric vessels, 5 and 11 mm trocars are inserted, via suprapubic incisions, as needed.

The initial inspection of the peritoneal cavity is done prior to attaching the video camera. We feel this allows a better assessment of fine detail and color differentiation. The upper abdomen and pelvis are inspected for obvious carcinoma, excrescences, and ascites. Pelvic and abdominal washings are saved for staging in the event that carcinoma is found. If excrescences are noted, they are biopsied with a 5 mm biopsy forceps and sent for frozen section. Adequate biopsies should be taken, since small amounts of tissue may be difficult for the pathologist to interpret. If an unsuspected malignancy is found at the time of laparoscopic management of an adnexal mass, the patient should have complete and timely surgical exploration. Maiman found appropriate staging laparotomy was performed immediately after laparoscopy in only 17% of cases studied, and was delayed an average of almost 5 weeks. However, another study of patients who had surgical staging of ovarian cancer by laparotomy found incomplete surgical staging in 95% of the early ovarian cancers and 65% were subjected to a second laparotomy to complete the staging. Thus, *delay* characterizes poor patient management, and not the laparoscopic approach per se. In addition, Maiman reported that

only 40% of the patients had a frozen section done at the time of surgery, adding to the delay in diagnosis and appropriate surgery. Frozen section should be done for all postmenopausal patients, because of the greater likelihood of malignancy. It should also be performed for premenopausal patients if suspicious areas are noted in the peritoneal cavity at the time of laparoscopy, or within the cyst after removal.

If obvious carcinoma, ascites, or a frozen section is found to be positive, then we proceed with immediate staging laparotomy through a midline incision. Once a decision has been made to proceed with laparoscopic surgery, the video camera is attached, allowing the assistant and the nurse to participate. The type of procedure is determined by the operative findings.

TECHNIQUES

1. Aspiration and fenestration
2. Cystectomy
3. Salpingo-oophorectomy
4. Oophorectomy
5. Salpingectomy
6. Paratubal cystectomy
7. Paraovarian cystectomy
8. Management of adnexal torsion
9. Minilaparotomy

PROCEDURES

Aspiration and Fenestration

Aspiration of adnexal cysts, either via operative laparoscopy or with a transvaginal sonographically guided needle, has been performed to diagnose benign and malignant adnexal masses. However, studies show that 10% to 66% of aspirates are interpreted as benign, when, in fact, malignancy is present. Therefore, reliance on negative cytologic analysis may delay appropriate surgery. In addition, needle puncture of a malignant cyst may seed the peritoneal cavity with malignant cells and, if appropriate surgery is delayed, may worsen the patient's prognosis. Also, many ovarian cysts contain functional epithelium and, if not removed, may reoccur. One study investigated 36 patients with ovarian cysts that appeared sonographically benign, who were subjected to transvaginal ultrasound-guided cyst aspiration. Recurrence was found in 48% of premenopausal patients and 80% of postmenopausal patients. Therefore, we do not recommend aspiration alone as treatment for an adnexal mass. Cystectomy, or, in appropriate cases, oophorectomy, allows complete removal of the cyst lining, which provides adequate tissue for pathologic analysis and prevents recurrence.

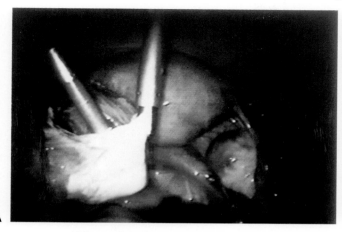

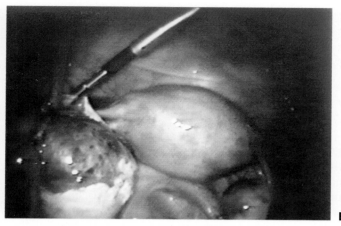

Figure 6-3 A, B. Ovarian cystectomy. The outer ovarian capsule is dissected away from the cyst wall with aquadissection.

Fenestration has been described as the removal of a window from the cyst wall. This allows pathologic analysis of a portion of the cyst wall and provides an opening in the cyst for drainage. Aspiration followed by fenestration of the cyst wall may be applicable when a cyst >5 cm, with benign ultrasound characteristics, is found in a premenopausal woman. Visualization of the entire cyst lining should also be performed in order to assess the cyst wall completely. If excrescences are found, they are biopsied and sent for immediate frozen section. Frank carcinoma or suspicious cells demand immediate staging laparotomy.

Procedure

The ovary is stabilized by grasping the utero-ovarian ligament with an atraumatic grasping forceps. The ligament is rotated laterally in order to bring the ovary into full view. A 1 cm avascular site on the cyst is chosen and the tissue blanched with the point endocoagulator at 120°, thus assuring hemostasis.

Using the 5-mm aspirating needle via a suprapubic trocar, the cyst is punctured and the contents aspirated with a syringe. The cyst wall is incised along the endocoagulated area with the endo-scissors. The irrigating instrument is used to fill the cyst with Ringer's lactate. The optics are then inserted inside the cyst and the lining is inspected for excrescences or solid parts. Suspicious areas should be biopsied and sent for frozen section. A 1 cm by 1 cm window of tissue is cut from the ovarian capsule with endo-scissors and the removed tissue is sent for pathologic analysis. This fenestration of the cyst wall, which allows drainage until the ovary heals, has been shown to decrease recurrence. The cyst lining is endocoagulated in its entirety with the point coagulator at 120°. This destroys the epithelium, thus decreasing the possibility of recurrence. The edges of the remaining cyst wall are endocoagulated to decrease bleeding and eliminate exposed raw surfaces.

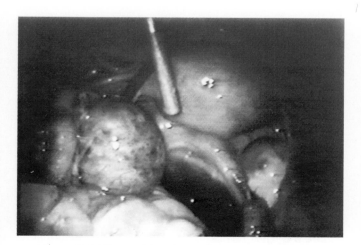

Figure 6-4 The cyst has been dissected entirely free.

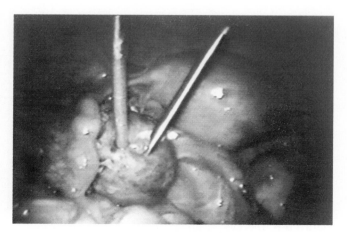

Figure 6-5 The cyst is incised with the hook scissors.

Cystectomy

This technique may be used for removal of dermoids, functional cysts, hemorrhagic cysts, and endometriomas.

Procedure

The utero-ovarian ligament is grasped with an atraumatic grasper and rotated laterally to expose the ovary. The antimesenteric portion of the ovarian capsule is then endocoagulated in a line approximately one half the length of the cyst. This provides an adequate avascular area through which the cyst may be removed.

Using an endo-scissors, the ovary is incised superficially along the endocoagulated area, exposing the cyst wall below. The edge of the ovarian capsule is grasped with a 5-mm grasping forceps. The irrigating instrument, attached either to a pump or a bag of Ringer's lactate within an inflated blood pressure cuff, is inserted between the cyst wall and the ovarian capsule. Using the high-pressure stream and the blunt edge of the instrument, the cyst is dissected away from the ovary. This technique is called aquadissection (Figure 6-3).

The cyst should be kept intact as long as possible, since this facilitates dissection. When the cyst is dissected to be as free as possible (Figures 6-4 and 6-5), or when it ruptures, it is emptied of its contents by repeated suction and irrigation until the effluent is clear (Figure 6-6). The cyst wall is then grasped with the 5-mm ovarian biopsy forceps and teased away from the ovarian capsule (Figure 6-7).

Dr. Semm has described a "hair curler" technique that we have found useful. The cyst is twisted around the grasping instrument repeatedly, which gently pulls the cyst wall away from the ovary (Figure 6-8). The cyst can then be removed intact from the abdominal cavity through a 5- or 11-mm suprapubic trocar (Figure 6-9). If necessary, the cyst may be

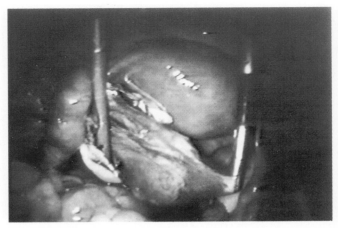

Figure 6-7 The decompressed cyst is teased away from the ovary.

grasped with claw forceps and the trocar sleeve slid out of the incision allowing more room for removal. If too large, the cyst may be bisected prior to removal.

Removal of dermoid cysts is often associated with spill of cyst contents, necessitating prolonged irrigation of the peritoneal cavity to prevent chemical peritonitis. Placing the cyst in an endo-bag as soon as feasible will help to limit spill of solid and sebaceous material contained within the cyst. The neck of the bag can be brought out of an 11-mm incision and the contents removed with suction and morcellation.

After removal, the cyst should be carefully inspected for papillations, septa, or thickening of the wall. If suspicious for malignancy, it should be sent for frozen section. If malignancy is found, the surgeon should proceed immediately with laparotomy. Excess ovarian tissue may be trimmed so that the edges of the ovary approximate each other (Figure 6-10). The internal portion of the ovary is then endocoagulated, with the

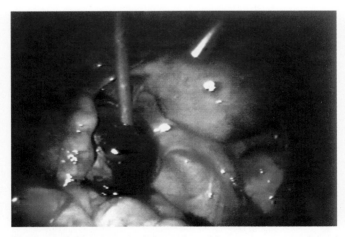

Figure 6-6 The cyst is irrigated and its contents suctioned from the cyst.

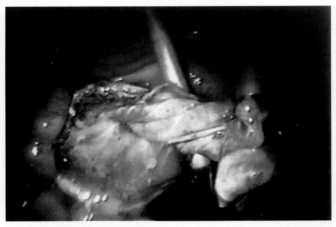

Figure 6-8 The "hair curler" technique is used to further remove the cyst.

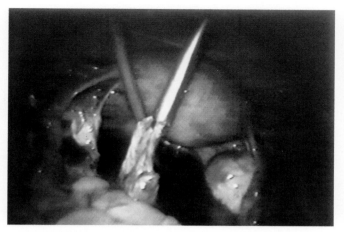

Figure 6-9 The cyst is removed through the 11-mm trocar sheath.

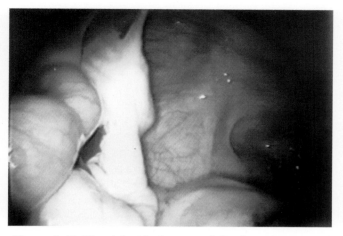

Figure 6-10 The defect in the ovary following cystectomy.

point endocoagulator at 120° for hemostasis (Figure 6-11). Bipolar desiccation is used for larger vessels. Endocoagulating the edges of the ovary causes them to invert and may decrease adhesion formation. There is some experimental evidence that suturing the ovary increases the likelihood of adhesions. Therefore, this is done only when the ovary can not be reapproximated by endocoagulation alone. We have found the intra-abdominal instrument tie with 4-0 Dexon to be most effective. As few sutures as possible are used.

The abdomen is copiously irrigated with Ringer's lactate. Suctioning of the sebacious material found in dermoid cysts is facilitated by warming the solution. This emulsifies the fat, allowing it to flow more freely through the suctioning instrument. Hair and other solid tissue is removed with the 11-mm spoon forceps. Care should be taken to irrigate both the upper abdomen and pelvis and to suction with the patient in the reverse Trendelenberg position. This avoids leaving debris in the peritoneal cavity, which might cause an inflammatory reaction. As many as 5 liters of fluid may be necessary for this final irrigation.

Salpingo-Oophorectomy

In premenopausal patients, laparoscopic salpingo-oophorectomy may be done in cases where the adnexa is not salvageable. In carefully selected postmenopausal patients, using the strict criteria described above, the adnexa should be removed for complete pathological diagnosis.

Procedure

An 11-mm trocar is placed in the suprapubic midline and a 5-mm trocar placed laterally on the side of the adnexa to be removed. Pelvic washings should be obtained and saved for staging should a malignancy be found. If

necessary, lysis of adhesions with the endo-scissors is done to free the adnexa. For safety, the ureter should be visualized near the infundibulopelvic ligament. If adhesions obscure the ureter, dissection of the ureter or isolation of the vessels away from the ureter should be accomplished.

If a cyst is present, needle aspiration is done carefully to reduce spill. The adnexa is then grasped with the 11-mm claw forceps and pulled medially to expose the infundibulopelvic ligament. The Endoloop is then inserted through the lateral 5-mm trocar. The claw is released and passed through the loop, and the adnexa is grasped and pulled medially again. The loop is then worked around the tube and ovary toward the infundibulopelvic ligament. If necessary, to place the loop properly, an atraumatic grasping instrument may be inserted through an additional contralateral 5-mm trocar. Three Endoloops, as per Semm, are placed, cinched down, and cut. Experimental evidence suggests that two pulls of ten seconds each gives maximum strength to

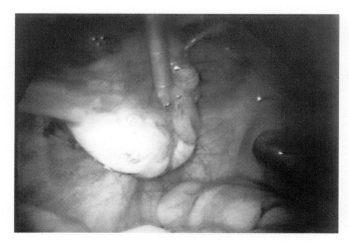

Figure 6-11 Good hemostasis has been obtained.

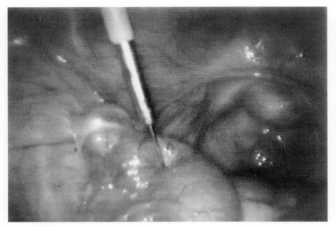

Figure 6-12 Salpingectomy for hydrosalpinx. The fluid is drained from the hydrosalpinx.

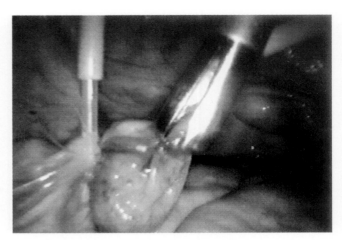

Figure 6-13 The decompressed hydrosalpinx is pulled medially while the Endoloop is applied.

the knot. Added pulls fray the suture, resulting in loss of tensile strength.

With the adnexa pulled medially with the 11-mm claw forceps, the 5-mm endo-scissors is passed throught the ipsilateral trocar so that the pedicle may be cut at a right angle to the vessels. Care should be taken to remove the entire ovary, while leaving enough of a pedicle to prevent slippage of the Endoloop. The adnexa is then removed via the 11-mm trocar, using the claw or spoon forceps. If necessary, it is bisected prior to removal. If inspection of the adnexa reveals suspicious areas, immediate frozen section is done. Frozen section is done for all postmenopausal women. In postmenopausal women, if the cyst is benign, consideration should be given to removing the contralateral ovary with the same technique. If malignancy is found, the pelvis should be filled with distilled water to lyse malignant cells and an immediate staging laparotomy done through a midline incision.

Oophorectomy

This technique may be employed when tubal preservation is desired or if the fallopian tube has been previously removed.

Procedure

Three Endoloops, as described above, are placed around the mesovarium and tightened. An additional instrument is used to hold the tube away from the loop, thus preventing inadvertent tubal injury. The ovary is separated from the pedicle with the endo-scissors. It may then be morcillated or bisected prior to removal through an 11-mm trocar sleeve.

Salpingectomy

Removal of the fallopian tube is indicated in patients with a large hydrosalpinx, an ectopic pregnancy with a diameter greater than 5 cm, or a ruptured ectopic pregnancy.

Procedure

The proximal portion of the tube, near the cornua, is endocoagulated with the crocodile endocoagulator and cut with the hook scissors. An Endoloop is then placed in this space, carried around the entire tube and cinched down (Figures 6-12, 6-13). The mesosalpinx, distal to the Endoloop, is then incised, taking care to leave an adequate pedicle (Figure 6-14). The incised tube is removed through the 5-mm trocar (Figures 6-15, 6-16).

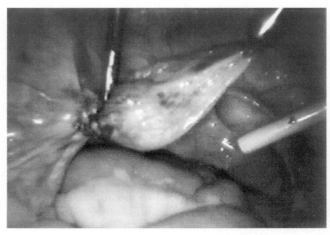

Figure 6-14 The tube is cut away from the secured pedicle.

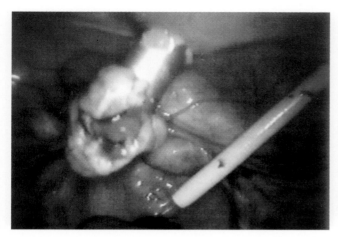

Figure 6-15 The tube is removed via the 11-mm trocar sheath.

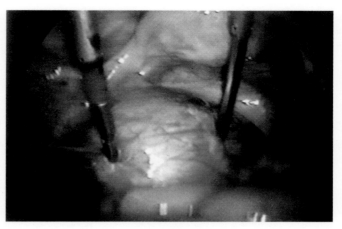

Figure 6-17 Paraovarian cystectomy. The peritoneum over the paraovarian cyst is endocoagulated.

Paratubal Cystectomy

Paratubal cysts, which are benign, are remnants of the Wolffian duct system. Removal may be considered to prevent future torsion.

Procedure

Paratubal cysts are usually on a pedicle, which facilitates removal. The pedicle is grasped and endocoagulated at 120° with the crocodile endocoagulator. The 5-mm endo-scissors are used to cut the pedicle. Aspiration of the cyst with the aspirating needle may be necessary to decompress the cyst and allow removal through the 5-mm trocar.

Retroperitoneal Paraovarian Cysts

Most commonly found in women of reproductive age, 2% of paraovarian cysts have been reported to be malignant. Strict ultrasound criteria, as used for ovarian masses above, should therefore be applied prior to surgery.

Procedure

The peritoneum over the cyst is endocoagulated until blanched and then incised with a hook scissors (Figures 6-17 and 6-18). Care is taken to stay away from the fimbriae of the fallopian tube, thus preventing inadvertent injury and postoperative adhesion formation. Aquadissection is used to separate the peritoneum from the underlying cyst wall. Aspiration, incision, and inspection of the cyst wall are then

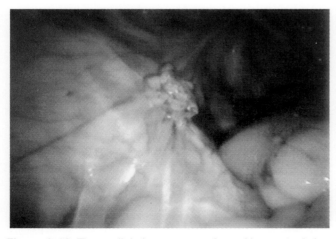

Figure 6-16 The pedicle is secure, and good hemostasis has been obtained.

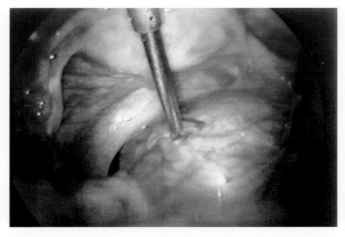

Figure 6-18 The hook scissors are used to incise the peritoneum overlying the cyst.

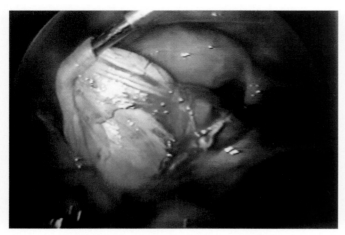

Figure 6-19 The hair curler technique is used to pull the cyst away from the retroperitoneal space.

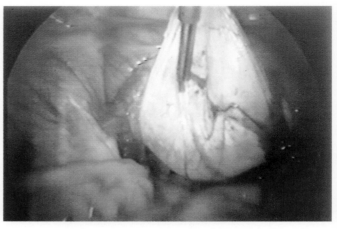

Figure 6-21 The cyst is incised with the hook scissors.

done as described above. The presence of papillations requires laparotomy.

The cyst is then removed by the hair curler technique (Figures 6-19, 6-20, 6-21, 6-22, and 6-23). It may be necessary to endocoagulate and excise adherent tissue near the base of the cyst prior to removal. The cyst is extracted through the 5-mm trocar and inspected (Figure 6-24). If any suspicious areas are seen, the specimen is sent for frozen section. Bleeding areas in the cyst bed are controlled with the endocoagulator. The peritoneal defect is left open.

Management of Adnexal Torsion

Patients with adnexal torsion present often with acute pain and the presence of a pelvic mass. Early laparoscopic intervention may offer the opportunity to untwist the adnexa prior to irreversible tissue damage. One study of 61

women treated with untwisting of a torsed adnexa, followed by conservative surgery, found excellent results and no evidence of postoperative embolism.

Procedure

A probe or grasping forceps may be used to untwist the adnexa. If observation reveals a return of circulation to the tissue, the adnexa may be preserved. Often, the torsion is the result of some pathology, (e.g., an ovarian or paratubal cyst), which should then be treated by the appropriate procedure. If the utero-ovarian ligaments appear too long, they may be shortened by triplicating them with an O-plain endosuture.

If the tissue is irreversibly damaged as evidenced by lack of circulation, it should be removed by the Endoloop technique as described above.

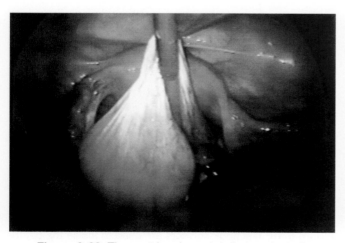

Figure 6-20 The cyst has been totally enucleated.

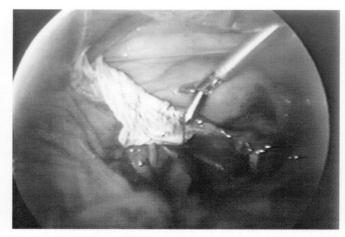

Figure 6-22 The collapsed cyst is teased away from the retroperitoneal space.

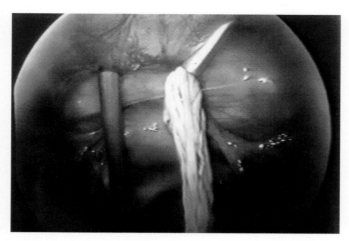

Figure 6-23 The cyst is removed via the 11-mm trocar sheath.

Minilaparotomy

In some cases, difficulty may be encountered during the procedure and it may be prudent to convert the operation to a minilaparotomy. A small, lower abdominal incision approximately 3 to 4 cm will provide enough room in most cases to complete the procedure. This is usually best accomplished by extending the suprapubic trocar incision. Some authors have described extending the infraumbilical incision for removal of tissue. We, however, have preferred colpotomy for this purpose. When done in a limited fashion, minilaparotomy is associated with only slightly greater morbidity and hospital stay than operative laparoscopy.

SUMMARY

Careful patient selection can choose patients who are appropriate for management of an adnexal mass via operative laparoscopy. Proper intraoperative assessment and liberal use of rapid frozen section are also important. Reported studies show that laparoscopic management can be safely performed. The short hospital stay and rapid return to normal activity benefit patient care. However, when invasive cancer is found at the time of surgery, the surgeon should be prepared to proceed with staging laparotomy for appropriate treatment.

SUGGESTED READING

Bouvier-Colle MH, Varnoux N, Breart G. Maternal deaths and substandard care: the results of a confidential survey in France. *Eur J Obstet Gynecol Reprod Biol* 1995;58:3–7.

Canis M, Mage G, Pouly J, Wattiez A, Manhes H, Bruhat M. Laparoscopic diagnosis of adnexal cystic masses: A twelve-year experience with long-term follow-up. *Obstet Gynecol* 1994;83:707–12.

Crane S, Chun B, Acker D. Treatment of hemorrhagic emergencies. *Curr Opin Obstet Gynecol* 1993;5:675–82.

Dembo A, Davy M, Stenwig A, Berle E, Bush R, Kjorstad K. Prognostic factors in patients with stage 1 epithelial ovarian cancer. *Obstet Gynecol* 1990;75:263–72.

Granberg S, Norstrom A, Wikland M. Tumors in the lower pelvis as imaged by vaginal sonography. *Gynecol Oncol* 1990;37:224–9.

Herrman U, Locher G, Goldhirsch A. Sonographic patterns of ovarian tumors: prediction of malignancy. *Obstet Gynecol* 1987;69:777–81.

Kurjak A, Predanic M, Kupesic-Urek S, Jukic S. Transvaginal color and pulsed Doppler assessment of adnexal tumor vascularity. *Gynecol Oncol* 1993;50:3–9.

Maiman M, Seltzer V, Boyce J. Laparoscopic excision of ovarian neoplasms subsequently found to be malignant. *Obstet Gynecol* 1991;77:563–5.

Neiman H, Mendelson E. Ultrasound evaluation of the ovary. In: Callen P, ed. *Ultrasonography in Obstetrics and Gynecology.* Philadelphia: WB Saunders; 1988:423–46.

Parker W, Levine R, Howard F, Sansone B, Berek J. Laparoscopic management of selected cystic adnexal masses in postmenopausal women: A multicentered study. *J Am Col Surg* 1994;179:733–7.

Parker W, Childers J, Canis M, Phillips D, Topel H. Laparoscopic management of benign cystic teratomas during pregnancy. *Am J Obstet Gynecol* (in press).

Reich H, McGlynn F. Treatment of ovarian endometriomas using laparoscopic surgical techniques. *J Repro Med* 1986;31:577–82.

Semm K. *Operative Manual for Endoscopic Abdominal Surgery.* Chicago: Year Book Medical Publishers; 1987.

Vasilev S, Schlaerth J, Campeau J, Morrow P. Serum CA-125 levels in preoperative evaluation of pelvic masses. *Obstet Gynecol* 1988;71:751–6.

Operative Laparoscopy, Second Edition
The Masters' Techniques in Gynecologic Surgery
Lippincott–Raven Publishers, Philadelphia © 1998.

7

Management of Adhesions via Laparoscopy

Anthony A. Luciano and Eugenio Solima

Peritoneal adhesions may give rise to bowel obstruction, pelvic pain and infertility. The adverse effects of postoperative adhesion formation on fertility potential following pelvic surgery have been recognized since 1935, when Stein and Leventhal reported the results of their classic studies on bilateral ovarian wedge resection for the treatment of infertility in patients with polycystic ovaries. Although normal ovulatory cycles were restored in 90% of patients, only 50% conceived successfully. Subsequent experience using microsurgical techniques reported similar results. Second-look laparoscopy of these patients revealed the presence of periovarian adhesions, which gave rise to mechanical infertility as well as hormonal dysfunction. Ovarian adhesions from previous ovarian surgery have been reported to give rise to compromise in ovarian responses to ovulation induction, luteal insufficiency, and luteinized unruptured follicle syndrome, as well as entrapped oocytes within luteinized, ruptured follicles (Figure 7-1).

Since one of the major determinants of the success of infertility surgery is postoperative adhesion formation, it is important for the gynecologic surgeon to understand the mechanism of adhesion formation, to implement optimal surgical techniques for adhesiolysis and to apply agents or devices appropriately that may reduce postoperative adhesion formation. In this manuscript, we review the pathophysiology of adhesion formation, the role of the various surgical tools, techniques and adjuvants that have been used in the management and prevention of pelvic adhesions, and describe our approach to laparoscopic adhesiolysis.

Adhesion Formation

Tissue trauma from infection, endometriosis or surgery results in the mobilization of the immunologic defenses that lead to the immediate formation of fibrinous attachments between adjoining structures covering the peritoneal defect. Normal fibrinolytic activity usually lyses these fibrinous attachments (fibrinous exudate), within 72 to 96 hours of the injury. Simultaneously, connective tissue cells carry on mesothelial repair so that within 5 days following injury a single cell layer of mesothelium covers the injured raw area, replacing the fibrinous exudate. However, if the fibrinolytic activity of the peritoneum is suppressed, fibroblasts will migrate, proliferate and form fibrous adhesions with collagen deposition and vascular proliferation.

The factors that suppress fibrinolytic activity and promote postoperative adhesion formation (Table 7-1), must be kept to a minimum by applying microsurgical principles, avoiding the use of reactive material (sutures) and by implementing hormonal manipulation and/or barriers with proven efficacy in reducing postoperative adhesion formation.

Unfortunately, even when used properly, adhesiolysis by microsurgical techniques is frequently followed by adhesion reformation as well as de novo adhesion formation. De novo adhesion formation is here defined as adhesions that were not present at the initial surgical procedure, but developed anew as a result of the surgical trauma itself. Adhesion reformation involves the reoccurrence of adhesions at the same anatomic sites, after they had been removed.

POSTOPERATIVE ADHESION FORMATION AND REFORMATION

Microsurgery connotes not only the use of magnification, but the whole concept of delicate surgery which embodies gentle handling and constant irrigation of tissues, meticulous hemostasis, the use of microsurgical instruments, fine sutures and precise tissue approximation. The discipline of microsurgery was specifically developed for the purpose of minimizing those factors that contribute to the development of postoperative adhesion formation and reformation. Although microsurgery has been successful in utero-tubal anastomosis, failures persist at disappointing rates, especially for distal tubal disease.

Hoping to provide infertile women with better pregnancy rates, newer and more sophisticated surgical tools and tech-

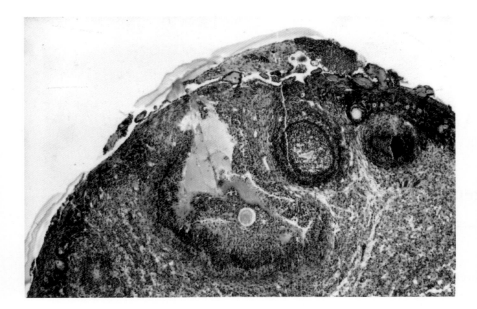

Figure 7-1 Photomicrograph of a luteinized "ruptured" follicle in which the oocyte has been trapped, presumably by the overlying adhesions. Notice the very thin layer of fibrous membrane (velamentous adhesions) covering the "stigma," suggesting that the microscopic adhesions prevented the release of the oocyte, thereby entrapping it within the luteinized follicle ($\times$40). (From Luciano AA, Marana R, Kratka S, Peluso JJ. Ovarian function after incision of the ovary by scalpel, CO_2 laser, and microelectrode. *Fertil Steril* 1991;56:349–53.)

niques have been introduced in our specialty, with varying degrees of acceptance and efficacy. The new tools involve various surgical lasers, and the new surgical technique involves the impressive expansion of operative endoscopy. The relative efficacy of these new developments will be discussed to define their role in gynecologic surgery.

Surgical Tools: Electrosurgery versus Lasers

For many years, the application of electrosurgery in operative laparoscopy had been limited to destructive rather than reconstructive procedures. The occurrence of unexpected complications, like bowel burns and ureteral injuries, kept the laparoscopic use of electrosurgery from popularity with reproductive surgeons, despite the fact that these complications are more often the result of faulty use of instrumentation than a flaw in the surgical theory itself. The introduction of the CO_2 laser in laparoscopic surgery during the late 1970s was met with great acceptance. However, like all innovations, the laser has had its strong advocates who have made glowing and sometimes unrealistic claims regarding its benefits, and its skeptics who have too quickly dismissed it as just another gimmick. Several authors have evaluated and compared thermal tissue injury, adhesion formation and healing patterns following scalpel, versus lasers and electrosurgery. Although variable results

Table 7-1 *Factors that contribute to adhesion formation*

Ischemia	Traction of Peritoneum
Drying of Serosal Surfaces	Instrumentation of Adnexae
Excessive Suturing	Prolonged Operating Time
Omental Patches	Blood Clots in Peritoneal Cavity

have been obtained, the general consensus is that thermal tissue injury is inversely proportional to the power density of the energy used, regardless of which laser or which electrical generator is delivering it. Moreover, when each surgical tool is optimally used, postoperative adhesion formation and healing patterns are similar. Therefore, although useful and versatile in adhesiolysis, lasers do not seem to have significant advantages over the more traditional microsurgical tools.

Surgical Techniques: Laparoscopy versus Laparotomy

The concomitant development of improved endoscopic instrumentation, optics and video systems, has allowed the gynecologic surgeon to perform progressively more complex operative procedures via laparoscopy for the treatment of pelvic disease, causing pain and/or infertility. Several animal and clinical studies have been conducted to evaluate and compare the efficacy of the laparoscopic treatment of pelvic disease versus laparotomy. In most cases, the results from the laparoscopic approach were equal to or better than those obtained by laparotomy.

The initial studies were conducted in laboratory animals, which were controlled and randomized. In the first study, by Filmar et al., a standardized injury was inflicted with sharp scissors on the uterine horn of rats, either by laparoscopy or by laparotomy. No significant difference in postoperative adhesion formation was found between the two surgical procedures, suggesting equal efficacy by laparoscopy and laparotomy. In the second study, Luciano et al. inflicted standardized injuries on the uterine horn and peritoneal surface of the abdominal wall of rabbits, with CO_2 laser delivered either by laparoscopy or laparotomy. Three weeks after the initial procedure, the animals with significant intra-abdominal adhesions were randomized to laser adhesiolysis either by laparoscopy or laparotomy. To ascertain that the injury was the same with both surgical procedures, similar power densities of the laser energy were used for both laparoscopy and laparotomy. With such power density (approximately 6,000 W/cm^2) the laser injury resulted in ablation of the full thickness of the antimesenteric uterine wall and excellent hemostasis by both laparoscopy and laparotomy.

After the initial procedure, when standardized injuries were inflicted on the uterine horn and peritoneal surface of the anterior abdominal wall, de novo adhesions were present in every rabbit that had undergone laparotomy but were totally absent in the laparoscopy group. These results are consistent with the observations, initially made a century ago by Von Dembrowski, and by Franz, and later confirmed by Ellis, who reported that peritoneal injury healed without adhesion formation when left untreated, as in our laparoscopy group. However, with ''meticulous repair'' or in association with tissue-drying, bleeding, or ischemia, significant adhesion formation follows peritoneal injury, as in our laparotomy group. These historical perspectives, which are summarized in Appendix 1, hold as true today as they did nearly a century ago when they were first published.

Postoperative adhesion reformation and the relative efficacy of adhesiolysis between the two surgical approaches were evaluated in the second part of these studies. Adhesiolysis by both techniques effectively reduced the intraperitoneal adhesion scores. However, a significantly greater reduction of intraperitoneal adhesions was accomplished by laparoscopy than by laparotomy (Figure 7-2; Table 7-2). Perhaps the most conclusive demonstration of the advantages of operative laparoscopy over laparotomy in postoperative adhesion formation and reformation was published by Lundorff et al. in patients with ectopic pregnancy. In this well-designed study, the authors stratified with regard to age and risk factors 105 women with ectopic pregnancy and

Table 7-2 *Mean (±SD) adhesion scores at all surgical sites, before and after laser adhesiolysis by laparoscopy versus laparotomy*

	Pre-lysis	Post-lysis	*p*[a]
Laparoscopy	2.8 + 0.1	0.9 + 0.4	*p* < 0.001
Laparotomy	2.6 + 0.3	1.8 + 0.6	*p*[a] = 0.04
p[a]	*p* > 0.05	*p* = 0.02	

[a] Wilcoxon signed test.

prospectively randomized them to surgery by either laparoscopy or laparotomy. Second-look laparoscopy revealed significantly more adhesions in the laparotomy than the laparoscopy group.

These well-controlled, prospectively-randomized studies demonstrate a major advantage of laparoscopic surgery over laparotomy in postoperative adhesion formation and reformation, and support the clinical reports in the literature that reproductive surgery by laparoscopy results in greater reduction of peritoneal adhesions and decreased de novo adhesion formation than when performed by laparotomy.

ADJUVANTS TO MINIMIZE ADHESION FORMATION/REFORMATION

Although the value of microsurgical techniques and endoscopy has been widely recognized, the benefits derived from medical adjuvants remain controversial, despite their widespread use by reproductive surgeons. The most commonly used agents aimed at preventing postoperative adhesion formation include:

- **Corticosteroids/Antihistamines** to inhibit fibroblast migration, to stabilize lysosomal membranes, and to decrease vascular permeability.
- **Antibiotics** to reduce the risk of infections.

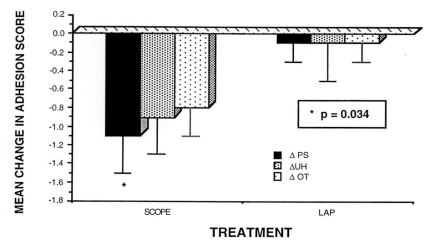

Figure 7-2 Changes in the mean (± SD) postoperative adhesion scores at the surgical and incidental sites following laser adhesiolysis by laparoscopy versus laparotomy. Δ PS = peritoneal surface; Δ UH = uterine horn; Δ OT = Other.

- **Nonsteroidal, anti-inflammatory agents** to decrease foreign body reaction.
- **Barriers (liquid or solid membranes)** to separate opposing peritoneal surfaces.
- **Hormonal manipulation** to induce a hypoestrogenemic and/or progestational milieu.

As yet, none have been found with the efficacy and the safety that is required for general acceptance. Hyskon is absorbed slowly from the peritoneal cavity, over a period of 7 to 10 days, during which time its osmotic effect draws sufficient fluid into the peritoneal cavity to float mobile, peritoneal organs, avoiding close contact and reducing adherence between intraperitoneal structures. Several studies, both in experimental animals and humans, have demonstrated therapeutic effects of Hyskon in postoperative adhesion reduction. However, inconsistent results have also been published, suggesting limited efficacy, with the more favorable effects being reported on the more dependent portions of the pelvis. Besides its questionable efficacy, reports of allergic reactions, infections, disseminated intravascular coagulation and complications of fluid overload, have tempered the use of Hyskon in reproductive surgery. The search for safer and more efficacious adjuvants continues.

Recent studies involving laboratory animals have found that the preoperative treatment with either medroxyprogesterone acetate (MPA) or GnRH-analogues (depo-Lupron) results in a significant reduction in postoperative adhesion reformation when compared to nontreated control animals. Both therapies are associated with gonadotropin suppression and hypoestrogenemia. However, MPA, which also has immunosuppressive and anti-inflammatory activity, was found to have significantly greater suppression of adhesion reformation than depo-Lupron.

Studies recently conducted on barrier methods, using either absorbable or nonabsorbable surgical membranes, also seem promising. The mechanism by which barriers may reduce adhesion formation relates at least in part to the physical separation of interposing peritoneal surfaces by preventing fibrous bands from binding different structures. In several prospectively randomized clinical studies, the application of Interceed (a new preparation of oxidized regenerated cellulose) was associated with significantly less adhesion reformation than the nontreated control side. Although the reformation of postoperative adhesions was not completely eliminated, it was reduced by 35% to 50% by Interceed in the majority of cases.

Gore-Tex (W. L. Gore and Associates, Inc., Flagstaff, AZ) is a nonabsorbable, nonreactive surgical membrane that has been used extensively for the repair and reconstruction of the pericardium or peritoneum where minimal adhesions are desired. Animal studies by Boyers et al. demonstrated that the Gore-Tex surgical membrane was effective in reducing primary adhesions following pelvic injuries. In a recent multicenter prospectively randomized study, uterine surgical incisions that resulted from multiple myomectomies were either covered with Gore-Tex membrane or left uncovered. At second-look laparoscopy 56.6% of the covered sites but only 7.6% of the uncovered sites were free of adhesions. The mean adhesion scores were significantly less for the Gore-Tex membrane group than the control [1.88 ± 0.46 vs 7.55 ± 57 ($p < 0.0001$)]. In a different study, the relative efficacy of reducing postoperative adhesion reformation by Gore-Tex membrane versus Interceed was tested in a multicenter randomized clinical trial. Although both barriers effectively decreased the mean adhesion scores, the patients randomized to the Gore-Tex membrane treatment had significantly lower adhesion scores [0.97 ± 0.30 vs 4.76 ± 0.61 ($p < 0.0001$)].

It appears from these studies that barrier methods, using either the absorbable Interceed or nonabsorbable Gore-Tex, are both safe and effective in the prevention or reduction of postoperative adhesion formation. It is our opinion that postoperative adhesions may be reduced significantly by:

- Utilizing a minimally invasive approach, such as laparoscopic microsurgery, to decrease the surgical trauma.
- Performing surgery in a hypoestrogenemic environment, following the preoperative administration of either MPA or GnRH-analogues.
- Using barriers, such as Interceed or Gore-Tex membranes, to separate interposing peritoneal surfaces and prevent them from adhering to each other.

Although we may never be able to achieve ''adhesion-free surgery,'' we may be able to keep them to a bare minimum by following microsurgical principles and the suggestions outlined above.

LAPAROSCOPIC ADHESIOLYSIS

To perform laparoscopic adhesiolysis adequately, a three-puncture technique is required in most cases; the intra-umbilical incision for the operative laparoscope and two suprapubic punctures, one on either quadrant. Seldom will two punctures be sufficient, and occasionally four punctures may be required, especially when there is a complete cul-de-sac obliteration (Figure 7-3). With the three-puncture technique, atraumatic grasping forceps are placed through the suprapubic port on the side of the assistant, to grasp the adhesion and stretch it to identify its boundaries and avascular planes. The opposite suprapubic port, on the side of the surgeon, should be used either for microscissors to cut or for the irrigator-aspirator to serve as a manipulator and as a backstop when the laser is used.

Adhesions should be cut close to the affected organ at both ends, and totally removed whenever possible. Vascular adhesions can be coagulated and ablated simultaneously with either lasers or microelectrodes. When scissors are used, the blood vessel should first be coagulated with bipolar current and subsequently severed with sharp scissors. We recommend a systematic approach whereby bowel ad-

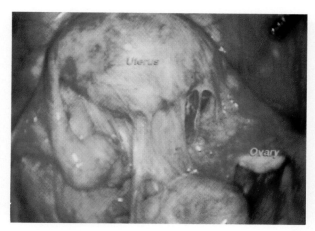

Figure 7-3 Complete cul-de-sac obliteration.

hesions are severed first, followed by adhesiolysis of the ovaries and then freeing the fallopian tubes. This approach allows for progressive exposure of the pelvic structures as the surgery unfolds. Once the bowel is freed from the uterus and adnexa, it can be gently pushed cephalad, away from the operative field, allowing for subsequent exposure of the uterus, ovaries, tubes and cul-de-sac. The ovaries are then freed from the pelvic sidewall or from the broad ligament. The grasping forceps are essential for applying traction on the ovary so that a plane of dissection can be identified and cut. Bleeders are immediately coagulated with laser or bipolar energy, so that one's vision is never compromised by a bloody operative field. Whenever possible, either the adhesions or ovarian ligaments should be grasped instead of the ovarian cortex to reduce trauma to ovarian tissue. Once the ovaries are lifted from the cul-de-sac and completely freed, the ipsilateral fallopian tube is relieved of adhesions throughout its length.

Adhesions can be effectively coagulated and incised with either carbon dioxide laser, superpulse or ultrapulse ($\geq$ 25 w), fiber lasers (15–20 W), or microelectrode (15–20 watts cutting mode). When there are dense, cohesive adhesions among different organs (bowel, uterus, adnexa or pelvic side walls), hydrodissection with the suction irrigator probe is useful in creating tissue planes before dissection.

Once the pelvic structures are freed and hemostasis is successfully achieved, the cul-de-sac is filled with fluid (Ringer's lactate) and the adnexae are allowed to float in the clear fluid. Filmy adhesions which are usually difficult to identify on the surface of the ovary will be clearly visible, as they float away from the ovarian cortex in the water (Figure 7-4). These adhesions can now be grasped with the forceps, sharply cut and removed from their attachments, preferably using laparoscopic microscissors (Figure 7-5), since they are generally filmy and avascular coagulation is not required. Under fluid, because of excellent visualization, microsurgical adhesiolysis with sharp scissors can be precise, effective and totally atraumatic; only the floating filmy adhesions will be grasped (manipulated) and resected.

Fimbrioplasty, where the fimbrial folds are agglutinated by fine avascular adhesions without tubal obstruction, is also best performed under fluid (Figure 7-6). As the fimbrial folds float and disperse in the water, the adhesions between them become clearly visible and are grasped, stretched, and sharply cut with fine scissors. The laser beam delivered through the laparoscope is 0.5 to 1 mm in diameter, which is too wide for these narrow bands of adhesions and frequently injures the involved fimbrial folds. Similar thermal damage may be inflicted with electricity and to a greater extent with the fiber lasers (YAG, KTP or argon). Thus, for the most delicate microscopic procedure of fimbriolysis and salpingo-ovariolysis, the laparoscopic microscissors work best in our hands. Fol-

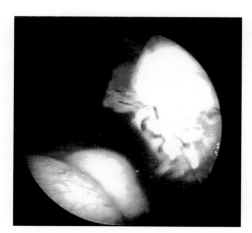

Figure 7-4 By filling the pelvis with fluid, filmy adhesions covering the adnexa (ovary in figure) float away from the ovarian surface and are easily visualized. These filmy adhesions must be removed to prevent entrapment of oocytes, as illustrated.

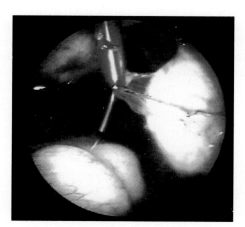

Figure 7-5 Floating adhesions are easily grasped, stretched with forceps and subsequently resected from their attached ovarian surfaces using scissors. The isolated bands of adhesions are removed from the peritoneal cavity.

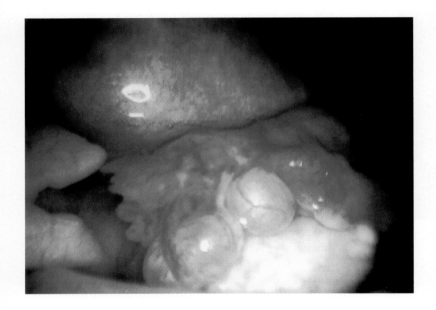

Figure 7-6 Hydroflotation of the tube and fimbria allows for better detection of fimbrial adhesions.

lowing adhesiolysis, pregnancy rates vary according to the extent of adnexal damage and, to a lesser degree, according to the severity of the adhesions.

CONCLUSION

Postoperative adhesion formation continues to be the ''bogey'' of the reproductive surgeon. Although significant progress has been made toward understanding the pathophysiology of postoperative adhesion formation, our efforts at their prevention by the use of medical adjuvants, barriers, and microsurgery, have only improved but not eliminated the problem. Until we discover the ideal adjuvant, which should prevent adhesions without impeding healing or inducing adverse effects, the reproductive surgeon must continue to rely on the time-honored microsurgical principles outlined above. Given the recent data from both animal studies, and clinical reports that operative laparoscopy is more effective than laparotomy in reducing peritoneal adhesion formation and reformation, we may conclude that when possible, adhesiolysis and most benign gynecologic surgical procedures may best be performed by the minimally invasive approach of laparoscopic microsurgery.

SUGGESTED READING

DiZerega GSD, Holtz G. Cause and prevention of postsurgical pelvic adhesions. In: Osofsky, H., ed. *Advances in Clinical Obstetrics and Gynecology,* Williams and Wilkins; Baltimore, MD: 1982:277–89.

Diamond MP, DeCherney AH. Pathogenesis of adhesion formation/reformation: application to reproductive surgery. *Microsurgery* 1987; 8:103–7.

Luciano AA. Prevention of postoperative adhesions in endometriosis-advanced management and surgical techniques. Nezhat CR, Berger GS, Nezhat FR, Buttram VC, Nezhat CH, eds. New York: Springer-Verlag Inc.; 1996:193–9.

Luciano AA, Hauser KS, Benda J. Evaluation of commonly used adjuvants in the prevention of postoperative adhesions. *Am J Obstet Gynecol* 1983;146:88–92.

Luciano AA, Maier DB, Koch EI, Nulsen JC, Whitman GF. A comparative study of postoperative adhesions following laser surgery by laparoscopy versus laparotomy in the rabbit model. *Obstet Gynecol* 1989;74:220–4.

Lundorff P, Hahlin M, Kallfelt B, Thorburn J, Lindblom B. Adhesion formation after laparoscopic surgery in tubal pregnancy: a randomized trial versus laparotomy. *Fertil Steril* 1991;55:911–15.

Montanino-Oliva M, Metzger DA, Luciano AA. Use of medroxiprogesterone acetate in the prevention of postoperative adhesions. *Fertil Steril* 1996;65:650–4.

Tulandi T. Salpingo-ovariolysis: a comparison between laser surgery and electrosurgery. *Fertil Steril* 1986;45:489.

APPENDIX 7-A

Historical Perspective of Peritoneal Adhesions: List of Major Articles

Von Dembrowski T. Peritoneal defects in dogs heal mostly without adhesions. *Arch Klin Chir* 1898;37:745; Franz K. *Geburtshilfe Gynaekol* 1902;47:64.

Benzi and Boeri. Ischemia is a major etiologic factor in adhesion formation. *Berl Klin Wochenschr* 1903;40:773.

Thomas J. et al. Oversewing serosal defects increase rather than decrease adhesion formation. *Proc Soc Exp Biol Med* 1950; 74:497.

Ellis H. Excision of parietal peritoneum from rats healed without adhesion formation in 52/58 experiments. But ''meticulous'' repair of peritoneal defects resulted in fibrous adhesions in 16/19 experiments. *Surg Gynecol Obstet* 1971;133:497.

Ryan et al. The combination of tissue drying and bleeding is a major promoter of adhesion formation. *Am J Path* 1971; 65:117–48.

Luciano et al. Postoperative adhesion formation and reformation occur much more frequently when surgery is performed by laparotomy than by laparoscopy. *Obstet Gynecol* 1989;74:220–4.

Operative Laparoscopy, Second Edition
The Masters' Techniques in Gynecologic Surgery
Lippincott–Raven Publishers, Philadelphia © 1998.

8

Abdominal Intrauterine Device Removal

Richard M. Soderstrom

Though the use of intrauterine devices (IUDs) has dropped substantially since the 1970s, a steady resurgence of IUD use has been noted in the 1990s. At one time it was suggested that intraabdominal IUDs could be declared ''asymptomatic'' and need not be removed. With experience, complications became apparent; today patients should be offered the opportunity of surgical removal. In particular, copper-containing IUDs cause a severe reaction once they find their way into the peritoneal cavity. Though the progesterone-containing IUD is not irritative, spontaneous bowel perforation from inert IUDs left within the abdominal cavity has been reported.

With few exceptions, intraabdominal IUDs can be located and removed by operative laparoscopists. It was once thought that ultrasound examinations could identify the ''wandering IUD.'' It was soon learned that an IUD outside of the uterus could easily be missed. Therefore, it is recommended that imaging studies used to search for intraabdominal IUDs should be limited to full abdominal anteroposterior (AP) and lateral radiographic explorations. It is sometimes helpful to insert a radiopaque substance or object into the uterus as a reference point when the radiographs are taken. This can easily be accomplished by giving the patient a paracervical block and inserting a sound or radiopaque dye in the uterus, as one does for a hysterosalpingogram (Figures 8-1, 8-2).

In cases where partial perforation is suspected, office hysteroscopy may solve the problem. If, however, the cavity is empty and the radiograph confirms an intraabdominal IUD, operative laparoscopy should be scheduled. Though any of the laparoscopic equipment can be used, it is helpful to use an operative laparoscope. With this combination, the IUD, once free of its adhesions and ready for retrieval, can be removed through the laparoscopic trocar sleeve, after securing the IUD with the grasper, removing the grasper, the IUD, and the laparoscope as a unit from the trocar sleeve.

Remember that intraabdominal IUDs are frequently embedded in the omentum. If the abdominal radiograph

series was performed with the patient flat and you place the patient on the operating table in Trendelenburg position, the omentum will fall into the upper abdomen, making a search for the IUD more difficult. On occasion, if the IUD cannot be seen through a standard laparoscopic search, be prepared to take an abdominal AP and lateral film while in the operating room. Leave the *metal* trocar sleeves in place as the x-ray film is exposed. This gives one a good spatial reference, improving accuracy in locating the intraabdominal IUD.

As previously mentioned, copper IUDs cause a profound tissue reaction and may be difficult to dissect away from their attachment. Here, the multiple-trocar approach may be the only way of dissecting the IUD free. If an operating laparoscope is not available, it is not difficult to push the IUD, with a secondary accessory grasping instrument, up into the main laparoscopic trocar sleeve, on out past the trocar for easy removal.

My colleagues and I have removed 99 intraabdominal IUDs since 1970. Aerobic and anaerobic cultures were done on 20 of these IUDs, revealing contamination with anaerobic bacteria in 10 cases. It would seem prudent, therefore, to give prophylactic antibiotics for patients undergoing laparoscopic removal of intraabdominal IUDs.

CONCLUSION

As long as IUDs are used for contraception, on occasion uterine perforation will occur. Today the hysteroscope plays a new role in the diagnosis of the ''wandering IUD'' and in many patients will prevent the need for further endoscopic exploration if only the string is lost or if only partial perforation occurs. Contamination of the intraabdominal IUD, which occurs at the time of insertion, can often be contained by normal intraabdominal inflammatory responses, which lead to adhesion formation. However, these

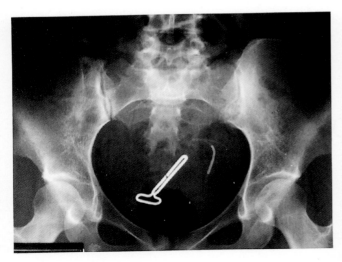

Figure 8-1 A posteroanterior lateral view of an intraabdominal copper IUD. A sterile metal marker lies within the uterine cavity.

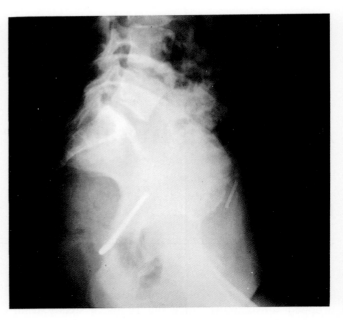

Figure 8-2 A lateral view revealing that the copper IUD is located anterior to the uterus.

same bacteria can and do survive in their inflammatory cocoon until host resistance is altered. On rare occasion, viscus perforation by intraabdominal IUDs has occurred. Laparoscopic retrieval of intraabdominal IUDs has proven to be remarkably safe when performed by the experienced operator. Compared to laparotomy for IUD removal, it is far safer and speeds recovery to perform laparoscopy. All intraabdominal IUDs, symptomatic or asymptomatic, should be removed by a laparoscopist experienced in operative laparoscopy.

SUGGESTED READING

Safety of intrauterine contraceptive devices symposium. *Infectious and Medical Disease Letters for Obstetrics and Gynecology.* 1989;11.

Soderstrom RM. IUD perforation—What to do? *Infect Dis & Gynecol* 1989;11:109–111.

Operative Laparoscopy, Second Edition
The Masters' Techniques in Gynecologic Surgery
Lippincott–Raven Publishers, Philadelphia © 1998.

9

Suturing and Ligation

Ronald L. Levine and Resad P. Pasic

Many operations that have traditionally been performed by laparotomy now may be primarily accomplished by laparoscopy, and some of the procedures may require the utilization of laparoscopic suturing. Laparoscopic ligation and suturing is used for approximation of tissue planes, and it is an effective way of providing hemostasis and preventing arterial hemorrhage in laparoscopic surgery.

The adaptation of tissue and suturing for hemostasis and reformation of anatomic structures has been considered one of the most demanding of endoscopic technical skills. The need for techniques to repair defects created by laparoscopic surgery has long been recognized. Endoscopic procedures are performed by looking at a bidimensional TV screen with up to 6 times magnification, eliminating depth perception and the tactile feeling of the tissue; this requires significant hand-eye coordination. Operative laparoscopy frequently creates large open areas that may necessitate closure. Defects can occur from removal of leiomyomas and large ovarian cysts and from lymph node dissection. The use of endoscopic suturing has been described in repair of inguinal hernias, uterine suspension, bladder suspension, pelvic reconstruction, and appendectomy. In the hands of the most expert operative endoscopists, even repair of the bowel and bladder has been described. At times, suturing, but most often ligation, is used for hemostasis. The advanced endoscopic procedures will require the laparoscopic surgeon to master suturing and learn techniques which will add to his level of comfort and performance. Each surgeon performing laparoscopic procedures should be thoroughly familiar with basic principles of suturing and instrumentation, and the limitations of this technique.

Aside from the usual laparoscopic equipment and instruments, for laparoscopic suturing you need the following instruments:

- laparoscopic needle holders
- laparoscopic graspers
- knot pusher
- laparoscopic scissors
- ligatures and sutures

INSTRUMENTS

The surgeon must be familiar with different suturing instruments and their capabilities and limitations before engaging in clinical suturing.

The primary purpose of needle holders is to hold the needle securely, not allowing it to slip, while placing the endoscopic stitch. Two important features of each needle driver are the handle and the jaw mechanism. The handles vary in shape, size, and the orientation of the handle to the shaft. The handle can be aligned in the same axes with the shaft, or it can be in an offset position. The in-line handles are ergonomically designed and may be easier to use. Most needle drivers also have some kind of locking mechanism that keeps the jaws closed, fixing the needle in place. The jaws of the instrument are the most important feature: they can be standard articulating alligator-jaws or spring-loaded, side-loading fixed jaws, or they can be magnetic to facilitate easier needle handling (Helmed Corporation, South, Easton, MA.) The Wisap needle holder has a round handle that permits suturing in any angle and also has a positive grip; i.e., the stronger one's grasp on the handle, the stronger is the grip on the needle. The Levine needle holder has a positive grip. The jaws have a notch that holds the needle in correct orientation not allowing the needle to slip. The Cook handle is spring-loaded and has a hook-held end that pulls into a sleeve, thus securing the needle. This type of hook-end needle holder is superior in driving a needle through tissue, particularly if the tissue is thick, as may be found in repairing the myometrium during a myomectomy, or placing sutures through Cooper's ligament. The disadvantage of a fixed locking jaw as opposed to grasping mechanisms with standard articulating jaws, is that the spring is very stiff, and the needle can be loaded at only one angle. This type of instrument will not allow instrument-tying and suture-grasping. Different types of needle holders are presented in Figure 9-1.

A variety of graspers are available to be used for tissue manipulation and stabilization during laparoscopic procedures. They come in different shapes and lengths and are divided into two categories: atraumatic and traumatic. Atraumatic graspers produce no tissue injury, while traumatic instrumentation can cause tissue injury where applied. Graspers can be used for tissue stabilization, needle holding or internal knot tying.

In 1972, Dr. H. Courtenay Clarke reported on instruments for suturing and ligating endoscopically. He described a ligator that could be used to push a knot into place. Having used this technique frequently, we think that it is one of the easiest methods of knot placement to master. One may use the Clarke-Reich Ligator (Marlow Surgical Technologies, Inc., Willoughby, OH) or a simple pusher of the slot type (Levine Knotguide, Resnick Instrument Co., Skokie, IL) (Figure 9-2). The Clarke-type ligator is less likely to lose the suture during the push; however, we have used both instruments.

Scissors are used for tissue dissection and suture-cutting. Care must be taken to keep the blades sharp. We use semi-disposable scissors (Marlow Surgical Technologies, Inc., Willoughby, OH) quite often, because they are sharp and

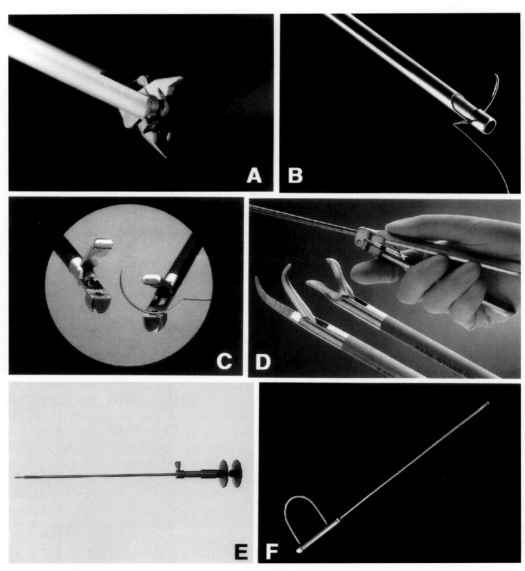

Figure 9-1 Needle holders. **A.** Diamond jaws of Levine needle holder **B.** Side-loading fixed jaws of Cook needle holder. **C.** Magnetic jaws of MAG needle driver. **D.** Standard articulating jaws and inline handle of Stortz needle holder. **E.** Handle of the Wisap needle holder. **F.** Spring-loaded handle of the Cook needle holder.

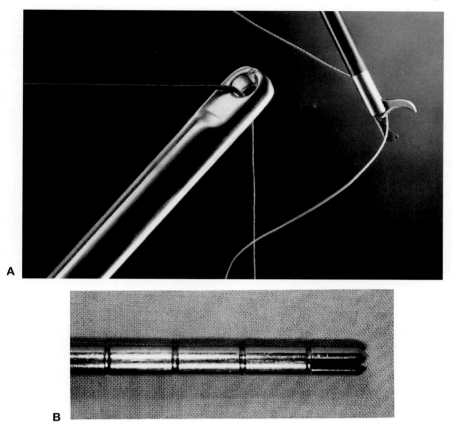

Figure 9-2 Knot pushers. **A.** The Clark-Reich ligator. This is an enlarged view of the end of the ligator. Instrument may be either a 3-mm or a 5-mm size. Each throw of the knot can be pushed with little effort. (Courtesy of Marlow Surgical Technologies, Inc., Willoughby, OH.) **B.** The Levine Knot Guide is a 3-mm or 5-mm rod with 1-cm markings and a slotted end. It can be used to slide a knot into place, but is mainly used to guide the loop ligature into place. (Courtesy of Resnick Instrument, Inc., Skokie, IL.)

can be used in combination with monopolar current, and the blades can be rotated.

Three basic steps in laparoscopic suturing are:

1. Introduction of the needle and suture into the abdominal cavity.
2. Placement of the suture ligature.
3. Knot tying, which can be intra corporeal or extracorporeal.

When performing laparoscopic suturing and knot-tying a two-handed manipulation is necessary, requiring an assistant to hold the camera and laparoscope and to stabilize the laparoscopic ports. A zero degree laparoscope should be used to permit a direct view. Proper placement of ancillary trocars is imperative for optimal suturing and knot tying. The instrument ports should not be too close to one another, and they must be positioned to ensure that the working tips of the instruments meet in the operative field at oblique angles to one another. The tips of the instruments must be in front of the laparoscope, and should enter the field of view tangentially, rather than along the shaft of the lapa-

roscope, in order to prevent obscuring the operative field. Therefore, four ancillary 5-mm ports are optimal, of which the lower two are placed lateral to the deep inferior epigastric vessels, and the upper two are placed lateral to the rectus muscle at the level of the umbilicus.

Laparoscopic surgeries can be performed using 5-mm trocar sleeves, but many surgeons use 10/11 disposable trocars, or if a linear stapler-cutter is to be used, a 12-mm trocar may be selected. Positions of the secondary puncture sites vary depending on the anticipated surgical procedure.

INTRAABDOMINAL NEEDLE INTRODUCTION

For laparoscopic surgery, the same principles of suture choice and suturing materials are applied as for conventional surgery. A majority of surgeons use CT-1, CT-2, HS or ski needles, since they can be introduced into the peritoneal cavity through 10/11 trocar sleeves. If extracorporeal knot tying is to be utilized, a long ligature thread of 70 cm should be used. If an intracorporeal technique is utilized, the preferable ligature length is 10 to 12 cm. Under no circumstances should a pop-off needle be used for laparoscopic suturing, since the needle can easily be lost in the abdomen. The CT-1 or CT-2 needle can be introduced into the peritoneal cavity through a 10/11 trocar sleeve by grasping the suture near the needle hub with a 5-mm grasper and introducing it into the peritoneal cavity.

Dr. Harry Reich's technique—putting any size of curved needle into the abdominal cavity—utilizes a 5-mm lower quadrant trocar placement. A needle holder or grasper is inserted through the trocar sleeve, after withdrawing it from the abdominal wall. The suture end is grasped and backloaded into the sleeve, and the suture regrasped about 3 to 4 cm away from the needle hub, then reinserted into the peritoneal cavity through the same incision. The trocar sleeve is then pushed over the grasper, using it as a guide to seal the incision in the abdominal wall (Figure 9-3). After the suturing is completed, it is important that the needle should be tagged to the anterior abdominal wall, and the suture cut about 2 to 3 cm away from the needle. The suture is then grasped and brought out through the same port for extracorporeal knot tying. The needle is subsequently removed from the peritoneal cavity by grasping the suture about 2 cm away from the needle and pulling it together with the 5-mm cannula, or extracting it through a 10/11 trocar sleeve. A potential complication of this method is the risk of losing the needle in the abdominal wall, and surgeons should have practiced the method on laboratory trainers and animal models before using it on patients.

LIGATURE PLACEMENT

Loop Ligature

Some closures are amenable to the use of a loop ligature. The loop ligature originally was demonstrated by Dr. Kurt Semm and was based on the Roeder Loop. The originally described ligature continues to be the one most commonly in use; it is made of chromic gut and has a preformed loop. Ligatures are now available that are composed of synthetic absorbable material that has low tissue reactivity. Although it is desirable to have little tissue reaction, some loops are slightly more difficult to use, because the material is more

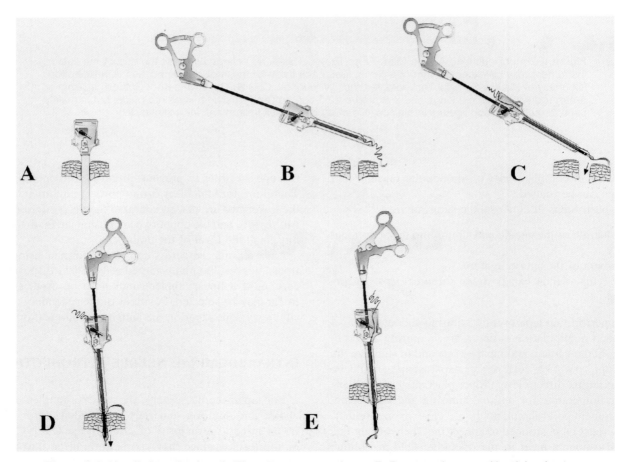

Figure 9-3 Needle introduction. **A.** Place 5 mm trocar sleeve. **B.** Remove sleeve and back load suture. **C.** Grasp suture 2–3 cm from the needle. **D.** Reintroduce the needle holder back through the original incision. **E.** The sleeve is pushed over the needle holder. **F.** Ready for suturing.

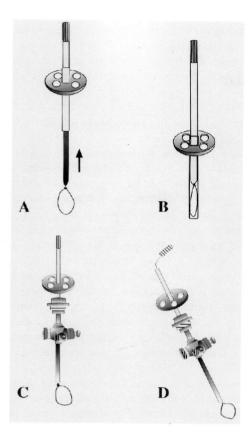

Figure 9-4 Endoloop placement. **A.** Roeder loop is loaded into the applicator from below. **B.** The loop is inside the applicator. **C.** Applicator is introduced through the sleeve. **D.** Plastic end of the loop is broken and pulled back, tightening the loop.

pliable and the loop is less formed. The loop is closed when the distal portion is pulled while pushing the knot into place with the plastic slide. Ligation with the preformed loop has certain limitations, since it is restricted to open-ended pedicles and utilizes a slip knot which may be prone to slipping, and requires a special introducer.

The loop ligature is backloaded into a hollow 3-mm tube called an applicator. The tube is then placed through a 5-mm trocar sheath. The edges of the tissue to be coapted, such as the capsule of an ovarian cyst, are then grasped through the loop with an appropriate instrument, and the loop is tightened. This is the simplest way to close this type of defect; however, it may be more likely to produce adhesions. Most often it is not necessary to close an ovarian capsule, as it frequently just falls together. If prepackaged loop ligature is not available, a loop can be improvised by tying a Roeder knot extracorporeally, and using a suture applicator to push the knot into the abdominal cavity (Figure 9-4).

Stitch Ligature

Often the endoscopic surgeon is faced with a situation in which it is not technically possible to use the Endoloop and

a suture must be placed with a needle in the traditional manner. Laparoscopic suturing may also be used to close a uterine defect after myomectomy, or in urogynecologic surgery. To place laparoscopic stitch ligatures, a grasper and a needle holder should be used. The grasper is used to load the needle into the needle driver, and to hold the tissue being sutured. Often it is pushed against the tissue to create a counter force while the needle is driven from the other side, and the grasper is also used to help grasp the needle from the needle holder after it is through the tissue. To attain this objective, the suture is grasped by the needle hub, while the needle holder, driven by dominant hand, is grasping the needle. The needle holder is used to drive the needle through the tissue being sutured. It holds the needle at a 90° angle to the needle holder shaft; therefore the needle may rotate around an axis perpendicular to the instrument shaft. Due to the restricted instrument mobility in laparoscopic surgery, passing the needle through a tissue is often limited by the trocar placement to a single rotating movement around the axis of the needle holder. Because of these limitations, it is crucial that the needle holder secure a firm grip onto the needle to avoid needle displacement and rotation in the needle holder's jaws. This is one advantage of the Levine needle holder.

An important principle of endoscopic suturing is to approach the tissue as close to 90° as possible, which makes the line of suture parallel to the shaft of the needle holder. If the surgeon is right-handed, the suture should be placed from right to left in a rotating motion (Figure 9-5). Once the needle is passed through the tissue, the ligature is fed around the pedicle with the help of a grasper which is introduced through the second sleeve. The needle is grasped

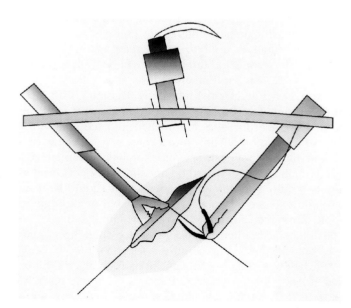

Figure 9-5 Ligature placement. The needle is at 90° angle to the wound. The needle is rotated around the axis parallel to the needle holder while the grasper holds the tissue.

with the needle holder and brought out of the peritoneal cavity through the same trocar sleeve where it was originally introduced. While the suture is drawn out of the abdomen, the rest of the ligature should be simultaneously fed into the peritoneal cavity to prevent pulling or sawing on the pedicle. Once both ends of the suture are secured, the extracorporeal knot can be tied.

KNOT TYING

Secure knot formation is essential to laparoscopic suturing procedures. Knot tying can be divided into two general categories: intracorporeal knots that are tied inside the abdominal cavity using laparoscopic instruments, and extracorporeal knots formed outside of the body and pushed into the peritoneal cavity through the trocar sleeve by the knot pusher. Both techniques are safe and reliable and can be used in different clinical situations, although the extracorporeal technique is used more often.

Extracorporeal Knots

Frequently we prefer to use an external knot technique. External knot tying does not require as much skill; however, it usually does require some extra instrumentation in the form of a "pusher" to slide the knot into place. Dr. Courtenay Clarke described the technique of extracorporeal surgical knot tying and developed the knot pusher that could be used to push the knot into place. According to this technique, a single throw is made extracorporeally and is pushed into the abdomen using the knot pusher thus forming a knot, similar to the knots performed during open surgery. The knot is advanced onto the pedicle, and tightened by holding and maintaining the constant tension on both ends of the suture with one hand. The other hand is used to apply traction on the knot pusher. The second and third throw can be used to secure the first knot. If monofilament sutures like Polyglyconate (Maxon, Davis and Geck Endoscopy, Danbury, CT), PDS or Polypropylene (Prolene) are used, a surgical knot can be tied extracorporeally and pushed into the abdominal cavity. The knot pusher sometimes may become dislodged during knot pushing, since some polyfilament materials such as silk or catgut do not slide easily. This technique is quite simple and reliable, but it should be used through a sleeve without a trumpet valve or through an applicator, since a trumpet valve may damage the suture. The assistant should prevent a gas leak by placing a finger over the suture exit site (Figure 9-6).

If a 10/11 cannula is used, an extracorporeal knot can be tied utilizing the laparoscopic Babcock grasper to push the knot. In this technique, a single throw is tied extracorporeally and the suture ends are passed outside in through the fenestrations at the tip of the Babcock grasper. The ends of the suture are held together in one hand and the grasper is passed through the trocar sleeve into the peritoneal cavity, thus driving the knot into place. When the knot is advanced to the pedicle, the Babcock tips are opened, applying additional tension to set the knot (Figure 9-7). Additional knots may be placed on top of it for security.

The Roeder knot, or external fisherman's knot, can be tied extracorporeally and passed into the peritoneal cavity with the help of a threaded plastic knot pusher or notched knot pusher. One trick we use is to load a plastic pusher with either 2-0 or 0 synthetic suture. The suture is loaded into the sterile plastic pusher by passing a 2-0 orthopedic-type wire into the pusher. A loop is formed on one end, and the suture is placed through the loop and then pulled back through the pusher. In this fashion we can quickly load a suture and then pass the needle as previously described, suture the tissue, and then make an external fisherman's knot and slide it into place (Figure 9-8). The advantage of this technique is that only one knot is necessary to secure the pedicles. There are many prepackaged products on the market that include suture with the knot pusher and the applicator such as Endoknot Suture (Ethicon Inc., Somerville N.J.). The disadvantage of this knot is that it is a sliding knot which may be subject to possible slippage; therefore 2 or 3 stitches may be placed over possible bleeding site. If an extracorporeal knot is tied, the slipping strength of the Roeder knot can be increased by adding a simple half throw intracorporeally to the knot, after the loop has been applied.

Intracorporeal Knots

The laparoscopic surgeon may choose to tie knots intraperitoneally. This technique involves instrument tying and requires a great deal of skill and patience. Intracorporeal knots are most often used for tissue fixation, and less often for hemostasis, since they cannot be tied with the same strength as extracorporeal knots. They are also used for anchoring a running suture, such as used for peritoneal closure, repair of bladder lacerations, or on tissue that is more likely to tear if tension is applied. For intracorporeal knot tying, a short ligature of about 10 to 14 cm is used, unless a running suture is placed, in which case a longer ligature is required. If the suture is too long, it can be very difficult to control the knot formation and potential for creating iatrogenic injuries may increase. The suture is passed into the peritoneal cavity as described above, and, following the suture placement, an instrument tie is performed within the peritoneal cavity. There are two types of intracorporeal knot tying: the classic tying which is similar to the technique used in microsurgery, a procedure more difficult to perform in the video-endoscopic setting, and the twist technique, which is somehow easier to perform with laparoscopic instruments.

Square Knot (Classic Knot)

The square knot is a series of two half hitches, where the second is formed on top of the first but in the opposite

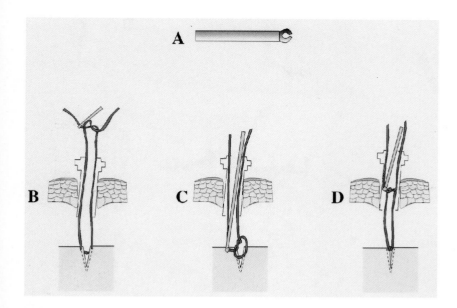

Figure 9-6 Extracorporeal knot. **A.** Clarke knot pusher. **B.** Simple knot is tied extra corporeally. **C.** Knot pusher is holding the knot and pushing it through the sleeve. **D.** Second knot is advanced in the same fashion.

direction. This knot is tied utilizing the classic microsurgical technique of instrument tying. After the needle is passed through the tissue, the suture is pulled almost all the way through, leaving only 1 to 2 cm of the suture tail at the site of the needle insertion. The long tail of the suture is grasped with the needle holder and rotated counterclockwise, forming the loop around the distal end of the grasper. Holding the jaws of the grasper open may help prevent slipping of the formed loop off of its tips. The short tail of the suture is grasped with the grasper and pulled back through the formed loop in the opposite direction of the needle holder, creating the first flat knot. The same procedure is repeated again clockwise, loosely wrapping the suture around the distal end of the grasper, forming a second locking knot. A third, optional, opposing flat knot can be added in the same manner as the first knot (Figure 9-9).

Thompson's Knot

Another method of internal knot tying that simplifies the process has been described by Dr. Robert Thompson of Anchorage, Alaska. Dr. Thompson is an avid fisherman who uses the clinch knot that has been popular for years among fishermen. This knot has rapidly become

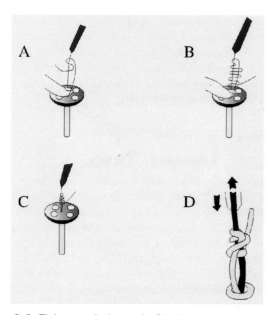

Figure 9-8 Fisherman's knot. **A.** Single-throw knot is made. **B.** Three revolutions around both suture strands are made with the free end of the suture. **C.** Tail of the suture is inserted through the first loop above the assistant's finger. **D.** Knot is tied by pulling the suture tail and sliding the knot with the plastic introducer.

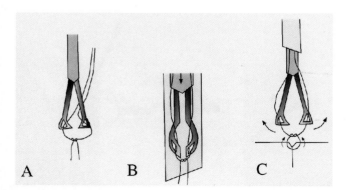

Figure 9-7 Babcock knot. **A.** A knot is tied extra corporeally, and suture ends are introduced through fenestrations of the Babcock grasper outside in. **B.** The grasper is introduced through the sleeve. **C.** Opening of the tips applies additional tension to the knot.

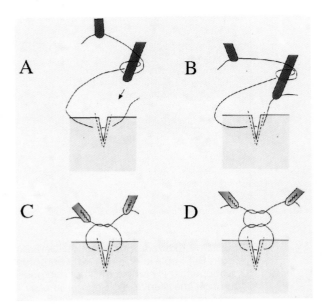

Figure 9-9 Internal square knot. **A.** Holding the long tail of the suture with the needle driver a counterclockwise C-loop is formed around the grasper. **B.** Suture tail is grabbed and pulled back through the loop. **C.** Knot is tied by pulling both ends in opposite directions. **D.** Second clockwise loop is made and the knot tied in the same fashion.

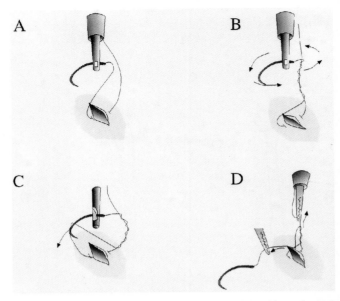

Figure 9-10 Thompson's knot. **A.** The needle is driven through the tissue. **B.** The needle is twirled around the suture tail three to four times. **C.** The needle is passed through the loop. **D.** The knot is tightened by pulling both ends of the suture.

one of our favorite methods of knot tying because of its simplicity. After suturing with a ski or straight needle, the needle is grasped close to its base. The tail of the suture is held through the applicator on the outside of the abdomen. The needle is then twirled at least three or four times around the suture. The needle is then passed back through the loop that was formed, and each end of the suture can be grasped and pulled to tighten the knot. This tie utilizes twist technique to form a slipping knot. The round-handle needle holder can facilitate the twirling part of the clinch knot (Figure 9-10).

Twist Knot (Topel Knot)

Dr Howard Topel, of Chicago, has described a variation of internal knot tying that he has named the "intra abdominal endoscopic 'twist' suturing technique." This technique may also be expedited by using a round-handle needle holder (Figure 9-11). After passing the needle through the incision, the needle end of the suture is grasped about 2 cm away from the needle hub, with the needle holder held in the right hand and rotated around its axis. After three loops are formed the suture is released, and grasped at the same place with the grasper held in the left hand, while the needle holder that has suture loops around it grasps the short tail of the suture pulling it back through the formed loops, thus forming a surgical knot. Applying tension on both ends of the suture ties the knot that is resistant to slippage, and can be secured with an additional square knot.

Noose Slip Knot

This knot is an extracorporeally tied jamming slip loop knot employed intra-corporeally to form a slip knot that can be used to start a running suture, or it can be secured with

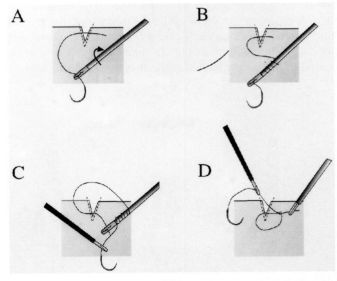

Figure 9-11 Twist knot. **A.** The needle end of the suture is grasped with the needle holder and rotated around its axis. **B.** Three loops are formed. **C.** The suture is gripped with the second grasper. The needle holder that has suture loops around it grasps the short tail of the suture. **D.** Pulling back on both suture ends forms a surgeon's knot.

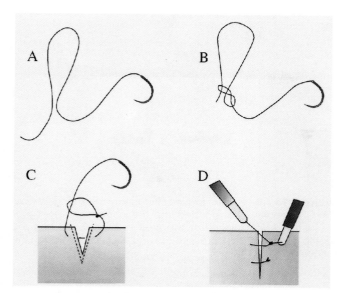

Figure 9-12 Noose slip knot. **A** and **B.** The loop is tied extracorporeally and introduced into the peritoneal cavity. **C.** The needle is then passed through the tissue, and back through previously formed loop and pulled. **D.** The suture tail by the loop is grasped with the grasper and pulled in the opposite direction, constricting the knot.

an additional knot for single suturing. The advantage of this suture is that the knot may be cinched with a minimal number of movements.

The jamming slip knot is tied extracorporeally by forming a loop of about 1 cm at the free end of the suture line. The entire length of the suture is introduced into the peritoneal cavity through one of the trocar sleeves, and the nee-

dle is passed through the tissue to be sutured. The needle is then passed through the previously formed loop, pulling the suture with it, and applying traction until the loop closes (Figure 9-12). After the knot is tightened, it can be further secured with a square slip throw tied intracorporeally in order to avoid slipping of the knot. There are commercially available preformed loop knot instruments on the market that may make suturing techniques less frustrating.

Aberdeen Knot

This type of intracorporeal knot is used to finish a running suture. Running stitches are not frequently used in laparoscopic surgery, but they may be utilized for closure of peritoneal defects after laparoscopic bladder suspensions or for closure of bladder injuries or uterine defects after laparoscopic myomectomies. The beginning of the running suture may be formed using a standard square knot, or twist knot, and a finishing knot may be tied utilizing the Aberdeen knot.

The Aberdeen tie contains a double slip knot that is tied around the last running stitch. The suture is folded and it is pulled back underneath the last stitch, forming a loop. The end of the suture is folded again and introduced back through the first loop that was formed. The needle end is then pulled back through the second loop, pulling the suture with it, and tightening the knot (Figure 9-13).

MECHANICAL SUTURING DEVICES

Alternative method of laparoscopic suturing, or passing suture through the tissue by automated devices, have been designed in order to simplify the suturing process. These devices

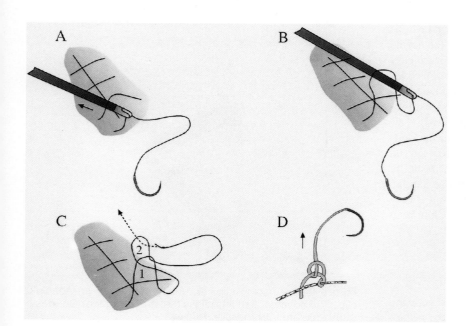

Figure 9-13 Aberdeen Knot. **A.** The grasper is introduced underneath the last running suture and the needle end of the suture is grasped and pulled back to form the loop. **B.** The grasper is then introduced through the primary loop, repeating the same procedure to form a secondary loop. **C.** The grasper is reintroduced through the secondary loop, and the needle is pulled back through the loop forming a knot. **D.** The knot is tightened by pulling the needle end of the suture.

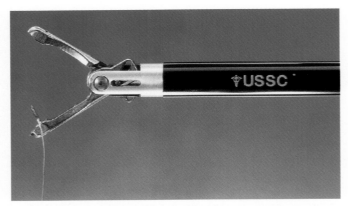

Figure 9-14 Endostitch. The needle with the suture attached in the middle is passed from one jaw to another by pressing the handles and flipping the toggle lever.

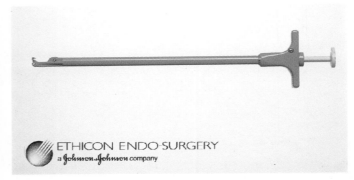

Figure 9-15 The Laurus In-Line Endoscopic Suturing Device. The SH needle is backloaded into the instrument. The tip of the instrument is placed at the area to be sutured and the needle driver button is pressed, driving the needle through the tissue.

may provide certain advantages when the surgeon is not familiar with suture introduction and ligature placement.

The Endostitch (U.S. Surgical Co., Norwalk, CT) suturing apparatus is a 10-mm disposable suturing device designed to make laparoscopic suturing less frustrating and more user-friendly. The instrument is like a hand-operated sewing machine, with two jaws and a suturing needle loaded from the disposable loading unit. The needle is straight, about 1 cm long, has two pointed ends, and the suture attachment in the middle. It is held in one jaw, and can be passed to the other jaw by closing the handle and flipping the toggle levers located on the handle. The Endostitch has application for the placement of running or interrupted stitches in the soft tissue during laparoscopic surgery. The tissue to be sutured is positioned inside of the Endostitch jaws. By pressing the handles, the jaws are closed, driving the needle through the tissue, and by flipping the toggle lever, the needle is passed to the opposite jaw. Releasing the handle opens the jaws, and pulls the suture through the tissue, leaving the tail. At this point a knot can be tied or the interrupted stitch continued, by passing the needle back to the other jaw. Suturing with this device may be easy and fast, and there are a number of ways to use the device for knot tying. The potential disadvantage of this instrument may be in placing the stitch through large pedicles and hard-to-access areas such the Cooper's ligaments (Figure 9-14).

The Laurus medical device is designed by Laurus Medical Corp. and Ethicon Endo-surgery Inc., to place a curved needle of a predetermined configuration through tissue by simple pressure on the plunger located in the in-line handle. This device fits through a 10-mm trocar sleeve and it may be particularly advantageous for placement of suture in Cooper's ligament (Figure 9-15).

CLIPS AND STAPLES

In an effort to save time and avoid complicated suturing during operative laparoscopic procedures, a number of lap-

aroscopic clip and stapling devices have been developed. They are used to secure adequate hemostasis and tissue fixation during various endoscopic procedures. However, they are not intended to replace all suturing techniques. Sutures may be necessary to ligate large blood vessels, to close defects in staple lines, closure of the vaginal cuff, and in some laparoscopic urogynecologic procedures.

As mentioned previously, clips and staples may be used both for coaption of tissue and for hemostasis, and occlusion of skeletonized vessels when a well-defined pedicle is established. The clips are prone to possible dislodgement and are not considered to be as safe for hemostasis as suturing. The Absolok clip (Ethicon Inc., Somerville, NJ) which is made of absorbable material (polydioxanone), is available in several sizes, from small to large. The Absolok may be used to bring tissue together; however, it is only practical if the tissue is thin (Figure 9-16). The Absolok is loaded individually into a 10-mm clip applicator. Dissolv-

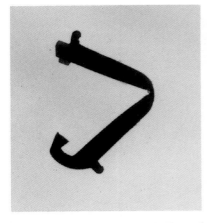

Figure 9-16 Absolok clip. An enlarged view of an Absolok clip. One advantage of this clip is that is absorbable. (Courtesy of Ethicon, Inc., Somerville, NJ.)

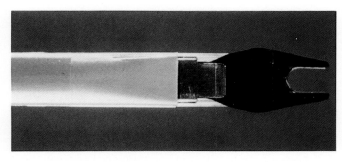

Figure 9-17 Clip applicator. The end of an Endoclip applier. The opening holds a titanium clip. Twenty clips may be fired without withdrawing the instrument. The applier requires a 10-mm port. (Courtesy of United States Surgical Corporation, Norwalk, CT.)

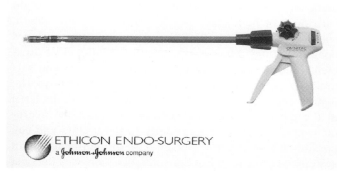

ETHICON ENDO-SURGERY
a *Johnson-Johnson* company

Figure 9-18 Endopath EAS II, Endoscopic articulating stapler. This is a 10-mm disposable instrument that stores 20 titanium staples. The tip of the instrument articulates, and can rotate in different directions. By squeezing the handle instrument will fire one staple at the time. (Courtesy of Ethicon Endo-surgery Inc., Cincinnati, OH.)

able clips made of polydioxanone PDS are also available in 5- and 10-mm sizes. It takes about 6 months for the clips to dissolve, and they can secure the pedicles in a fashion similar to their metal counterparts. Latching can sometimes limit their use, since proper latching is not possible with larger pedicles. The specially designed absorbable clips Laparotie by Ethicon can be used to anchor the continuous suture line, by placing one clip at each end of the running suture ligature, thus avoiding complicated knot tying procedures.

Most clips are made of metal and are designed to maintain hemostasis in vessels up to 3 mm in diameter. They can be loaded singly into a reusable applicator, or can be applied using a disposable applicator with multi-firing clips (Endoclip, US Surgical Corp., Norwalk, CT). The Endoclip has a great deal of use for hemostasis, and it has been the mainstay for ligating the cystic artery during cholecystectomy. Many surgeons use this method when performing appendectomies, using the clip to secure the appendiceal artery. The clips are titanium, and there are 20 clips in a disposable instrument. The instrument requires a 10-mm sheath (Figure 9-17). There are also 5-mm disposable clip appliers available.

Staples are used most frequently in disposable 10-mm multi-firing applicators, and they operate on the same principle as paper staples. They may be used for inguinal hernia repairs in general surgery and retropubic bladder suspension in gynecologic surgery. The Endopath EAS II (Ethicon Endo-Surgery Inc, Cincinnati, OH), has 20 staples in a reloadable cartridge, and the articulating tip that can rotate in different directions making it easier to apply staples in hard to reach areas such as Cooper's ligaments (Figure 9-18).

The linear stapler cutter Endo G.A. (United States Surgical Corp., Norwalk, CT), and Endoscopic linear cutter AZ. 35 (Ethicon Endo-surgery Inc., Cincinnati, OH), apply parallel rows of titanium hemostatic staples for a distance of 3 to 6 cm in length and cut the tissue between the staples by pushing a sharp knife between the staple

lines (Figure 9-19). Both instruments are passed into the abdomen via a 12-mm cannula. You can then take a 3.5-cm long bite of tissue between the jaws. After the jaws are closed, you inspect all around to make sure that only the tissue that you wish to incise is encompassed by the jaws. If you are not satisfied that the area is free and clear, then the jaws may be opened and the instrument moved. When you are sure of the application, you fire the instrument. By squeezing the trigger, two triple-staggered rows of titanium staples are laid down, and the instrument simultaneously divides the tissue between the two innermost rows. If one bite is not adequate, a new cartridge may then be loaded and used for another bite. We have used this to perform a salpingo-oophorectomy, with excellent results. A more recently introduced instrument, called the Multi-fire Endo-Powered GIA 60, takes a 6-cm bite. These instruments are available only in disposable form and require a cannula of 12 to 18 mm in

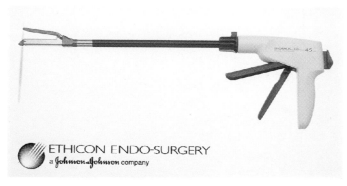

ETHICON ENDO-SURGERY
a *Johnson-Johnson* company

Figure 9-19 Endoscopic linear cutter. The Endoscopic linear cutter EZ 35 is a 12-mm instrument. The jaws when closed will produce a 3.5 cm long bite. When the jaws are closed, squeezing the trigger will fire the two lines of three rows of titanium staples and simultaneously cut between them. (Courtesy of Ethicon Endo-surgery, Inc., Cincinnati, OH.)

diameter. The applicator is designed to fire four to eight cartridges of hemostatic staples of 1 to 1.5 mm depth, and 1.2 cm in width. The linear stapler cutter reduces operating time when used for infundibulopelvic ligaments during oophorectomy, or uterine arteries and cardinal ligaments during laparoscopic hysterectomy. The instrument should be used with great caution at the level of the uterine arteries, because the width of the instrument places it in close proximity to the ureters and can possibly cause ureteral damage. Use of the linear stapler system saves time, but it considerably increases the cost of surgery, and its use should be critically planned for selected cases. For economic reasons, surgeons should consider laparoscopic suturing or electrosurgery to maintain hemostasis during operative laparoscopic procedures. Should the cost of disposable products decrease in the future, the economic possibilities of linear staples will increase.

The ability to perform endoscopic surgery is limited not only by the skill and training of the surgeon and the availability of the appropriate equipment but also by the judgment of the operator. One must spend time developing the skill necessary for the previously discussed techniques and also for honing the faculty of good clinical judgment.

SUGGESTED READING

Clarke HC. Laparoscopy—new instruments for suturing and ligation. *Fertil Steril* 1972;23:274–7.

Gunn GC, Cooper RP, Gordon NS, Gagnon L. Use of new device for endoscopic suturing in the laparoscopic Burch procedure. *J Am Assoc Gyn Laparosc* 1994;2:65–70.

Lee C, Soong Y. Laparoscopic hysterectomy with the Endo GIA 30 stapler. *J Reprod Med* 1992;38:582–6.

Liu CY. Laparoscopic hysterectomy, report of 215 cases. *Gynecol Endosc* 1992;1:73–7.

Marrero MA, Corfman RS. Laparoscopic use of sutures. *Clin Obstet Gynecol* 1991;34:387–94.

Ou C, Presthus J, Beadle E. Laparoscopic bladder neck suspension using hernia mesh and surgical staples. *J Laparendosc Surg* 1993;3:563–6.

Pasic R, Levine RL. Laparoscopic suturing and ligation techniques. *Journal Am Assoc Gynecol Laparosc* 1995;3:67–79.

Reich H, Clarke HC, Sekel L. A simple method for ligating with straight and curved needles in operative laparoscopy. *Obstet Gynecol* 1992;79:143–7.

Semm K. New method of pelviscopy for myomectomy, ovariectomy, tubectomy, and appendectomy. *Endoscopy* 1979;11:85–93.

Semm K. Tissue-puncher and loop-ligation: new ideas for surgical therapeutic pelviscopy (laparoscopy) endoscopic intra-abdominal surgery. *Endoscopy* 1978;10:119–24.

Senagore AJ. Tissue approximation and ligation techniques. In: *Laparoscopic Surgery.* Ballantyne GH, Leahy PF, Modlin IM, Cheadle WG, and Polk HC, eds. Philadelphia: W.B. Saunders, 1994:107–113.

Soper NJ, Hunter JG. Suturing and knot tying in laparoscopy. *Surg Clin N Am* 1992;72:1139–52.

Topel H. *The Video Encyclopedia of Endoscopic Surgery for the Gynecologist.* Gerald S. Shirk, ed. Tape 1, Medical Video Productions, 1994.

Woodland MB. Ureter injury during laparoscopy-assisted vaginal hysterectomy with the endoscopic linear stapler. *Am J Obstet Gynecol* 1992;167:756–7.

Operative Laparoscopy, Second Edition
The Masters' Techniques in Gynecologic Surgery
Lippincott–Raven Publishers, Philadelphia © 1998.

10

Myomectomy and Appendectomy

10-1   Laparoscopic Myomectomy

Harrith M. Hasson

Uterine leiomyoma is the most common gynecologic tumor, occurring in 20% to 25% of all women. In 1988, more than 200,000 surgical operations were performed in the United States for such a diagnosis: > 170,000 hysterectomies; 33,000 myomectomies. Any change in the operative approach of treating leiomyoma from traditional laparotomy to operative laparoscopy will have a significant impact on the quality of health care for women. When compared to laparotomy, an adequately performed laparoscopic myomectomy is associated with less blood loss, a shorter hospital stay and recovery time, fewer complications, fewer postoperative adhesions, better documentation for follow-up, and better cosmetic scar. Despite these apparent advantages, most gynecologists have been reluctant to adopt this technique, citing the following concerns:

1. fear of perioperative complications (especially hemorrhage) and intraoperative technical difficulties
2. apprehension concerning the ultimate status of the uterine scar (in cases of intramural tumors)
3. uncertainty about the extent of postoperative adhesions
4. doubt concerning the reproductive outcome and operative efficiency relative to relief of symptoms, recurrence, and reoperation.

INDICATIONS AND CONTRAINDICATIONS

With few exceptions, the indications for myomectomy by laparoscopy are identical to those for myomectomy by laparotomy:

1. bleeding, pain, and pressure symptoms of significant nature and duration
2. infertility with or without associated factors
3. recurrent abortion (usually categorized as a subgroup of infertility)

4. pelvic mass, uterine size > 12 weeks gestational size, dominant myoma > 8 cm, rapid change in myoma size.

The exceptions are outlined in the exclusionary criteria.

The contraindications fall under two categories:

1. Medical: Patient's medical condition and/or degree of obesity makes it inadvisable to keep her in Trendelenberg position with a pneumoperitoneum for a prolonged period of time.
2. Surgical: See exclusion criteria.

PREOPERATIVE PATIENT SELECTION AND PREPARATION

Successful outcome of laparoscopic myomectomy depends upon proper patient selection and preoperative preparation. With increasing experience the surgeon may extend the limits of application of the laparoscopic approach. The surgical exclusion criteria include:

1. diffuse leiomyomas or adenomyosis
2. submucous myoma > 50% into cavity
3. size > 15 cm
4. patient desire for hysterectomy.

Intraligamentary and cervical leiomyomas require precise technique; large, deep intramural tumors demand a two-layer closure with sutures. These types of leiomyomas should not be taken lightly. If the number and/or size of the tumors is greater than a given value, to be determined by each individual surgeon, open laparotomy is indicated. It is important to know when to proceed with laparoscopy and when to stop proceeding with it.

The clinical diagnosis of uterine leiomyoma is confirmed by ultrasound. Further anatomic data concerning number, size, location, and presence of degeneration are best obtained with magnetic resonance imaging (MRI). Preoperative MRI studies are most helpful in evaluating the type of surgery required and the need for drug therapy. For instance, patients with a submucous myoma protruding > 50% into the endometrial cavity are suitable for hysteroscopic resection. Patients with combined submucous and intramural/subserous myomas are treated with hysteroscopic resection and laparoscopic removal, but not at the same sitting. The more significant lesion is treated first. Patients with diffuse leiomyomas of the uterus or adenomyosis are not candidates for laparoscopic treatment.

Preoperative medical therapy is usually limited to patients with leiomyomata larger than 6 cm. The drugs are administered for 3 to 6 months and their efficacy monitored with serial determinations of estradiol levels, pelvic examinations, and ultrasound. Alternative medications include Depot Luprolide 3.75 mg intramuscularly monthly, Danazol 800 mg orally daily, and Nafarelin 0.4 mg nasally daily.

INSTRUMENTATION

An electronic high-flow insufflator, a high-resolution laparoscope, a video camera, and a monitor are essential requirements for this operation, as in other procedures of operative laparoscopy. Energy sources available for performing a laparoscopic myomectomy include unipolar and bipolar cautery, CO_2 laser, fiberoptic lasers, endocoagulation according to Semm, and mechanical energy such as scissors. These are all substantially equivalent. Usually more than one energy type is needed to effect optimal sharp dissection and hemostatic coagulation. I prefer to use the open laparoscopy entry method and the following special instruments while performing laparoscopic myomectomy: (1) stable access cannula (Marlow), (2) holding forceps with teeth, (3) 5-mm myoma drill (Reznik), (4) bulldog grasping forceps (Linvatec), (5) vaginal speculum with fiberoptic light (Reznik) (Figure 10-1.1).

The stable access cannula (SAC) provides optimal stability during instrument exchanges and manipulations with

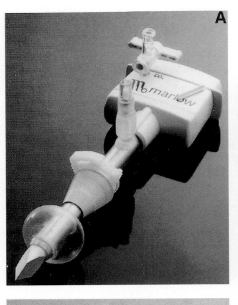

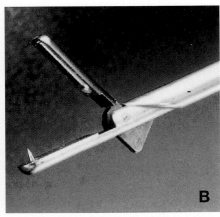

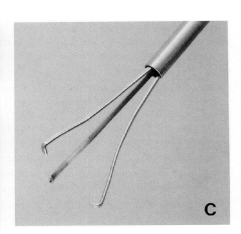

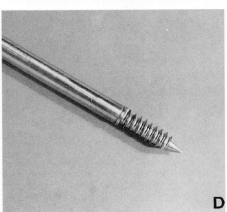

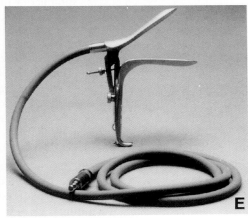

Figure 10-1.1 Special instruments for laparoscopic myomectomy. **A.** SAC (stable access cannula). **B.** Holding forceps with teeth. **C.** Bulldog grasper. **D.** Myoma drill, 5 mm. **E.** Vaginal speculum with fiberoptic light.

minimal protrusion into the abdomen and eliminates occurrences of subcutaneous emphysema. The bulldog grasper and toothed forceps hold tissues securely during various steps of the procedure. The myoma drill is most useful for manipulation of the tumor before it emerges out of its uterine bed. The vaginal speculum with attached fiberoptic light provides excellent illumination of the cervix and vaginal apex during vaginal procedures.

TECHNIQUE

A capable associate surgeon or assistant is indispensable. Many of the technical steps of this operation require movements coordinated precisely between two knowledgeable and able individuals. By and large, if the laparoscopic myomectomy is very easy to perform, it is probably not indicated. Laparoscopic myomectomy requires three ancillary access points in the suprapubic region and the right and left lower quadrants of the abdomen. The position of the points of access should be consistent with the size of the dominant myoma; the larger the tumor, the higher the points of entry. Essentially, the operative technique involves carrying out three distinct tasks:

1. disengaging the myoma from its uterine bed
2. managing the uterine defect
3. removing the myoma from the abdomen.

Disengaging the Myoma

Diluted vasopressin is a useful adjuvant in achieving hemostasis. Currently, I use a solution of 20 U (one ampule) of vasopressin in 50 mL of saline. Although we had no problems using a more concentrated solution of 20 U in 20 mL of saline, we decided to use the more dilute solution after hearing of complications from our European colleagues. I inject the vasopressin solution superficially (raising a wheal) into the base of the myoma and/or along the site of the proposed incision (Figure 10-1.2) and repeat the dose after 30 minutes, as needed. The next step is to incise the pseudocapsule of the myoma down to the characteristic pearly white substance of the tumor. This is done with the energy source of the surgeon's choice. The incision should only be large enough to permit extraction. I prefer to remove more than one myoma through a single vertical incision, if possible. If not, I do not hesitate to make additional vertical incisions, as needed. I do not use transverse incisions; as these appear to be associated with a greater incidence of adhesion formation. Pedunculated myoma are excised at the base of the pedicle.

Once I identify the myoma, I fix it by turning the myoma drill into its substance or otherwise holding it with the bulldog grasper or toothed forceps. While pulling on the myoma and moving it to and fro, I start developing the cleavage plane between the myoma and uterus, using blunt and

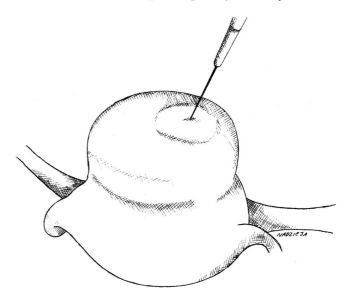

Figure 10-1.2 Vasopressin injection.

sharp dissection. One method for blunt dissection is to place a probe (or any instrument that functions as a probe) in the cleavage plane and leverage the tumor against the uterine wall to pry it out of its bed. This prying technique should be performed firmly but not with excessive force, to avoid rupturing vascular bridges between the tumor and uterus and subsequent bleeding. Cleavage planes between various tissues or between tissues and benign tumors consist of a potential space containing a small amount of loose areolar tissue as well as small and large bridges connecting the two sides. These bridges contain various amounts of strong connective tissue fibers, bands, blood vessels, lymphatics, and nerves. Some resist gentle blunt dissection and require sharp dissection. Larger bridges usually require prior coagulation to prevent bleeding. As the myoma begins to emerge from its bed, I favor using the bulldog grasper to hold the tumor, move it, and apply tension on the tissue planes in various directions, for optimal exposure of connecting bridges. When proper technique is used, dissection proceeds with surprising ease and with minimal to no bleeding. Once the vascular pedicle is identified, I coagulate it thoroughly with bipolar cautery and cut it with sharp scissors to free the myoma (Figure 10-1.3). The absence of bleeding is explained by the fact that individual vessels are easily identified with the magnification obtained with video laparoscopy, and coagulated individually before they are cut.

Managing the Operative Defect

Over the last 3 years, this procedure has evolved into the following current practice: Edges of the operative site of pedunculated, subserosal, and intraligamentary leiomyomas

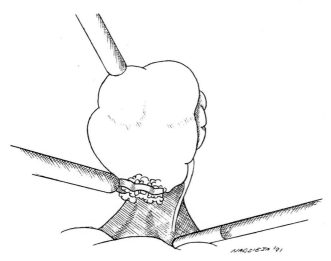

Figure 10-1.3 Bipolar coagulation of vascular pedicle.

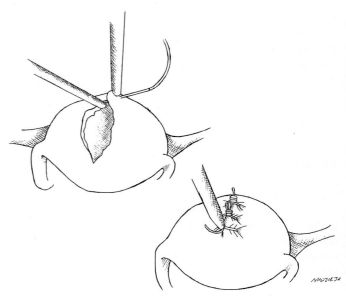

Figure 10-1.4 Uterine closure with interrupted sutures.

are coagulated so as to achieve meticulous hemostasis, and the site is covered with TC7 (Interceed, Ethicon), as indicated. Following meticulous hemostasis of the wound edges, the uterine defect resulting from a superficial intramural tumor is approximated with one layer of continuous or interrupted suture, including the serosa and a thin segment of the adjacent myometrium (Figure 10-1.4). The suture site is then covered with TC7. In cases of deep intramural myomas with or without submucous component, bleeding from the wound edges is first controlled with detailed coagulation. The defect is then closed in two layers: a deep layer using interrupted polyglactin-O sutures bound with extracorporeal Roeder loop knots, and a superficial layer including the serosa, using a continuous fine suture and intracorporeal knot tying. Again, the dry, sutured site is covered with a layer of TC7.

Removing the Myoma

Following excision, individual myomas are stored in the cul-de-sac and then removed jointly by an abdominal or vaginal route. If the tumors are small (≤ 5 cm) and few in number I employ the orange peel technique associated with abdominal removal. The myoma is held with the bulldog forceps on one side and the toothed forceps on the other side, and the mass is converted into a long narrow strip of tissue (Figure 10-1.5). The 5-mm incision in the suprapubic region is enlarged to accommodate a 10/11-mm cannula, and the myoma strip(s) are picked up and removed through the sleeve. A morcellator is not used.

Larger myomas are removed vaginally, if vaginal elasticity is not compromised. Using the bulldog forceps, the dominant myoma is held, positioned in the middle of the cul-de-sac, and pushed from above to create a bulge in the vaginal apex. When viewed from below, this bulge estab-

lishes a landmark for safe vaginal incision, usually with a unipolar needle. Because of vaginal elasticity, a small incision in the apex can accommodate masses of larger diameters without additional cutting. If indicated, the transverse incision is enlarged bilaterally to within safe limits. Exceedingly large myomas are first divided with scissors into two or three pieces before attempting vaginal extraction, to avoid the occurrence of a disproportion between the dimensions of the tumor mass and that of the incision. Vaginal removal of large myomas is one area where perfect coordination between two capable operators is essential. The surgeon working from above presents the tumor to the operator working from below in the middle of the vaginal

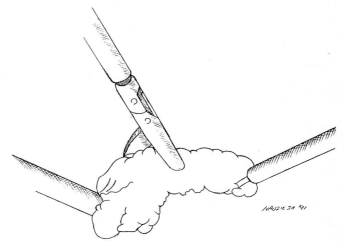

Figure 10-1.5 Converting the myoma into a narrow strip of tissue—the orange peel technique.

apex slightly below the cervix. When the vagina is incised, the surgeon slides the tumor into the vaginal defect to prevent escape of the gas. The operator working from below causes the field to be cleared of accumulating blood and fluids and quickly identifies the anterior and posterior edges of the vaginal incision and grasps each with a long Allis clamp. The operator's assistant holds the vaginal edges open and apart. The speculum with attached fiberoptic light is used at this stage, for optimum visualization of the vaginal apex. The surgeon working from above pushes the tumor further into the vagina and moves it to and fro. This movement aids the operator working from below in identifying the tumor prior to grasping it with a tenaculum. Once the myoma is grasped firmly, the operator gradually pulls it down with one tenaculum applied on top of the other. The process is repeated, using well-directed traction and rotation maneuvers to effect delivery. Careful positioning of the tumor from above and judicial use of well-applied traction from below are the ingredients for success. To regenerate the pneumoperitoneum following vaginal withdrawal of a myoma, the Allis clamps are repositioned on the vaginal apex to close the incision temporarily. Additional clamps are applied as needed.

Other myomas stored in the cul-de-sac are similarly extracted, one at a time. Alternatively, all of the tumors can be collected in a pouch and withdrawn at one time. To further facilitate vaginal removals, a specialized stable access cannula (Marlow) is being developed to prevent loss of the pneumoperitoneum during this process. Following removal of the myomas, the vaginal incision is closed from below, using a continuous running suture. Constant irrigation washes the vaginal mucosa in a one-way lavage. The pressurized fluid and gas in the pelvis moves in one direction only—toward the vagina. Under such circumstances, abdominal contamination with vaginal flora is not expected.

If the tumor(s) is (are) large and vaginal elasticity is compromised, or if conditions are not suitable for vaginal delivery for other reasons, the mass is withdrawn through a suprapubic minilaparotomy incision. The myomas are positioned under the incision for identification and extraction with a tenaculum. Collecting all the tumors within a pouch makes for easier withdrawal from the abdomen. The abdomen is then closed in layers.

CLINICAL EXPERIENCE

Our experience with laparoscopic myomectomy in more than 60 cases performed during the last 3 years confirms the safety and efficacy of the procedure and permits us to address the concerns voiced at the beginning of the chapter. The mean estimated blood loss (EBL) was 75 mL in the first 56 patients. No blood transfusions were given. In a study by Daniell and Gurley involving 17 cases of laparoscopic myomectomy, the mean EBL was 78 mL. Studies reporting on myomectomy by CO_2 laser laparotomy report higher mean blood loss (150 mL [Starks], 200 mL [McLaughlin]), while those involving conventional laparotomy report even higher values (300 mL [Smith and Uhlir], 311 mL [McLaughlin]). Thus it would appear that the EBL is smaller in cases of myomectomy performed by laparoscopy, as compared to laparotomy. The reason is better hemostasis, as discussed earlier.

The length of hospital stay was less than 1 day for all except three of our patients. One extremely obese nulliparous patient had two large myomas removed through a minilaparotomy incision. In this patient, following detachment of the myomas from the uterus, we could not maintain an adequate pneumoperitoneum due to gas leakage around the secondary sleeves, which led to significant subcutaneous emphysema. We elected the minilaparotomy approach for removal, as previously discussed, and kept the patient 1 extra day. The second patient also stayed a second day to have bladder polyps removed by a urologist. The last patient stayed 4 days. She developed febrile morbidity associated with upper respiratory tract infection and significant subcutaneous emphysema, which subsided within that time.

In total, we had four instances of significant subcutaneous emphysema, making this the most frequent complication. The subcutaneous emphysema resulted from leakage of the pneumoperitoneum gas around loose ancillary sleeves into the subcutaneous compartment; with repeated instrument exchanges and manipulations over an extended period of time the secondary incisions became larger than the ancillary sleeves, permitting CO_2 gas to leak around them, as well as causing instruments to be pulled out of the abdomen with each unguarded exchange. Replacing the sleeves into the abdomen with or without a trocar further compromised the integrity of the fascia and increased the rate of gas leakage into the subcutaneous tissues.

There were no other immediate complications, and no late complications other than adhesion formation. Problems with subcutaneous emphysema ceased when we began using the stable access cannula (SAC). The abdominal wall in the area of application is captured between the cone and balloon of the cannula. This arrangement prevents the SAC from slipping in or out of the abdomen and eliminates the possibility of gas leaks around the sleeve.

The integrity of the uterine scar following laparoscopic myomectomy for deep intramural leiomyomas is a cause of concern. Nezhat et al. noted six uterine fistulas posteriorly in patients with deep intramural leiomyomas. In three of the six patients, the uterine defect was not sutured. In the remaining three, only the serosa was reapproximated. We have not noted any instances of uterine fistula or weak scar in 26 second-look procedures, including one cesarean section for obstetric indications. Nine patients have had normal vaginal deliveries, two had a cesarean delivery, and two are continuing pregnancy without problem. We advocate a two-layer closure of the uterine defect, as described previously, and believe that such a closure is substantially equivalent to that performed at laparotomy in terms of uterine tensile strength. However, until this controversy is settled, it is prudent to test the integrity of the uterine scar, especially in reproductive women, with a hysterosalpingogram at 4 months postsurgery in patients with deep intramural tumors.

The occurrence of postoperative pelvic adhesions is a multifactorial phenomenon. Some of the factors involved are unrelated to type of surgery. Our data indicate that laparoscopic myomectomy is associated with less adhesion formation than myomectomy by laparotomy. There were no adhesions in the cul-de-sac after vaginal removal of the leiomyomas in any case. Comparative data are difficult to find because no one performed second-look laparoscopy or second-look laparotomy after conventional laparotomy. However, in one recent study of 20 patients where second-look procedures consisting of ten laparoscopies and ten cesarean sections were performed following laparotomy and CO_2 laser myomectomy, Starks found that the incidence of postoperative adhesion formation was 100% (75% mild, 25% moderate +). In the study by our group, 30% of the patients had no postoperative adhesions and 67% did (21% mild, 46% moderate +). Currently, we advocate routine second-look laparoscopy at 3 weeks after surgery for all patients undergoing laparoscopic myomectomy. To minimize the occurrence of postoperative adhesions, it is essential to secure meticulous hemostasis at the operative site and to cover the site with an adhesion barrier such as TC7, especially if sutures are applied.

The presence of pelvic adhesions does not appear to affect the efficiency of myomectomy as a reproductive procedure. The conception rate in infertile patients in our study was 71%; Starks reported a rate of 63%. The general figure for conception rate following myomectomy by laparotomy is 40%, according to the review of Buttram and Reiter. The incidence and severity of adhesions following myomectomy by conventional laparotomy has not been reported. Satisfactory relief of symptoms related to bleeding, pain, and pressure symptoms associated with myomas was obtained in all patients following laparoscopic myomectomy. Clinical recurrences without significant symptomatology have occurred, but none have required reoperation for recurrent symptoms. This is not surprising, given the short period of follow-up in our series. However, we expect rates of recurrence and reoperation following laparoscopic myomectomy to be comparable to rates following myomectomy by laparotomy, since these rates are independent of the type of surgery performed.

CONCLUSION

Laparoscopic myomectomy is a relatively simple procedure that requires the combined skills of two surgeons or a surgeon and a well-trained assistant. Observing appropriate technique and patient selection criteria, the procedure is at least as effective as myomectomy by laparotomy in terms of reproductive outcome and relief of symptoms. When compared to laparotomy, myomectomy by laparoscopy is associated with less blood loss, fewer complications, shorter hospital stay, shorter recovery time, fewer adhesions, better documentation for future follow-up, and a better cosmetic scar. Although the rate of postoperative adhesions following laparoscopic myomectomy is expected to be less than that of myomectomy by laparotomy, concerns about postoperative adhesions mandate the routine use of second-look laparoscopy at 3 weeks after initial laparoscopic surgery for therapeutic reasons. Awareness of the possibility of a weak uterine scar or fistula following laparoscopic removal of deep intramural tumors mandates the use of a two-layer closure in such cases and the performance of a hysterosalpingogram at 4 months after the surgery in order to test the integrity of the uterine scar before allowing the patient to get pregnant.

SUGGESTED READING

Buttram VC, Reiter RC. Uterine leiomyomata: etiology, symptomatology and management. *Fertil Steril* 1981;36:433–45.

Daniell JF, Gurley LD. Laparoscopic treatment of clinically significant symptomatic uterine fibroids. *J Gynecol Surg* 1991;7:37–40.

Dudiak CM, Turner DA, Patel SK, Archie JT, Silver B, Norusis M. Uterine leiomyomas in the infertile patient: pre-operative localization with MR imaging versus US and hysterosalpingography. *Radiology* 1988;167:627–30.

Friedman AJ, Hoffman DI, Comite F, et al. Treatment of leiomyomata uteri with leuprolide acetate depot: a double-blind, placebo-controlled, multicenter study. *Obstet Gynecol* 1991;77:720–75.

Hasson HM, Rotman C, Rana N, Sistos F, Dmowski WP. Laparoscopic myomectomy. Submitted for publication in *Obstetrics & Gynecology.*

McLaughlin DS. Metroplasty and myomectomy with CO_2 laser for maximizing the preservation of normal tissue and minimizing blood loss. *J Reprod Med* 1985;30:1–9.

Nezhat C, Nezhat F, Silfen SL, Schaffer N, Evans D. Laparoscopic myomectomy. *Int J Fertil* 1991;36:275–80.

Smith DC, Uhlir JK. Myomectomy as a reproductive procedure. *Am J Obstet Gynecol* 1990;162:1476–9.

Starks GC. CO_2 laser myomectomy in an infertile population. *J Reprod Med* 1988;33:184–6.

Togashi K, Ozasa H, Konishi I, et al. Enlarged uterus: differentiation between adenomyosis and leiomyoma with MR imaging. *Radiology* 1989;171:531–4.

Operative Laparoscopy, Second Edition
The Masters' Techniques in Gynecologic Surgery
Lippincott–Raven Publishers, Philadelphia © 1998.

10-2 Laparoscopic Appendectomy, Myomectomy, Presacral Neurectomy and Treatment of Extensive Endometriosis of the Bowel, Bladder and Ureter

Camran R. Nezhat, Farr R. Nezhat, and Ceana H. Nezhat

Due to the rapid refinement of operative laparoscopy, we believe that laparotomy will become obsolete in managing a majority of benign and some malignant pelvic diseases in the near future. Over the past 15 years, we have devised a combination of techniques, which we call videolaparoscopy and videolaseroscopy (VLS), to expand the number of procedures possible through the laparoscope.

The subjects selected for this chapter represent the extremes of the spectrum of operative laparoscopy today. Laparoscopic appendectomy is a simple, straightforward procedure and has therefore become one of the starting points for general surgeons to embrace laparoscopy. As a result of this increased number of laparoscopists, we are seeing an explosion in laparoscopic technology, including the development of clip applicators and suture materials. In contrast, myomectomy represents the most tedious of laparoscopic procedures but mimics the procedure performed at laparotomy. Finally, laparoscopic treatment of endometriosis involving the rectovaginal septum, bowel, bladder, and ureter introduces a technique far superior to any available by laparotomy for managing these complex conditions.

Videolaseroscopy, as the name implies, combines the use of a high-resolution video camera, monitor, and recording system, using the CO_2 laser through the operative channel of an operative laparoscope, as a cutting modality and for hemostasis of small blood vessels and bipolar forceps for dessication of larger vessels. The principles used are those of microsurgery; we will review these principles briefly before presenting the specific procedures. The CO_2 laser, used via the operative channel of the laparoscope as a "long knife," and combined with the technique of hydrodissection, has enabled us to perform microsurgical intraperitoneal and retroperitoneal operations. For the past several years in our practice, we have been able to avoid almost all laparotomies for benign conditions.

VLS begins with placement of the infraumbilical operative laparoscope and three suprapubic ports. A miniature video camera (Circon-ACMI, Santa Barbara, CA) is attached to the eyepiece of the laparoscope, enabling the surgical team to observe the procedure on a monitor, thereby providing better assistance. The surgeon can operate in the upright position, allowing him/her more comfort while performing complicated surgery. The high-resolution video equipment available produces a magnified image on the monitor and, combined with the surgeon's ability to place the laparoscope close to the pelvic tissues, produces an image comparable to that obtained with surgical loupes.

The CO_2 laser set at powers between 30 and 80 W ULTRAPULSE (Coherent, Palo Alto, CA) is used as a precise cutting instrument, acting as a "long knife" while providing hemostasis in the surgical field. The laser is introduced into the abdomen by a direct lens system.

The recently introduced ULTRAPULSE 5000L (Coherent, Palo Alto, CA) combined with the Coherent-Nezhat direct laparoscope coupler further improves the precision and accuracy of the videolaseroscopy system. This laser produces short duration, high energy pulses with up to 5 times more energy per pulse than a conventional superpulsed laser. This high pulse energy is sufficient, for the typical spot size delivered through the laparoscope, to produce clean tissue ablation with each pulse. In addition, this new generation CO_2 laser uses a carbon-13 isotope rather than the conventional carbon-12. This change, or "tuning" of the laser energy, avoids the resonant absorption of the laser beam by the CO_2 insufflation gas. Preventing this absorption and the resulting "thermal blooming" of the laser beam enables the ULTRAPULSE 5000L to deliver power densities and energy fluences up to 20 times that of conventional superpulsed CO_2 lasers when used through a laparoscope. Char formation is minimized, resulting in less opportunity for foreign body reaction and less potential for adhesion formation.

Because this laser has been fitted with separate, independent controls for setting energy per pulse and average power, the operator is able to select a constant pulse energy ranging from 1 to 200 millijoules. Adjusting the average power changes only the pulse repetition rate, not the pulse energy. The average power delivered to tissue, which is equal to the pulse energy multiplied by the pulse rate, determines the speed at which the laser produces an effect upon tissue. The control panel of the ULTRAPULSE laser allows the operator to select average power levels from 1W up to 80W. Because tissue effect is determined predominantly by pulse energy level, changes in pulse rate or average power change only the operating speed.

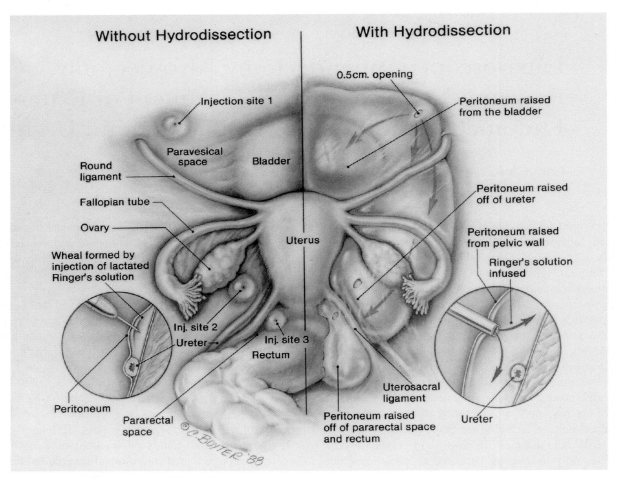

Figure 10-2.1 Hydrodissection technique. (Drawing courtesy of Fertility and Endoscopy Center, Inc., Atlanta, GA.)

A suction-irrigation cannula (Bard Reproductive Systems, Tewksbury, MA) is one of the most important accessory instruments in VLS. The cannula is introduced through the left suprapubic port and manipulated by the surgeon's left hand (for the right-handed person). It evacuates smoke and fluids, irrigates the pelvis, and serves as a backstop for the laser beam.

Because CO_2 laser cannot penetrate fluid, a technique known as hydrodissection has been developed for use in VLS (Figure 10-2.1). Lactated Ringer's (Baxter Healthcare Corp., Deerfield, IL) is injected into subserosal tissues, using a 22-gauge needle or suction-irrigator, permitting laser incisions in delicate areas such as above the ureter or bowel blood vessels.

Additional instruments are used as needed in VLS. In the following procedures, bipolar forceps are used for desiccation, Endoloop sutures (Ethicon, Cincinnati, OH) with applicator are necessary for appendectomy, and laparoscopic or regular sutures on the straight or curve are used for repair.

APPENDECTOMY

The suction-irrigator, bipolar forceps, and Endoloop sutures or atraumatic grasping forceps (Karl Storz, Culver City, CA) are introduced into the left, midline, and right suprapubic portal, respectively. Prophylactic antibiotics are suggested. We use cefoxitin (Mefoxin; Merck, Sharp & Dohme, West Point, PA) 2 g or doxycycline (Vibramycin; Pfizer, New York, NY) 100 mg preoperatively. Lysis of periappendiceal and pericecal adhesions is accomplished by VLS techniques, allowing the distal appendix to be grasped. Bipolar desiccation of the mesoappendix must be carried out above the cecum, allowing a margin of viable tissue at the appendiceal-cecal junction. The desiccated area is incised with the CO_2 laser or scissors, and a chromic or PDS (Ethicon, Somerville, NJ) Endoloop suture is passed through a suprapubic port, applied at the base of the appendix (5 mm from the cecum), tied securely using the applicator, and cut. A second Endoloop suture can be applied over the first; a third is placed 5 to 10 mm distally on the appendix to close off the lumen, and is held for later specimen retrieval. The appendix is then transected above the suture, and the stump is sterilized by superficial vaporization with laser and is generously irrigated. The appendix is removed from the abdominal cavity by introducing a grasping forceps through the operating channel of the laparo-

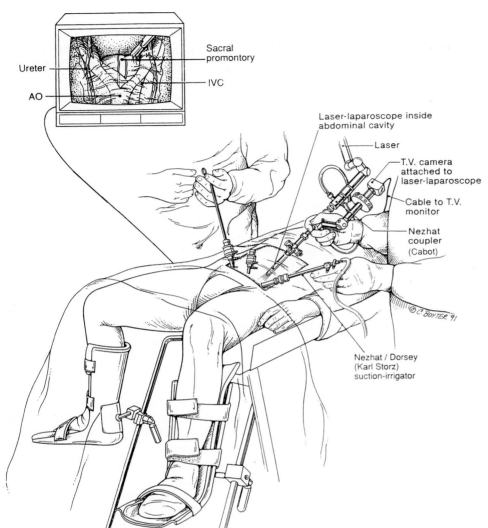

Ureter

AO

Sacral promontory

IVC

Laser-laparoscope inside abdominal cavity

Laser

T.V. camera attached to laser-laparoscope

Cable to T.V. monitor

Nezhat coupler (Cabot)

Nezhat / Dorsey (Karl Storz) suction-irrigator

Figure 10-2.2 Room set up. (Drawing courtesy of Fertility and Endoscopy Center, Inc., Atlanta, GA.)

scope, then removing the appendix, forceps, and scope as a unit, or through a 10-mm suprapubic trocar. An Endobag (Ethicon, Cincinnati, OH) can be used for containing the appendix before removal. Another technique for removal of the appendix is using an endoscopic stapler. The stapler is introduced via a 12-mm trocar. It can be applied to the mesoappendix and appendix, which is then stapled, cut and removed in one bite (Figures 10-2.2 to 10-2.6).

MYOMECTOMY

The surgical procedure of laparoscopic myomectomy can be viewed as occurring in two stages. The first, removing the tumor from the uterus, is generally straightforward, while the second, repairing the uterine defect and removing the tumor from the abdomen, can be long and tedious. A pedunculated

myoma is simply tied and then excised at the stalk using a high-power laser; bleeding is controlled with bipolar electrodesiccation. For intramural or subserosal myomata, 5 to 10 mL of dilute vasopressin (20 U in 100 mL of sterile saline) is injected under the capsule. The capsule is then incised with the CO_2 laser between 60 and 80 W (or electrosurgical knife or scissors) and gradually dissected away, using a combination of Nezhat-Dorsey Probe (Bard Reproductive Systems, Tewksbury, MA), hydrodissection, and laser. When CO_2 gas is used for pneumoperitoneum, the high-power CO_2 laser (except the 5000L) creates a large spot between 2 and 3 mm that is hemostatic for vessels with diameters of 2 to 3 mm. Traction on the myomas can be produced with a small hook or claw forceps. Once the myoma is removed, the base is thoroughly irrigated, and hemostasis generally requires bipolar electrodesiccation rather than low power laser. Extensive coagulation of tissue should be avoided, because it can compromise heal-

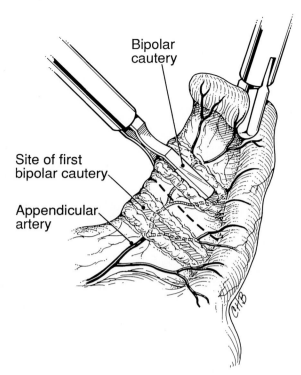

Figure 10-2.3 Mesoappendix is being desiccated with bipolar electrocautery. (Drawing courtesy of Fertility and Endoscopy Center, Inc., Atlanta, GA.)

ing of the uterus and cause possible subsequent fistula formation. The myometrial defect is repaired using 2-0 or 0 Vicryl (Ethicon, Somerville, NJ) sutures. Attempts should be made to repair the defect in layers. Intraligamentous myomata are approached by incising the anterior leaf of the broad ligament after identifying the location of large vessels, the ureters, and the bladder. Excision is then accomplished as described for subserosal myomata.

The excised myoma can be removed from the abdomen by morcellation, using scissors, manual Semm morcellator, or electronic Steiner morcellator (Karl Storz, Culver City, CA) until the fragments are small enough to fit through a 10-mm suprapubic port. Laser is unnecessary in this instance, because hemostasis is no longer a factor. Posterior colpotomy, with or without morcellation, or mini-laparotomy incision, is performed if morcellation is technically impossible. Postoperative ecchymosis of the abdominal wall can result.

LAPAROSCOPICALLY ASSISTED MYOMECTOMY

The technique of LAM allows conventional multi-layer suturing and is less technically demanding and less time-consuming. The procedure can thus be performed by less experienced endoscopic surgeons and may be more cost-effective. The criteria for LAM are myoma larger than 5 cm, numerous myomas requiring extensive morcellation, deep intramural

myoma, and removal that requires multiple layer uterine repair with sutures. After laparoscopic evaluation of the pelvic cavity and treating any associated pelvic adhesions and endometriosis, the location and number of myomas are evaluated. The leiomyoma (or most prominent one) is injected with diluted vasopressin subserosally. A vertical incision is made over the uterine serosa until the capsule of the leiomyoma is reached. A corkscrew manipulator is inserted into the leiomyoma and used to elevate the uterus toward the midline suprapubic puncture. With the trocar and manipulator attached to the myoma, this midline 5-mm puncture is enlarged to a 4 to 5 cm transverse incision. The rectus muscles are then separated at the midline.

The peritoneum is entered transversely, and the leiomyoma is located and brought to the resulting incision, using the corkscrew manipulator. The uterine manipulator is replaced with two Lahey tenacula. The leiomyoma is shelled sequentially and morcellated, gradually exposing new areas. After complete removal of the leiomyoma, the uterine wall defect is seen through the incision. If uterine size allows, the uterus is exteriorized through the minilaparotomy incision to complete the repair. When multiple leiomyomas are found, as many as possible are removed through a single uterine incision. When the leiomyomas are in distant locations and identification is impossible, the minilaparotomy incision is closed temporarily by inserting a distended surgical glove. The laparoscope is reintroduced and the leiomyomas identified and brought to the incision. If a posterior leiomyoma is difficult to reach with the minilaparotomy incision, it is removed completely laparoscopically, allowing exteriorization of the uterus through the minilaparotomy incision. The uterus is reconstructed in layers using 4-0 to 2-0 and 0 polydioxanone suture. The uterus is palpated to make sure all leiomyomas are removed. The mini-laparotomy incision is closed, laparoscopic reevaluation of the pelvic cavity is performed, and any blood clots are removed. When hemostasis is completely adequate, we cover the uterus with Interceed absorbable adhesion barrier (Johnson & Johnson Medical, Inc., Arlington, TX) to decrease the chance of adhesion formation.

PRESACRAL NEURECTOMY

Presacral neurectomy offers a surgical alternative for the amelioration of intractable dysmenorrhea. Originally introduced in 1899, it fell into disfavor as a result of poor patient selection and with the introduction of nonsteroidal antiinflammatory drugs, oral contraceptives, danazol and GnRH analogues. Despite the overall success of medical therapy, approximately 30% of patients fail to obtain pain relief. Until recently, presacral neurectomy was performed by laparotomy, limiting its application to women who had incapacitating dysmenorrhea and central pain unresponsive to medical therapy, or who were undergoing laparotomy for other pelvic pathology. However, recent advances in en-

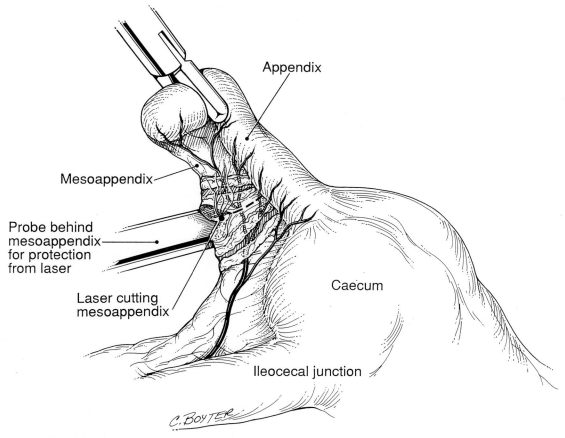

Appendix

Mesoappendix

Probe behind
mesoappendix
for protection
from laser

Laser cutting
mesoappendix

Caecum

Ileocecal junction

C. BOYTER

Figure 10-2.4 Mesoappendix is being cut with the CO_2 laser or scissors. (Drawing courtesy of Fertility and Endoscopy Center, Inc., Atlanta, GA.)

doscopic surgery now permit a laparoscopic approach to the classical presacral neurectomy in women with primary and secondary dysmenorrhea and in endometriosis-associated dysmenorrhea and central pelvic pain where medical therapy has failed to provide adequate relief.

Technique

Steep Trendelenburg positioning and tilting of the operating table to the left side are required to keep the bowel out of the operative field. The sacral promontory, ureters, and iliac vessels are identified. The peritoneum overlying the sacral promontory is elevated by smooth grasping forceps, and a small opening is made in the peritoneum. The peritoneum is incised vertically and horizontally and extended cephalad to just below the aortic bifurcation. Bleeding points are controlled using electrosurgery. The following landmarks are identified beneath the peritoneum: common iliac veins and arteries; ureters; inferior mesenteric, superior hemorrhoidal and midsacral arteries. The loose areolar tissue is excised as necessary to gain access to the plexus nerves. Care should be exercised to avoid

retroperitoneal major vessels, especially the left common iliac vein. The superior hypogastric (presacral nerve) bundle is identified, grasped, and skeletonized as necessary. A 3–4 cm segment of nerve tissue is excised, using the CO_2 laser or any other cutting modality. It is important to remove a wide portion of nerve between the two common iliac arteries laterally, bifurcation of aorta superiorly and sacral promontory inferiorly (triangle of Cote). Suturing the ends of the nerve bundle is not necessary. The retroperitoneal space is irrigated copiously and bleeding points are controlled with the laser or surgical electrode. The edges of the peritoneum are not sutured. Interceed (Johnson & Johnson Medical, Inc., Arlington, TX) is applied for adhesion reduction. The pain relief in our patient group has been around 90% (Figures 10-2.7 to 10-2.9).

LAPAROSCOPIC TREATMENT OF INFILTRATIVE ENDOMETRIOSIS INVOLVING THE RECTOSIGMOID COLON AND THE RECTOVAGINAL SEPTUM

The posterior cul-de-sac is the site most often involved with endometriosis. This area consists of the back of the

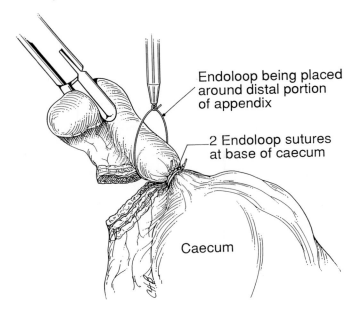

Figure 10-2.5 Endoloop suture is being placed at base of appendix. (Drawing courtesy of Fertility and Endoscopy Center, Inc., Atlanta, GA.)

cervix and vagina, anterior surface of the rectum, and the pararectals, along with the uterosacral ligaments and lower portion of the posterior aspect of the broad ligaments. Superficial endometrial implants on the peritoneum in this area can be easily treated by vaporization, excision or coagulation. However, infiltrative lesions are usually proximal to or involving structures such as ureters, uterine and lower pelvic vessels, and rectum. The recognition and thorough treatment of these implants is challenging and requires familiarity with anatomy and surgical skill, not only to remove the lesions completely, but also to manage injuries appropriately which may occur during treatment. Severe and infiltrative lesions result in anatomical distortion of the posterior cul-de-sac. Affected uterosacral ligaments are often retracted and attached to the cervix; the ureters are then retracted medially. When the posterior broad ligament is involved, it may result in periureteral fibrosis and stricture, and, rarely, partial or complete ureteral obstruction. Partial or complete posterior cul-de-sac obliteration occurs when endometriosis of the back of the vagina, pararectal area and lower rectum is present, and there is retraction and attachment of the rectum to the uterosacral ligaments, back of the vagina, cervix, and uterus, laterally or centrally. This attachment usually is associated with different degrees of infiltrative endometrial implants and nodules which are found after the rectum is separated from the cervix and vagina. The lesions may involve the different layers of the rectal wall and penetrate to the pararectal area below the uterosacral ligaments, toward the levator ani muscles and/or toward the rectovaginal sep-

tum, and occasionally may penetrate the entire vaginal wall.

Technique

The assistant should stand between the patient's legs and perform rectovaginal examination with one hand. With the other hand, he or she holds the uterus up with a rigid uterine elevator while both the assistant and surgeon observe the monitor. For rectovaginal septum and uterosacral ligament endometriosis, 5 to 8 mL of dilute vasopressin (10 units in 100 mL of lactated Ringer's) is injected into an uninvolved area with a 16-gauge laparoscopic needle. The peritoneum is opened and a plane is created in the rectovaginal septum using hydrodissection.

It is imperative that the ureters be located before continuing with this procedure. Any alteration in the direction of the ureters should be identified. Because ureters are lateral to the uterosacral ligaments, we stay between the ligaments as much as possible. Using hydrodissection and making a relaxing incision lateral to the uterosacral ligament allows the ureters to retract laterally. This increases the protection of the ureters. Ureterolysis often is necessary to free the ureters from the surrounding fibrotic diseased tissue and from endometriosis. Hydrodissection with the CO_2 laser and blunt dissection can be used for ureterolysis, enterolysis, and ovarian cyst resection.

While the assistant examines the rectum, the involved area is completely excised or vaporized until the loose areolar tissue of the rectovaginal space and normal mus-

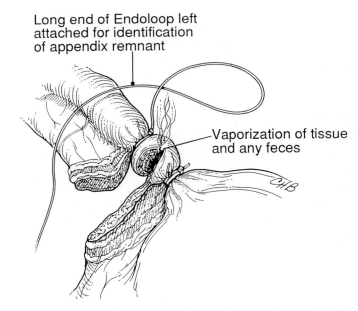

Figure 10-2.6 Tissue and any feces are being vaporized with the CO_2 laser. (Drawing courtesy of Fertility and Endoscopy Center, Inc., Atlanta, GA.)

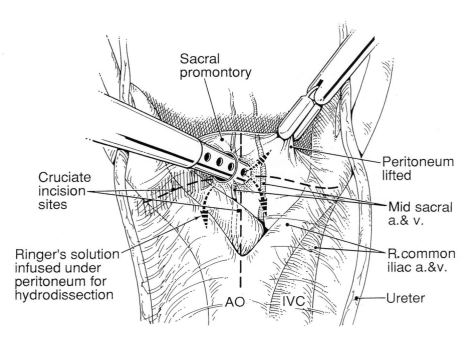

Sacral
promontory

Peritoneum
lifted

Cruciate
incision
sites

Mid sacral
a. & v.

Ringer's solution
infused under
peritoneum for
hydrodissection

R. common
iliac a.&v.

AO   IVC

Ureter

Figure 10-2.7 Hydrodissection and CO_2 laser are being used to expose the sacral promontory. (Drawing courtesy of Fertility and Endoscopy Center, Inc., Atlanta, GA.)

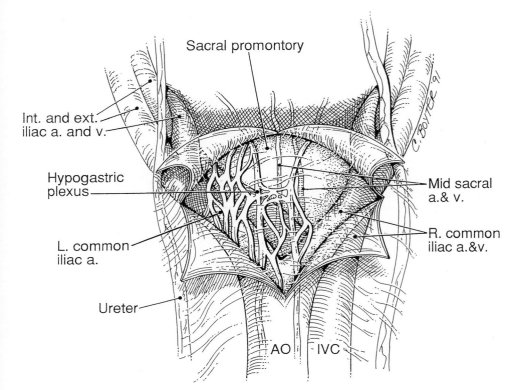

Sacral promontory

Int. and ext.
iliac a. and v.

Hypogastric
plexus

Mid sacral
a.& v.

L. common
iliac a.

R. common
iliac a.&v.

Ureter

AO   IVC

Figure 10-2.8 Hypogastric plexus has been exposed. (Drawing courtesy of Fertility and Endoscopy Center, Inc., Atlanta, GA.)

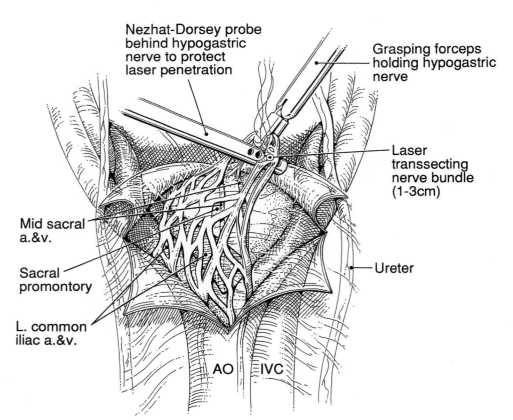

Nezhat-Dorsey probe
behind hypogastric
nerve to protect
laser penetration

Grasping forceps
holding hypogastric
nerve

Laser
transsecting
nerve bundle
(1-3cm)

Mid sacral
a.&v.

Sacral
promontory

L. common
iliac a.&v.

Ureter

AO   IVC

Figure 10-2.9 Hypogastric plexus is being removed. (Drawing courtesy of Fertility and Endoscopy Center, Inc., Atlanta, GA.)

cularis layers of the rectum are reached. In a woman whose rectum is pulled up and attached to the back of the cervix between the uterosacral ligaments, the uterus is anteflexed sharply and an incision is made at the right or left pararectal area, then extended to the junction of the cervix and the rectum. If the rectal involvement is more extensive and the assistant's finger is not long enough, a sigmoidoscope, a sponge on forceps, or a rectal probe is used. Two advantages of the sigmoidoscope are that it helps the surgeon identify the rectum and it aids in identifying or ruling out bowel perforation, because air bubbles can be seen passing from the air-inflated rectum into the posterior cul-de-sac when the latter is filled with irrigation fluid. The insertion of these devices should be done gently and cautiously to prevent rectal perforation. While the assistant guides the surgeon by rectovaginal exam, the rectum is completely freed from the back of the cervix. Generalized oozing and bleeding can be controlled with an injection of 3 to 5 mL dilute vasopressin (1 ampule in 100 mL), laser or bipolar electrocoagulator. Occasional bleeding from the stalk vessels, caused by dissection or vaporization of the fibrotic uterosacral ligaments and pararectal areas, is controlled with bipolar electrocoagulator.

Endometriosis rarely penetrates the mucosa of the bowel, but commonly involves the serosa, subserosa, fatty tissue, and the two muscularis layers. This involvement begins with an implant on the outermost surface, and progresses toward the mucosa, layer by layer. We use the ULTRA-PULSE CO_2 laser set between 40 and 80 W, and between 25 and 200 millijoules to excise or vaporize the lesion. When significant portions of both serosal and muscularis layers have been excised or vaporized and the mucosa is reached, the bowel wall may be reinforced by one to three 0 polydioxanone or polyglactin sutures. The rectum is thoroughly evaluated by a rectal examination and sigmoidoscopy, and if a perforation is detected, it is repaired laparoscopically in one layer. Consultation with a colorectal surgeon is usually recommended.

Postoperatively, the patient gradually advances her diet from clear liquids to a low residual diet and then to solid food. Oral laxatives are prescribed to avoid constipation, and rectal manipulation is avoided for 6 weeks.

LAPAROSCOPIC BOWEL RESECTION

When the lesion is deeper and full thickness of the rectum, sigmoid colon, or any other part of the large or small bowel is involved, or if the lesion has caused stricture, segmental or complete resection of a portion of the rectum or sigmoid colon is necessary in symptomatic patients. One of the following techniques is used, depending upon the location and extent of the disease.

DISK EXCISION AND PRIMARY REPAIR OF THE ANTERIOR RECTAL OR SIGMOID WALL WITH SUTURE

The following technique for total laparoscopic resection of part of the colon wall and repair is used to treat selected cases of infiltrative symptomatic intestinal endometriosis.

Technique

The extent of bowel involvement is evaluated and the need for full thickness disk excision is determined. We use a sigmoidoscope to clean the rectum completely, in order to further delineate the lesion and to guide the surgeon. If the lesion is low enough, an assistant can identify it by performing a rectal examination. After the ureters are identified in each side, the lower colon is mobilized. Depending on the location of the lesion, the right and/or left pararectal area(s) is (are) separated from adjacent organs. Any bleeding which is not controlled with the CO_2 laser is managed with bipolar electrocoagulation.

Full thickness excision begins above the area of visible disease. After identifying normal tissue, the lesion is held at its proximal end with grasping forceps inserted through the right lower quadrant trocar. An incision is made through the bowel serosa and muscularis, and the lumen is entered. The lesion is completely excised from the anterior rectal wall. Following complete excision of the lesion, the pelvic cavity is thoroughly irrigated and suctioned. The lesion is removed from the abdomen through the operative channel of the laparoscope or sigmoidoscope using a long grasping forceps, and is submitted for pathology.

The bowel is repaired transversely in one layer. Two traction sutures are applied to each side of the bowel defect, transforming it into a transverse opening. The stay sutures are brought out via the right and left lower quadrant trocar sleeves. The sleeves are removed, then replaced in the peritoneal cavity next to the stay sutures, and the sutures are secured outside the abdomen. The bowel is then repaired by placing several interrupted through-and-through sutures in .4 to .6 cm increments until it is completely repaired. We use 0 polyglactin laparoscopic sutures and a straight or curved needle with extracorporeal knot tying. For cases in which the bowel defect was less than 4 cm long and 1 cm wide, we have repaired the rectum vertically without causing bowel stricture.

At the end of the procedure, we carefully examine the rectosigmoid colon using the sigmoidoscope as described earlier to confirm that the closure is airtight and to ensure that there is no bowel stricture. Neither a Jackson-Pratt drain nor a nasogastric tube are used routinely. The Foley catheter is removed the day of surgery. Oral feeding is resumed after the spontaneous release of flatus, usually on the first or second postoperative day. All patients are released from the hospital between postoperative days two and four, when they are able to tolerate clear liquids well. Low residual diet is begun after the patient has a bowel movement.

PARTIAL TRANSANAL OR TRANSVAGINAL RESECTION

Technique

For small, isolated lesions in the lower rectum near the anus, the following technique can be used. The rectovaginal septum is delineated by the assistant who performs the simultaneous vaginal and rectal examination. The rectum is mobilized along the rectovaginal septum anteriorly to within 2 cm of the anus, using scissors and blunt dissection or the CO_2 laser and hydrodissection. Mobilization is continued along the left and right pararectal spaces by coagulating and dividing branches of the hemorrhoidal artery, if necessary.

When the rectum is sufficiently mobilized, the lesion is prolapsed to the level of the anus transvaginally or transanally (individualized based on the patient's condition), the perineal body is retracted and an RL 30 (Ethicon, Cincinnati, OH) multifire stapler is applied across the segment of the anterior rectal wall containing the nodule. Two staple applications usually are required to traverse the width of the involved mucosa. The affected area is excised and two additional interrupted 2-0 polyglactin sutures are applied along the staple line. Resection can be performed without the multifire stapler, instead using primary resection and suturing for repair.

The rectum is returned to the pelvis under direct observation. Integrity of the anastomosis is verified by insufflation of air into the rectum while the cul-de-sac is filled with lactated Ringer's.

COMPLETE SEGMENTAL RESECTION WITH TRANSANAL OR TRANSVAGINAL PROLAPSE

When there are multiple lesions or a larger portion of the bowel is involved, an entire segment of bowel is resected. The technique used depends on the location of the lesion. If the lesion is in the rectum or lower rectosigmoid colon, the bowel is mobilized by entering the pararectal area, rectovaginal septum, and posterior rectosigmoid colon from the presacral space to the levator muscles, as is done via laparotomy. The resection and reanastomosis are completed transvaginally or transrectally, using a circular stapler.

Technique

As in bowel resection at laparotomy, the rectum is mobilized, and the presacral space entered to the level of the levator ani muscles. The branches of the inferior mesenteric vessels are electrodesiccated and cut if necessary. In patients with rectal lesions, the rectum is transected distal to the lesion, and the proximal limb is prolapsed into the distal limb or through a posterior colpotomy, using Babcock clamps. The involved rectal segment is transected proximal to the lesion. The resected segment is sent for pathologic diagnosis, and a 2-0 polypropylene pursestring suture is placed around the circumference of the proximal limb of the bowel. The anvil of an ILS 29 or 33 stapler (Ethicon, Cincinnati, OH) is placed through the pursestring into the proximal bowel, and the proximal limb of bowel is replaced into the pelvis. Using Babcock clamps, the distal rectal segment is prolapsed through the anal canal and closed with an RL60, and the rectal stump is replaced through the anal canal into the pelvis. The ILS stapler is placed into the rectum, and the anvil trocar within the proximal bowel is inserted into the stapling device using the laparoscope. The device is fired, creating an end-to-end anastomosis. A proctoscope is used to examine the anastomosis for structural integrity and bleeding. The pelvis is filled with lactated Ringer's and observed with the laparoscope as the rectum is insufflated with air to check for leakage. Air leaks may be corrected using 2-0 polyglactin sutures placed transanally or laparoscopically. This technique is identical to resection at laparotomy, with the bipolar electrocoagulator and laser replacing suture and scissors.

A variation of this technique involves complete laparoscopic mobilization of the bowel, after which the involved area is prolapsed transvaginally or rectally and resection and application of the anvil is performed outside. The proximal end and rectal stump are reduced in the pelvis and reanastomosis is performed as described above.

Another method utilizes a 60-mm Endostapler (Ethicon, Inc., Cincinnati, OH) to resect the bowel intraabdominally after it is completely mobilized. The stapler is fired distal to the lesion. The proximal limb of the colon is delivered from the abdomen and exteriorized through a small incision. The lesion is amputated, and the anvil of the stapler is inserted into the lumen following placement of a pursestring suture. At this stage, anastomosis is completed with the stapler gun.

SEGMENTAL RESECTION THROUGH A MINILAPAROTOMY

When the lesion is high on the sigmoid or other part of the colon, or if a large portion of bowel must be removed (e.g. diverticulitis or cancer) this technique is utilized.

Technique

The portion of bowel to be resected is mobilized using the CO_2 laser or scissors for cutting and bipolar, surgical clips, or laparoscopic stapler (EZ35W, Ethicon, Inc., Cincinnati, OH) to desiccate or clip the mesocolon attachment and vasculature. The location and size of the ancillary incision is modified based on the area of the involved colon. A minilaparotomy is performed in the mid-suprapubic, left or right lower quadrant, by extending the corresponding ancillary incision. The bowel is guided to the minilaparotomy with grasping forceps. After resection and reanastomosis are completed, the bowel is returned to the abdominal cavity. The integrity of the repair is evaluated underwater by injecting air through a proctoscope as described.

We have used this technique for resection and reanastomosis for small bowel injuries with a trocar, during lysis of small bowel adhesions, or to correct small bowel strangulation through a Richter herniation. At times, in these situations, resection and reanastomosis can be done through an umbilical incision which is enlarged vertically or transversely.

TREATMENT OF ENDOMETRIOSIS OF THE BLADDER

Infiltrative endometriosis of the bladder wall is relatively uncommon. If the lesions are superficial, hydrodissection and vaporization or excision are adequate for removal. Using hydrodissection, the areolar tissue between the serosa and muscularis, beneath the implants, is dissected. The lesion is circumcised with the laser, and fluid is injected into the resulting defect. The lesion is grasped with forceps and dissected, using the laser. Traction allows the small blood vessels supplying the surrounding tissue to be coagulated as the lesion is resected. Frequent irrigation is necessary to remove char, ascertain the depth of vaporization, and ensure that the lesion does not involve the muscularis and the mucosa.

Endometriosis extending to the muscularis, but without mucosal involvement, can be treated laparoscopically and any residual or deeper lesions may be treated with postoperative hormonal therapy. When endometriosis involves full bladder wall thickness, the lesion is excised and the bladder reconstructed.

Simultaneous cystoscopy is performed and bilateral ureteral catheters are inserted. The bladder dome is held near the midline with the grasping forceps and the endometriotic nodule is excised 5 mm beyond the lesion. An incision is made with the CO_2 laser, using the suction-irrigation probe as a backstop. The specimen is removed from the abdominal cavity with a long grasping forceps, through the operative channel of the laparoscope. CO_2 gas distends the bladder cavity, allowing excellent observation of its interior. After identifying the ureters and examining the bladder mucosa again, the bladder is closed with several interrupted 4-0 polydioxanone or polyglactin through-and-through sutures, using extracorporeal or intracorporeal knotting. Cystoscopy is performed to identify possible leaks. Patients are discharged the following day and instructed to take trimethoprim and sulfamethoxazole for 2 weeks. The Foley catheter is removed 7 to 14 days later, after cystograms are done to be sure the bladder has healed and that there is no leakage or fistula.

TREATMENT OF ENDOMETRIOSIS OF THE URETER

Superficial implants over the ureter are generally treated by a combination of hydrodissection and CO_2 laser vaporization, or excision as described for superficial bladder endometriosis. Approximately 20 to 30 mL of lactated Ringer's is injected subperitoneally on the lateral pelvic wall. When the endometriosis has penetrated retroperitoneally and has caused partial or complete ureteral obstruction, the following techniques are utilized. Ureterolysis and mobilization of the ureter usually is required. The retroperitoneal space is entered at the level of the pelvic brim. The overlying peritoneum is opened with the CO_2 laser, and elevated by injecting irrigation fluid. The opening is enlarged, an irrigation probe is inserted, and more fluid is introduced into the retroperitoneal space along the course of the ureter. The fluid surrounds the ureter, moves it posteriorly, and allows safe superficial laser dissection or vaporization. If the endometrial implant is embedded and deeply scarred, the ureter is freed from surrounding tissue using hydrodissection and CO_2 laser, avoiding damage to the major pelvic wall blood vessels. Any bleeding which is not controlled by the CO_2 laser is managed with bipolar electrodesiccation.

After ureterolysis has been completed, endometriosis and fibrosis are vaporized or excised until the ureter is completely dissected and free of disease. At this point, if the ureter is obstructed partially or completely and requires resection, a retrograde ureteral catheter is placed via cystoscopy, with laparoscopic guidance. Partial wall resection is done over the catheter. Pinpoint entries to the lumen are not repaired.

When the lumen is invaded, the ureter is repaired with 1 to 3 interrupted 4-0 polydioxanone sutures. If the lumen is completely occluded and retrograde catheter placement is unsuccessful, we transect the ureter at that point using the laser and excise the obstructed section. Indigo carmine is injected antegrade to verify patency of the proximal lumen. Anastomosis is performed over the ureteral catheter with four interrupted through-and-through 4-0 polydioxanone sutures at 3, 6, 9, and 12 o'clock to approximate the proximal and distal ureteral segments, or to rejoin the ureter and bladder using intracorporeal or extracorporeal knot tying. The ureteral stents are removed 2 to 8 weeks postoperatively, after the integrity of the repair is confirmed by intravenous pyelogram (IVP).

CONCLUSION

Operative laparoscopy is an excellent alternative to laparotomy. The surgeon's eyes are within millimeters to centimeters from the tissue (via the videoscope), so the operative field is well-magnified. This allows the most tedious procedures to be performed microsurgically. However, the surgeon must be properly trained, then increase his skill level gradually to ensure that this method is used effectively and safely, without needless complications. Videoendoscopic procedures lack the three-dimensional perspective present with laparotomy. Successful utilization of videolaparoscopy requires that the previously trained surgeon relearn his operating skills. The time necessary to acquire the ability to perform advanced operative laparoscopy is typically longer than that for laparotomy (6 to 8 years). A lack of training or inexperience will be revealed by an unacceptable complication rate. This will impede the advancement of therapeutic laparoscopy, as did the problems and injuries which occurred during the use of the electrocoagulator for tubal ligation. However, future generations of surgeons can be taught the technique of operative videolaparoscopy without ever having to learn laparotomy.

SUGGESTED READING

Bryson, K. Laparoscopic appendectomy. *J Gynecol Surg* 1991;7:93–5.

Cornillie FJ, Oosterlynck D, Lauwernys JM, et al. Deeply infiltrating pelvic endometriosis: histology and clinical significance. *Fertil Steril* 1990;63:978–83.

Coronado C, Franklin RR, Lotze EC, Bailey RH, Valdes CT. Surgical treatment of symptomatic colorectal endometriosis. *Fertil Steril* 1990;53:411–6.

Dubuisson JB, Chapron C, Mouly M, et al. Laparoscopic myomectomy. *Gynaecol Endosc* 1993;2:171–3.

Hasson HM, Rotman C, Rana N, et al. Laparoscopic myomectomy. *Obstet Gynecol* 1992;80:545–6.

Koninckx PR, Martin DC. Deep endometriosis: a consequence of infiltration or retraction or possibly adenomyosis externa? *Fertil Steril* 1992;58:924–8.

Koninckx PR, Meuleman C, Demeyere S, Lesaffre E, Cornillie FJ. Suggestive evidence that pelvic endometriosis is a progressive disease, whereas deeply infiltrating endometriosis is associated with pain. *Fertil Steril* 1991;55:759–65.

Metzger DA, Montanino-Olivia M, Davis GD, et al. Efficacy of presacral neurectomy for the relief of midline pelvic pain. *J Am Assoc Gynecol Laparosc* 1994;1:S–22.

Nezhat CR, Nezhat FR, Luciano AA, Siegler AM, Metzger DA, Nezhat CH, Eds. *Operative Gynecologic Laparoscopy: Principles and Techniques.* New York: McGraw-Hill; 1995.

Nezhat CR, Berger GS, Nezhat FR, Buttram VC, Nezhat CH, Eds. *Endometriosis: Advanced Management and Surgical Techniques.* New York: Springer-Verlag, 1995.

Nezhat F, Seidman DS, Nezhat CR, Nezhat CH. Myomectomy: why, when and for whom? *Human Reprod* 1996;11(5):102–3.

Nezhat C. Videolaseroscopy: a new modality for the treatment of endometriosis and other diseases of reproductive organs. *Colposc Gynecol Laser Surg* 1986;2(4):221–4.

Perez JJ. Laparoscopic presacral neurectomy: results of the first twenty-five cases. *J Reprod Med* 1990;35:625–30.

Redwine DB. Laparoscopic en bloc resection for treatment of the obliterated cul-de-sac in endometriosis. *J Reprod Med* 1992;37:695–8.

Sharpe DR, Redwine DB. Laparoscopic segmental resection of the sigmoid and rectosigmoid colon for endometriosis. *Surg Lap Endosc* 1992;2:120–4.

Operative Laparoscopy, Second Edition
The Masters' Techniques in Gynecologic Surgery
Lippincott–Raven Publishers, Philadelphia © 1998.

11

Specimen Removal During Laparoscopic Surgery

Harry Reich

SPECIMEN REMOVAL DURING LAPAROSCOPIC SURGERY

Large puncture sites or incisions bordering on mini-laparotomy should be replaced by an umbilical extension or a laparoscopic culdotomy approach. Many surgeons dilate 5-mm lower quadrant puncture sites to 11 mm or more so that larger instruments, including morcellators, can be used to extract ovaries, tubes, and fibroids. Others routinely use 11-mm trocar sleeves through many sites. The number and size of puncture sites should be kept to a minimum, because deep fascia never fully regains its previous strength after division. Incisional hernias can occur when these sites are longer than 5 mm and the fascia is not closed directly. Primary repair of deep fascia at lower quadrant incisions is usually possible.

Techniques for umbilical incision enlargement and laparoscopic culdotomy were developed to remove ovaries, cysts, and myomas from the peritoneal cavity and to avoid large lower quadrant incisions when morcellation of myomas was too time-consuming with available instruments; recently released morcellators will be discussed which may overcome this difficulty. Post-menopausal cystic ovaries should be removed intact through the cul-de-sac if possible, preferably in impermeable sacks, as should peri-menopausal cystic ovaries that don't drain chocolate-like material upon mobilization from their respective pelvic sidewall or uterosacral ligament. Large endometriomas in women who do not desire future fertility usually are sufficiently cystic and pliable—once separated from the pelvic sidewall—to be removed through the umbilical incision.

SMALL SPECIMENS

Biopsies 8 mm or less in diameter are removed through laterally placed 5-mm lower quadrant incisions. These are made with a No. 11 blade near the top of the pubic hairline, lateral to the rectus abdominus muscle and the deep inferior epigastric vessels. These vessels, an artery flanked by two veins (venae comitantes), are located by direct vision of the inner abdominal wall, lateral to the umbilical ligaments (obliterated umbilical artery), as they generally cannot be found consistently by traditional transillumination. After grasping a specimen larger than the 5-mm trocar channel, the trocar sleeve is slipped upward on the biopsy forceps shaft out of the peritoneal cavity; the biopsy forceps with specimen are then pulled out in one motion through the soft tissue of the anterior abdominal wall. The biopsy forceps are then reinserted through their exit tract and the trocar sleeve pushed back into the peritoneal cavity over the forceps. Initial placement of the trocar sleeves lateral to the rectus muscle and the deep epigastric vessels facilitates this procedure, as it avoids going back and forth through the muscle. The trocar penetrates the external oblique, internal oblique, and transversalis fascia only, leaving an easily identifiable tract.

Fascial closure is not usually necessary for 5-mm incisions, though rare incisional hernias have been reported. Suture material is avoided in the lower quadrant 5-mm and 3-mm skin incisions, as their prolonged dissolution results in scarring. These incisions are loosely approximated with Javid vascular clamps (V. Mueller, McGaw Park, IL) and covered with collodion (AMEND, Irvington, NJ) to allow drainage of excess Ringer's lactate solution, should increased intraabdominal pressure be present. Patients are instructed to expect incision leakage for 24 hours and to wait one week for the collodion to slough off. These wounds heal by secondary intention as they are clean, free from pressure, surrounded by mobile tissue, and have good blood supply. Minimal scarring results.

A 10-mm operating laparoscope with 5-mm operating channel is used for 9- to 15-mm specimens, including small ovaries or ruptured cysts without any solid components, large fibrotic endometriosis biopsies, and the appendix. Biopsy forceps in the operating channel grasp the tissue, which is partially delivered into the tip of the umbilical trocar sleeve. The trocar sleeve and laparoscope are popped out of the umbilicus in one motion, after which the protruding tissue is grasped with hemostats or Kocher clamps and gently teased out of the peritoneal cavity. Alternatively, a 5-mm laparoscope can be used for visualization through the 5-mm lower trocar sleeve; tissue to be removed is then grasped with 11-mm grasping forceps inserted through the umbilicus and extracted.

UMBILICAL EXTENSION

With decompressed ovaries (benign pathology), fallopian tubes, and small fibroids, the 11-mm umbilical incision can be enlarged, especially if the initial skin incision is vertical midline through the deepest part within the umbilicus. This incision overlies the area where skin, deep fascia, and parietal peritoneum of the anterior abdominal wall meet, permitting little opportunity for the parietal peritoneum to tent away from the Veress needle. This vertical midline incision is made initially with a No. 15 blade (never a No. 11) on the inferior wall of the umbilical fossa extending to and just beyond its lowest point. In thin patients, this incision frequently traverses the deep fascia, but intraperitoneal injury is avoided by pulling the umbilicus onto the surgeon's forefinger, a maneuver that controls the incision's depth. Fol-

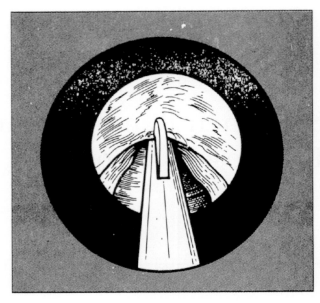

Figure 11-2 Scissors are in position to divide deep fascia. (Reprinted with permission from Reich H, Laparoscopic oophorectomy without ligature or morcellation. *Contemporary Ob/Gyn* 1989;34:9. Medical Economics Company, Inc.)

lowing CO_2 insufflation until the intraabdominal pressure is above 25-mm Hg, the trocar (usually a 10-mm Apple trocar) is seated vertically just inside the skin prior to a horizontal thrust. The result is a parietal peritoneal puncture directly beneath the umbilicus. Shielded trocars are never used, because this parietal peritoneal exit is too close to the

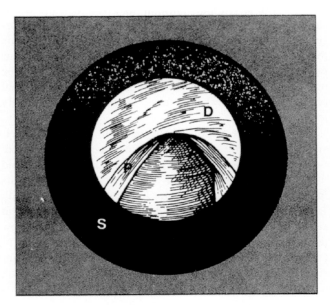

Figure 11-1 Visualize the peritoneum (P) and deep fascia (D) laparoscopically before incising them (S—scope). (Reprinted with permission from Reich H, Laparoscopic oophorectomy without ligature or morcellation. *Contemporary Ob/Gyn* 1989;34:9. Medical Economics Company, Inc.)

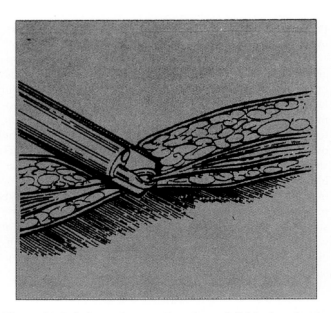

Figure 11-3 Scissors in operating channel divide deep fascia. (Reprinted with permission from Reich H, Laparoscopic oophorectomy without ligature or morcellation. *Contemporary Ob/Gyn* 1989;34:9. Medical Economics Company, Inc.)

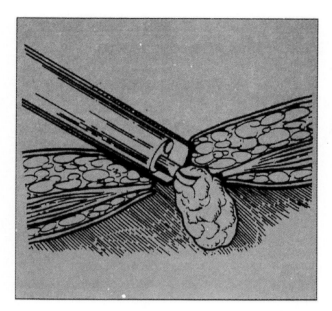

Figure 11-4 The ovary is removed through the umbilical incisions. (Reprinted with permission from Reich H, Laparoscopic oophorectomy without ligature or morcellation. *Contemporary Ob/Gyn* 1989;34:9. Medical Economics Company, Inc.)

aortic bifurcation; both sharp trauma from the trocar tip and blunt trauma from the shield could result.

The operating laparoscope is used with scissors in the operating channel. The tip of the laparoscope is placed one cm above the tip of the trocar sleeve, which is then carefully removed from the peritoneal cavity. The peritoneum is first visualized (Figure 11-1), and then incised downward in the midline, with the scissors in the operating channel of the operating laparoscope. Next, deep fascia is identified and incised to add another one cm or more to the incision (Figures 11-2, 11-3). Finally, the skin incision inside the umbilicus can be extended upward to incorporate the superior wall of the umbilical fossa. This umbilical incision is closed with a single 4-0 Vicryl suture opposing deep fascia and skin dermis. The knot is buried beneath the fascia by catching first the fascia and then the skin closest to the surgeon with the needle and then taking skin and finally fascia on the other side. Compressible ovaries and cysts and solid myomas less than 3 cm in diameter can be removed through this incision; this includes most benign cysts and normal ovaries removed for adhesive disease (Figure 11-4).

LAPAROSCOPIC CULDOTOMY

Solid lesions greater than 3 cm in diameter and ovarian cysts of unknown pathology separated intact from the pelvic sidewall are best removed through the cul-de-sac. A posterior *culdotomy* incision using CO_2 laser or electrosurgery through the cul-de-sac of Douglas into the vagina is preferable to a *colpotomy* incision with scissors through the vagina and overlying vagina because complete hemostasis is obtained while making the incision.

The anatomic relationship between the rectum and the posterior vagina must be confirmed to avoid cutting the rectum while making the laparoscopic culdotomy incision. A curette is placed in the uterus for elevation. A wet sponge in ring forceps is placed just behind the cervix to identify the posterior vaginal fornix by distending it. A rectal probe assures that the rectum is out of the way and aids in the dissection required, should the rectum cover the posterior vagina (Figure 11-5).

Alternatively, a Valtchev uterine mobilizer (Conkin Surgical Instruments, Toronto, Canada) can be inserted to antevert the uterus and delineate the posterior vagina. With this device, the cervix sits on a wide acorn that is readily visible in the vagina between the uterosacral ligaments when the cul-de-sac is inspected laparoscopically.

Before the rectal probe is removed, it may be necessary to reflect the rectum off the posterior vaginal fornix. This is done using either cutting current through a spoon electrode or the laparoscopic laser at 20 W ultrapulse. The peritoneum at the junction of the rectum and vagina is incised, and, using the aquadissector, the plane between rectum and vagina is developed and the rectum pushed downward.

Following these maneuvers, and when it is clear that the rectum has been separated off the posterior vaginal wall or vaginal apex if the uterus has been removed, the upper vagina or posterior fornix is distended by the wet sponge on ring forceps. The transverse laparoscopic culdotomy incision is made with the spoon electrode at 100 W of cutting current or the CO_2 laser with power set at 50 to 100 W continuous without the bleeding that accompanies a vaginal colpotomy incision made with scissors (Figure 11-6). The sponge in the posterior vagina comes rapidly into view. Some difficulty may be encountered maintaining adequate pneumoperitoneum once the vagina is entered, but the sponge in contact with the incision usually is adequate for this purpose. In addition, gas loss may be slowed if the assistant cups the labia to bring them together. Because of the sudden loss of pneumoperitoneum and field of view, there is the potential danger of grasping bowel with a sharp grasper through the vagina, after losing sight of the lesion to be extracted. Following culdotomy, a sponge, pack, or 30-cc Foley balloon should be kept in close contact with the vaginal incision to avoid the loss of pneumoperitoneum and to facilitate the extraction of large masses. A ring forceps, single-toothed tenaculum, or a laparoscopic biopsy forceps is inserted through the vagina and used to grasp the fibroid, ovary, or its attached tube, and pull it out through the culdotomy incision (Figure 11-7). Alternately, a 5-mm lower quadrant grasping forceps can be used to push the mass through the culdotomy incision. On occasion, the clinician's fingers can be inserted into the peritoneal cavity and used to grasp the ovary.

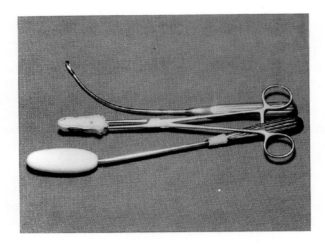

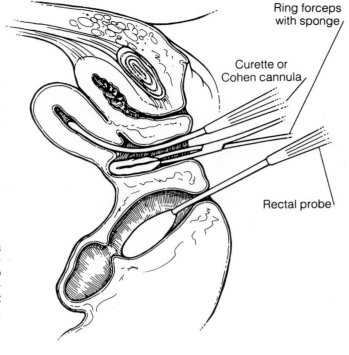

Ring forceps
with sponge

Curette or
Cohen cannula

Rectal probe

Figure 11-5 Laparoscopic culdotomy probes, consisting of a curette in the uterus, a ring forceps with sponge in the posterior vaginal fornix, and a rectal instrument in the rectum help avoid accidental cutting of the rectum. (Reprinted with permission from Reich H, Laparoscopic oophorectomy without ligature or morcellation. *Contemporary Ob/Gyn* 1989;34:9. Medical Economics Company, Inc.)

For large cystic masses a 14 to 18-gauge needle on a needle extension adapter (Crown Brothers, Decatur, GA) is directed through the vagina for cyst decompression, or, if a dermoid is present, the mass can be incised so that the thick cyst contents drain into the vagina until the mass is small enough to be pulled through the incision (Figures 11-8, 11-9). However, my technique of choice is to insert an impermeable sack (Lap Sac: Cook OB/GYN, Spencer, IN) intraperitoneally through the culdotomy incision. This 5 × 8 inch nylon bag has a polyurethane inner coating and a nylon drawstring. It is impermeable to water and dye. The ovary with intact cyst is placed in the bag, which is closed

by pulling its drawstring. The sack is delivered by the drawstring through the posterior vagina, the bag opened and the intact specimen visually identified, decompressed, and removed (Figures 11-10, 11-11).

For fibroids, the tenaculum or 11-mm corkscrew is inserted through the vagina by maneuvering it around the sponge to minimize loss of pneumoperitoneum. The fibroid is grasped under direct laparoscopic vision. In some cases, the fibroid can be pushed into the deep cul-de-sac and held there while a second surgeon identifies it from below and applies the tenaculum. An 11-mm corkscrew device is screwed into the myoma vaginally through the culdotomy incision, and the myoma is put on traction at the incision

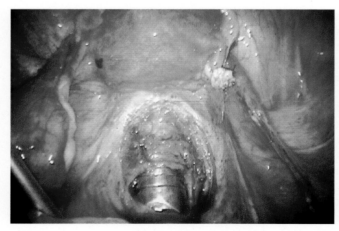

Figure 11-6 A posterior culdotomy incision is made with the CO_2 laser in the upper vagina over the Valtchev uterine mobilizer (Conkin Surgical Instruments).

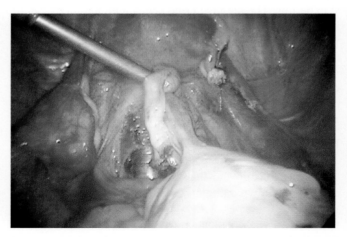

Figure 11-7 A ring forceps is inserted through the vagina to grasp the ovary.

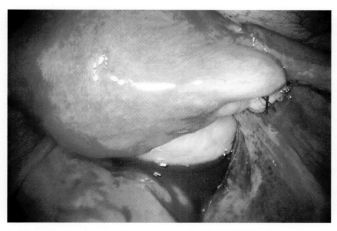

Figure 11-8 The mass is pulled into the deep pelvis to prevent leakage into the peritoneal cavity. An 18-gauge on a needle extension is directed into the vagina to decompress the cyst for removal through the culdotomy incision.

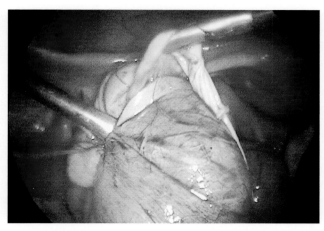

Figure 11-10 An intact cyst is removed from the ovary with the CO_2 laser.

and further morcellated vaginally with scissors or scalpel if necessary until removal is completed.

Following removal of the mass, the incision is closed vaginally or laparoscopically. Vaginal closure is done with interrupted, figure-of-eight, or running 0-Vicryl sutures. Vaginal suturing is aided by the use of a lateral vaginal retractor used to spread the lateral vagina adjacent to the culdotomy incision (Euro-Med, Inc., Redmond, WA or Simpson/Basye, Wilmington, DE). This device is self-retaining with a thumb-ratchet release that keeps it open and in place. Vaginal suturing can be difficult, because the vaginal incision frequently becomes edematous during the procedure, making exposure inadequate. I usually elect to close the culdotomy incision from above, using 1-3 curved

needle sutures (Vicryl on a CT-1 or CT-2) tied extracorporeally with the Clarke knot pusher; this method helps maintain laparoscopic suturing skills.

While culdotomy surgery offers an opportunity for invasion by organisms already present in the vagina, the use of an electrosurgical or laser incision, aspiration of all blood clots, and copious irrigation, after which at least 2L of irrigant is left in the peritoneal cavity at the close of the procedure, eliminates the environment necessary for proliferation of these organisms. Pelvic cellulitis and postoperative sepsis with laparoscopic culdotomy has not been reported when these techniques are used.

PROBLEMS ENCOUNTERED DURING CULDOTOMY

During multiple myomectomy procedures it is not uncommon to have difficulty locating all of the myomas after

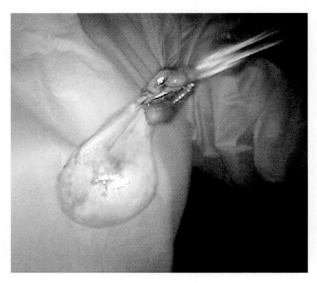

Figure 11-9 The intact mass is shown following removal.

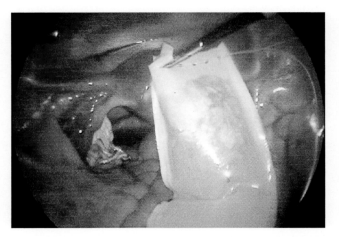

Figure 11-11 The intact cyst is placed into an impermeable sack (LapSac; Cook OB/GYN) for removal through the culdotomy.

excising them from the uterus. In most cases, excised myomas are placed in the deep cul-de-sac for later removal through a laparoscopic culdotomy incision. On occasion, myomas are placed in the right iliac fascia especially if cecal adhesions are present to prevent their egress into the upper abdomen. In cases where all of the myomas cannot be located, copious irrigation with Ringer's lactate is performed with the patient in a reverse Trendelenburg position. The area beneath the liver is searched by manipulating the laparoscope and the actively irrigating aquadissector tip, in unison, around the right lateral border of the liver and then beneath it. Foreign bodies in this area can then be visualized and grasped with biopsy forceps. Should the myoma be intertwined among loops of small bowel, the reverse Trendelenburg position, copious irrigation, and gravity will usually result in its return into the cul-de-sac from where it can be grasped and delivered. When multiple small myomas are encountered, the culdotomy incision can be made early, the Lap Sac introduced for fragment storage, and pneumoperitoneum maintained with a 30-cc Foley balloon in the vagina, or better, a vaginal delineator (Richard Wolf, Chicago, IL, USA). Small fibroids will usually resorb, though anecdotal reports abound of this necrosing tissue attracting a blood supply from surrounding organs.

After vaginal delivery of the last fibroid, the peritoneal cavity should be inspected for additional lesions prior to closing the culdotomy. It is very frustrating to have to take down this closure to extract an additional fibroid.

Large masses can be removed through a small culdotomy incision by morcellation. These large masses include 10-cm fibroids and large fibroid uteri. This can be a particularly time-consuming portion of the procedure and can last over one hour. During long procedures, it is wise to change from laparoscopic stirrups (Allan stirrups or knee supports) to candy cane stirrups to obtain better hip flexion to permit assistance with vaginal sidewall retractors. Self-retaining lateral vaginal wall retractors or Vienna retractors (Brisky-Navatril) are considered for shorter procedures.

Morcellation can be done laparoscopically or vaginally. For the laparoscopic technique, a No. 10 blade on a long handle is introduced gently through the left 5-mm trocar incision after removing the trocar. With care, the mass (uterus and/or large myoma) can be bivalved with the blade. The surgeon's fingers in contact with the skin prevent loss of pneumoperitoneum.

Using a small culdotomy incision, an 11-mm laparoscopic corkscrew (WISAP, Sauerlach, Germany) is inserted into the mass to be delivered to gain an initial grip. A second 11-mm corkscrew is then inserted alongside the first one, and using a scalpel, the myoma is divided between the two corkscrew devices. The leading corkscrew device with surrounding tissue is then wedged free with scalpel or scissors from the larger body of the lesion. With traction around the second corkscrew, an apple-coring technique can be performed, with the scalpel en-

circling the exposed myoma through 360° to remove a large core of it. The soft tissue of a uterus will often invert during this procedure, allowing delivery of much of the lesion. However, myomas rarely lose their shape unless degenerative changes have resulted secondary to menopause or GnRH analogs. Much morcellation is necessary, but the surgeon's patience and hard work will be rewarded by accomplishing removal of large size masses, sometimes exceeding 1000 grams.

During laparoscopic hysterectomy for large fibroids, vaginal morcellation is done after securing the ovarian arteries from above and the uterine arteries from above or below. A No. 10 blade on a long knife handle is used to make a circumferential incision into the fundus of the uterus while pulling outwards on the cervix and using the cervix as a fulcrum. The myometrium is incised circumferentially parallel to the axis of the uterine cavity and the serosa of the uterus. The knife is not extended through the serosa of the uterus. The incision is continued around the full circumference of the myometrium in a symmetrical fashion beneath the uterine serosa. Traction is maintained on the cervix, and the avascular myometrium is cut so that the endometrial cavity, with a surrounding thick layer of myometrium, is delivered with the cervix, bringing the outside of the uterus closer to the operator for further excision by wedge morcellation.

Wedge morcellation is done by removing wedges of myometrium from the anterior and posterior uterine wall, usually in the midline, to reduce the bulk of the myometrium. After excision of a large core, the fundus is morcellated with multiple wedge resections, around either a tenaculum or an 11-mm corkscrew. The remaining fundus, if still too large for removal, can be bivalved so that one half can be pulled out of the peritoneal cavity, followed by the other half.

ANTERIOR ABDOMINAL WALL MORCELLATION

Although morcellation of fibroids through anterior abdominal wall puncture sites has not been practical with instruments presently available, recent developments may solve this problem for the gynecologist. Professor Kurt Semm, who developed the first manual morcellator, has developed a manual circular saw to core out 2-cm cylinders of fibromyomatous tissue while the fibroid is still in or attached to the uterus. This device is inserted through a 2-cm lower abdominal trocar sleeve and depends on a corkscrew inside it to fixate the fibroid prior to twisting the circular saw into it. Loss of resistance during twisting indicates that the base of the fibroid has been reached, after which the cylindrical specimen is pulled free by traction, the specimen is removed, and the instrument is reinserted. After the bulk of the lesion is removed in this fashion, a claw forceps is substituted for the corkscrew in the device for traction and the compressible, fenestrated, remaining tissue is removed from the uterus through the 2-cm cannula. Semm accomplishes supracervical hysterectomy using this same device, after coring out the endocervical canal with a 1-cm circular saw. These 2-cm puncture sites require direct peritoneal or fascial closure with skin hooks to prevent hernias.

Cook Urological (Spencer, IN) has developed a 1-cm motorized circular saw with suction for laparoscopic nephrectomy. After placement of the kidney into the Lapsac, it is morcellated into small soft pieces that are sucked into the device until the LapSac is small enough to be pulled out of the umbilicus. I have used this instrument for myoma morcellation during laparoscopic hysterectomy and myomectomy and for fibroma oophorectomy. Currently I am working on 2- and 3-cm versions for culdotomy morcellation.

The Steiner Electromechanic Morcellator (Karl Storz, Tuttlingen, Germany) is a 10-mm diameter motorized circular saw that uses claw forceps or a tenaculum to grasp the fibroid and pull it into contact with the fibroid. Large pieces of myomatous tissue are removed piecemeal until the myoma can be pulled out through the trocar incision. With practice this instrument can often be inserted through a stretched 5-mm incision without an accompanying trocar.

I have developed the poor man's morcellator, a No. 10 blade on a long handle introduced gently through the left 5-mm trocar incision after removing the trocar. With care, the myoma can be bivalved with the blade. The surgeon's fingers in contact with the skin prevent loss of pneumoperitoneum. Multiple blades may be necessary.

SPECIMEN RETRIEVAL SACKS

In addition, there are also numerous organ/cyst retrieval systems available commercially that allow for specimen removal through the trocar sites without enlarging the incision. These systems allow for entrapment, fragmentation and retrieval of resected tissue.

They are available in various sizes ranging from 200 to 800 ml with special introducers that mostly fit through a 10-mm trocar sleeve. The retrieval bags are made of different materials including:

- **Polyurethane (PU) foil** (Endobag, Dexide Co.); (Endo Catch, Auto Suture Co.); (Extraction Bag, Karl Storz Co.): They are gas- and liquid-impermeable, but have limited tensile strength and mechanical resistance. The risk of perforation with morcellation of pathological tissue (cancer, infected tissue) and consequent peritoneal contamination limit their use to extraction of tissue without morcellation.
- **Special plastic foil** (Endopouch, Ethicon Co.): Main use is retrieval of small tissue that does not require morcellation. The material has a potential for instrument perforation which makes tissue morcellation potentially dangerous.
- **Polyamide textile and PU coating** (LapSac, Cook Co.); (Espiner Bag, Espiner Co.); (Lap Bag, Angiomed Co.):

Polyamide is a plastic material manufactured with nylon fibers of appropriate diameter that provides high tensile strength and mechanical resistance to perforation. Tears in the material also do not widen further. This combined with PU coating to make them waterproof ensures that they are safer for tissue morcellation.

For deployment, most devices have an introducer or tube with the sack packaged inside. This arrangement allows its placement in a 10-mm trocar without loss of pneumoperitoneum. They are also designed to stabilize the sack and to maintain contact in order to prevent its loss in the abdominal cavity. While some systems require the use of endoscopic forceps or dissectors to open the mouth of the bat, other designs use springs, wires and rubber rings that allow for spontaneous opening once deployed in the abdominal cavity. And some have designs that allow for easier capture of specimens. Others allow use of instruments while the sac remains open. This is particularly useful in performing cystectomy with the ovary in the sac to avoid spillage in case of cyst perforation (if one chooses not to drain the cyst). All these features, of course, increase sack bulk and limit its potential size.

For specimen removal, some sacks have incorporated a drawstring to close its mouth prior to extraction while others have a long extended tail so that it can be drawn into the mouth of the trocar. Extraction of the specimen from the abdomen (after the mouth of the bag is secured) requires the removal of the trocar from the body wall, along with the device. At this point, the mouth of the bag should be outside of the body wall, where it can be grasped with fingers and removed entirely by pulling. If the specimen is larger than the 10-mm incision, the incision can be extended or the specimen can be morcellated with fingers, forceps, scissors, or morcellators, within the bag. Smaller pieces of tissue are then removed until the entire specimen within the sack can be extracted through the 10-mm incision. Again, for morcellation of pathologic specimens, one should use a system made of polyamide textile in order to prevent perforation and spillage into the abdominal cavity.

Additionally, for endoscopic morcellation or dissection (e.g. cystectomy), it is advantageous to use a system that has an endoscopically visible transparent sack.

Moreover, these organ retrieval systems also afford protection of the exit wound from contamination by an infected or cancerous specimen.

As one can see, numerous options are now available for laparoscopic retrieval of specimen. In closing, the optimal device should be easy to deploy, endoscopically visible for manipulation/dissection, and easy and safe to extract with a sac that is strong, liquid-impermeable, resistant to tear and of sufficient size to capture the specimen.

FUTURE CONSIDERATIONS

Morcellators should get better and smaller; sacks should become easier to insert and to place specimens into them.

Directed-beam MRI or similar energy sources should become available to dissolve fibroids and probably the uterus without surgery. Photodynamic dye therapy may destroy endometriosis and ovarian tumors. Medicines may actually be developed that effectively treat endometriosis and fibroids, instead of the presently available useless drugs that do little beyond establishing hormonal deprivation and its sequelae.

SUGGESTED READING

Kadar N, Reich H, Liu CY, Manko GF, Gimpelson R. Incisional hernias after major laparoscopic gynecologic procedures. *Am J Obstet Gynecol* 1993;168:1493–5.

Levine RL. Pelviscopic surgery in women over 40. *J Reprod Med* 1990;35:597.

Reich H. Laparoscopic oophorectomy and salpingo-oophorectomy in the treatment of benign tuboovarian disease. *Int J Fertil* 1987;32:233.

Reich H. Laparoscopic oophorectomy without ligature or morcellation. *Contemporary Ob/Gyn* 1989;34:34.

Reich H. New Techniques in Advanced Laparoscopic Surgery. In: Sutton C, ed. *Bailliere's Clinical Obstetrics and Gynecology.* New York: Harcourt Brace Javonovich, 1989:655–81.

Reich H, Clarke HC, Sekel L. A simple method for ligating in operative laparoscopy with straight and curved needles. *Obstet Gynecol* 1992; 79:143–7.

Reich H, McGlynn F, Sekel L, Taylor P. Laparoscopic management of ovarian dermoid cysts. *J Reprod Med* 1992;37:640–4.

Reich H, McGlynn F, Sekel L. Total laparoscopic hysterectomy. *Gynaecological Endoscopy* 1993;2:59–63.

Operative Laparoscopy, Second Edition
The Masters' Techniques in Gynecologic Surgery
Lippincott–Raven Publishers, Philadelphia © 1998.

12

Laparoscopic Presacral Neurectomy

David B. Redwine and James J. Perez

HISTORY

First described in Europe in 1899, presacral neurectomy has enjoyed varying degrees of popularity since its introduction. Utilized for the management of pelvic pain, the procedure became less popular in the 1960s due to enthusiasm for treatment of pelvic pain by medical management, including use of non-steroidal anti-inflammatory drugs, oral contraceptives, danocrine, and gonadotropin-releasing hormone agonists. Although medical management has been rather successful in controlling patients with pelvic pain, there are many patients who do not respond to medical management, and many who have recurrent symptoms after cessation of successful medical therapy. Laparoscopic presacral neurectomy has been developed in an attempt to provide an outpatient surgical treatment of central pelvic pain.

ANATOMY AND PHYSIOLOGY

Pain impulses from the cervix, uterine corpus and proximal fallopian tubes are transmitted through afferent sympathetic neural fibers traversing cephalad from the central pelvis. These small, scattered, neural fibers exist in the true pelvis as the inferior hypogastric plexus and coalesce into the intermediate hypogastric plexus at approximately the level of the upper sacral and lower lumbar vertebral regions. The intermediate hypogastric plexus is composed of two or sometimes three separate trunks lying on the vertebral body of L-5. More cephalad, the neural fibers coalesce further into the superior hypogastric plexus which continues up and over the bifurcation of the aorta, lying slightly to the left of midline.

In performing a presacral neurectomy, the superior and upper intermediate hypogastric plexuses are the structures most commonly resected. As such, a presacral neurectomy is neither presacral (since it is largely performed in the region of the vertebral bodies of L-4 and L-5) nor a neurec-

tomy (since a plexus but no individually named nerve is involved). The neural tissue is imbedded in loose areolar tissue beneath the posterior peritoneum, traveling with small lymphatics. While performing the procedure, the surgeon will be able to appreciate the substance of the presacral plexus when it is grasped and elevated, but occasionally will be unable to distinguish neural from lymphatic tissue, even with magnification through the laparoscope.

Sensory fibers from the fundus of the uterus may travel through the more lateral ovarian and renal neural plexes and therefore may not be disrupted with a presacral neurectomy, leading to failure of pain relief in some patients.

INDICATIONS

The chief indication for performance of a presacral neurectomy is for relief of intractable central pelvic pain or uterine cramping with menses which has not responded to medical management.

Severe Uterine Cramping with the Menstrual Flow

Since endometriosis is a disease primarily of the peritoneal surfaces which infrequently involves the uterus, it is unsurprising that resection of endometriosis does not always alleviate uterine cramping. The observation has been made that patients with endometriosis may hurt severely with their menstrual flow. This does not necessarily mean that this increased pain is uterine in origin, or that the patients, if asked, would even describe it as uterine cramping in nature. Actually, when specific types of symptoms are examined, it is apparent that many patients with endometriosis may hurt throughout the month, with an *exacerbation* of this chronic pain at the time of menses. Nonetheless, if the clinician does not make an attempt to distinguish between various types of pain, the inference that could incorrectly be drawn is that uterine cramping with the menstrual

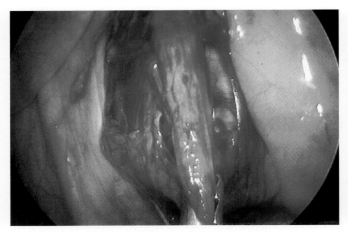

Figure 12-1 The intermediate hypogastric plexus.

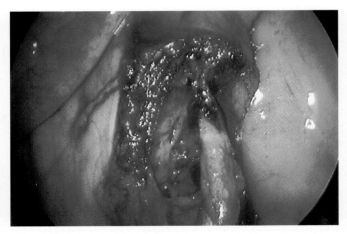

Figure 12-2 Superior hypogastric plexus after application of bipolar coagulation.

flow is the cardinal symptom caused by endometriosis. Only after removal of endometriosis will it become apparent what pain was due to that disease. In any event, a patient with severe uterine cramping with menses who is unsatisfactorily relieved by medical therapy is a candidate for a presacral neurectomy. Other types of midline pelvic pain may be relieved by laparoscopic presacral neurectomy.

TECHNIQUE

Suprapubic Approach

The suprapubic approach was developed at the Center for Operative Laparoscopy in Columbus, Ohio, and has the advantage of recreating the anatomic orientation the surgeon is familiar with at laparotomy. Although more time-consuming than is an umbilical approach, it is useful to master this approach while learning. In difficult cases, this approach may be necessary. After laparoscopic excision of endometriosis has been completed, a 10-mm trocar is passed through a third puncture suprapubically in the midline. A 5-mm trocar is placed suprapubically on the left and a 3-mm trocar on the right. The sacral promontory and overlying peritoneum is identified. Twenty mL of a solution containing 50 U of vasopressin diluted in 100 mL of normal saline is injected retroperitoneally. A vertical incision is made in the peritoneum, extending from the bifurcation of the aorta caudad toward the hollow of the sacrum. A laparoscope in the umbilical incision can be used to retract the sigmoid colon laterally. Observing through the suprapubic laparoscope and operating through the suprapubic sheaths, the retroperitoneal space is explored bluntly. If more exposure is needed, two 2.3-mm instruments 1 inch apart can be passed down through the abdominal wall halfway between the umbilicus and the pubic symphysis. These can be used to retract the cut edges of the peritoneum laterally by attaching a sterile rubber band between the external

sheaths of the instruments, so that the internal ends spring apart. Using only blunt dissection, the superior hypogastric plexus is identified, grasped, and elevated. The lateral margins of dissection are the right ureter on the right and the mesocolon on the left. Approximately 2 cm of the nerve is resected (Figure 12-1), in one of several ways. Once the superior and intermediate hypogastric plexes are isolated, an internal suture can be placed superiorly and inferiorly and the intervening tissue resected. Also, the bipolar coagulator can be used to coagulate the superior hypogastric plexus just distal to the bifurcation of the aorta, then the distal transection can be performed either by using bipolar coagulation and scissors transection or by the Nd:YAG laser with contact tip (Figures 12-2, 12-3, 12-4, 12-5). After resection, the retroperitoneal space is irrigated, bleeders bipolar coagulated, and then the peritoneum can be closed by gathering the cut edges within an Endoloop suture (Figure 12-6). When the peritoneum is left open, peritoneal regen-

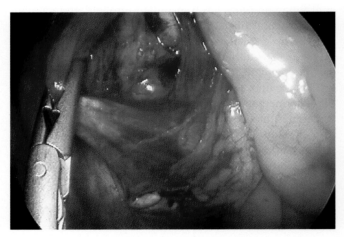

Figure 12-3 Presacral nerve grasped just above the bifurcation of the inferior hypogastric plexus.

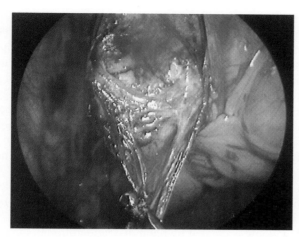

Figure 12-4 The retroperitoneal space with bifurcating inferior hypogastric plexus seen over the lower one-half of this frame.

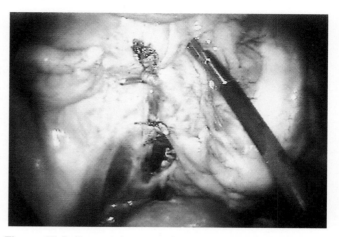

Figure 12-6 It may take several sutures to reperitonealize this space adequately. In this way the protective retroperitoneal fat is returned to its anatomic position.

eration has occurred without complication, although without a layer of retroperitoneal fatty tissue. The pelvis is irrigated copiously and, once good hemostasis is noted, the incisions are closed with subcuticular 3-0 vicryl suture.

Umbilical Approach

The umbilical approach was developed in 1988 at St. Charles Medical Center in Bend, Oregon. The patient is in steep Trendelenburg position and a triple puncture technique is employed, with a 10-mm operating laparoscope inserted through the umbilicus, a grasper in the left lower quadrant, and a suction-irrigator in the right lower quadrant. The patient is rolled slightly to the left to facilitate the lateral displacement of the sigmoid colon. After completion of any pelvic surgery, the laparoscope is drawn back slightly in order to gain a panoramic perspective of the sacral prom-

ontory. The pneumoperitoneum allows ample space for easy storage of the small bowel away from the operative site. This is in distinct contrast to the difficulty with visualization that is frequently encountered at laparotomy, particularly if a presacral neurectomy is performed through a low transverse incision. The most obvious visual landmarks that will be first encountered are the common iliac arteries, the sacral promontory, and the mesentery of the sigmoid colon (Figure 12-7).

Before surgery is begun, take the time to palpate the area between the common iliac arteries with a blunt probe. The structure that is most subtly hidden is the left common iliac vein. The left common iliac vein lies further down the sacral

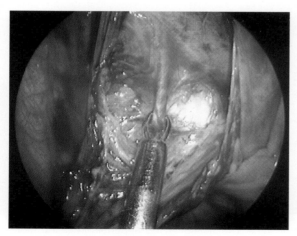

Figure 12-5 Great care must be exercised so as to not damage the middle sacral vessel (seen within the grasper).

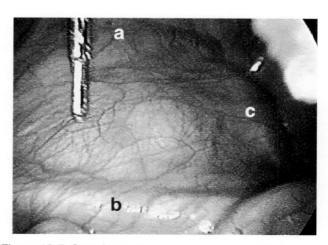

Figure 12-7 Seen from a laparoscope inserted at McBurney's point, the lateral margins of presacral neurectomy are **A.** the edge of the sigmoid mesentery and **B.** the right common iliac vessels. The transverse peritoneal incisions will be made between these two points. The sacral promontory is seen at **C.** while the atraumatic grasper is palpating the left common iliac vein, seen as a blue retroperitoneal structure.

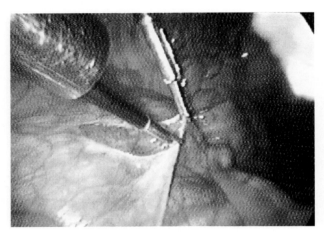

Figure 12-8 The peritoneum is grasped and elevated away from underlying structures and incised transversely, using 90 W of pure cutting current delivered through 3 mm monopolar scissors passed down the operating channel of a 10-mm laparoscope inserted through an umbilical port.

promontory than does the artery, but it is not very obvious due to the low pressure in the vein. The left common iliac vein has a quite variable location with respect to the artery, lying more caudad in some patients. There are two signs that can help identify this large vein. Percussive tapping of the peritoneum medial to the left common iliac artery with a blunt probe or by the closed scissors may elicit the ''waterbed'' sign: the low pressure of blood in the left common iliac vein, when percussed, will frequently cause the surface of the peritoneum to bounce and shake like a perturbed waterbed, whereas bare sacral promontory will react like percussing a rock, i.e., nothing happens. The second sign that can help identify this structure is the characteristic wave of the dicrotic pulsation associated with right atrial contraction, which may be visible during positive pressure ventilation. The increased thoracic pressure resulting from the anesthesiologist's ventilator will result in a temporary increased filling of the inferior vena cava and the common iliac veins. Transmission of the atrial contraction is sometimes visible in the left common iliac vein as a dicrotic pulsation. Identification of the left common iliac vein is important, since it is one of the largest vascular structures near the left margin of the upcoming dissection.

After the initial survey of the region of the sacral promontory, with identification of the area of the left common iliac vein, it is time to decide where to make the peritoneal incision. At laparotomy, the peritoneal incision over the sacral promontory usually is made vertically, with lateral retraction by stay sutures or retractors. At laparoscopy, it is advantageous to make the peritoneal incision transversely, because this will allow the peritoneum to separate and expose the area of dissection without further lateral retraction. A probe can be used to retract the sigmoid colon to the left, and the graspers now grasp the peritoneum in the midline

of the sacral promontory. The peritoneal incision is most commonly made about 2 or 3 cm above the angle of the sacral promontory. The scissors nick the elevated peritoneum (Figure 12-8), then incise it transversely toward the right and left margins of the dissection using either high current density electrosurgery or sharp dissection. The right margin of the dissection is marked by the right common iliac vessels, the left margin by the edge of the sigmoid mesentery and left common iliac vein. The left ureter is hidden by the vessels of the sigmoid mesentery and is not a logical endpoint for the left margin of the dissection. At this point, pay attention again to the location of the left common iliac vein, since retroperitoneal dissection will begin now.

A window is created by blunt dissection through the retroperitoneal areolar tissue at each lateral margin of the peritoneal incision. The goal of this dissection is to expose the periosteum of the sacral promontory. Once the periosteum is encountered, further blunt spreading will allow fuller visualization of the periosteum. Here is where the efforts to identify the location of the left common iliac vein pay off, since the window on the left will be created just medial to this structure and the edge of the sigmoid mesentery. Once the windows at the lateral margins of the dissection have been developed down to the periosteum, the intervening tissue of the superior presacral plexus is grasped and elevated away from the sacral promontory which allows any presacral vessels to avoid damage (Figure 12-9). With the presacral plexus elevated and well-defined, it sometimes resembles a wishbone, with the right and left inferior hypogastric plexuses below joining to form the intermediate and superior hypogastric plexuses above. The elevated presacral plexus is then transected in successively deeper layers, using 50 W of coagulation current. Transection of the presacral plexus in multiple, thin layers gives the surgeon a chance to identify any large vessels which may be lying

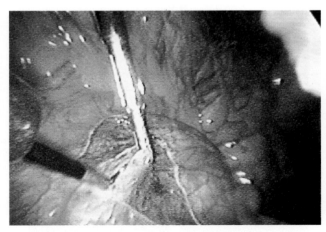

Figure 12-9 The tissue of the superior presacral plexus is grasped and elevated away from the sacral promontory and is being transected with 50 W of coagulation current.

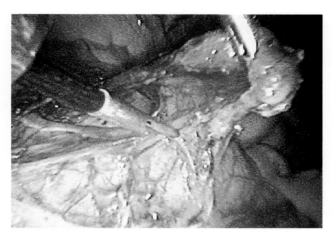

Figure 12-10 Following the complete transection of the presacral plexus, the presacral tissue is bluntly dissected off of the vertebral body of L-5 in a caudal direction.

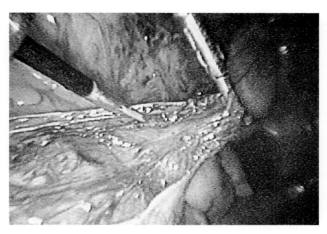

Figure 12-12 The isolated presacral tissue is transected distally using 50 W of coagulation current. Notice that the sigmoid colon lays behind the elevated peritoneum. It could potentially be injured if the undersurface of the peritoneum is burned during transection of the presacral tissue.

hidden on the periosteum. Sometimes neural tissue can be identified as a rather thick bundle of tissue. The wispy retroperitoneal neural and lymphatic tissue which remains over the sacral promontory can now be further transected, laying the sacral promontory bare except for any presacral vessels. It is not necessary to transect these vessels. Once the presacral plexus is completely transected at the superior margin of the dissection, it is dissected bluntly off the periosteum and presacral vessels for several centimeters (Figure 12–10). The overlying peritoneum is then grasped and elevated so the presacral tissue can be bluntly stripped from it (Figure 12-11). This results in isolation of the presacral tissue, which can now be grasped and transected transversely with 50 W of coagulation current (Figure 12-12) so the specimen can be removed. It is not necessary to interrupt the presacral vessels, as the neural tissue lies anterior to them (Figure 12-13).

Closing the peritoneum is optional, and there have been no apparent complications in more than 200 cases from leaving it open. Laparoscopic presacral neurectomy requires up to an additional 15 minutes of operating time, but can sometimes be performed much more quickly, especially in thin patients.

RESULTS

Trials with historical and randomized controls indicate efficacy of PSN as performed at laparotomy. Observational studies have suggested the efficacy of PSN at laparotomy or laparoscopy. A prospective multicenter study by Perry and Perez found that 79 of 87 consecutive patients (91%)

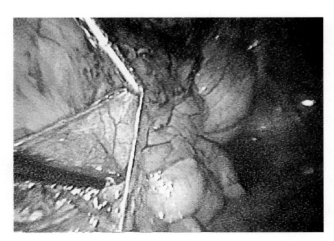

Figure 12-11 After the presacral tissue has been dissected off of the sacral promontory, it is bluntly stripped from the overlying peritoneum.

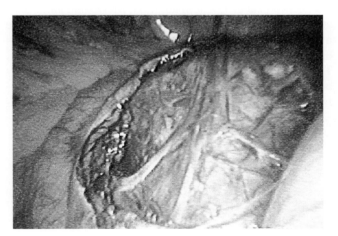

Figure 12-13 Presacral vessels are seen after removal of the presacral tissue. Presacral vessels are variably present, and are not always midline structures.

Table 12-1 *Central pelvic pain scale*

0. No pelvic pain.
1. Mild cramping.
2. Moderate cramping, completely relieved with BCP (birth control pills) or NSAID (non-steroidal anti-inflammatory drugs).
3. Mild cramping while on the BCP and/or NSAID.
4. Moderate cramping while on the BCP and/or NSAID. The patient can function adequately at work and school.
5. Severe cramping while on BCP and/or NSAID. Relieved with narcotics. Patient can function adequately at work and school most of the time.
6. Severe cramping and pelvic pain, patient intolerant to BCP, mild to moderate relief with NSAID and narcotics. The patient has missed work and/or school due to pelvic pain; however, can function at work and school most of the time.
7. Severe cramping and pelvic pain, patient intolerant to BCP, minimal relief with NSAID and narcotic medication. The patient frequently misses work and/or school due to pelvic pain.
8. Severe cramping and pelvic pain, moderate relief with NSAID, BCPs, narcotic medications. The patient has missed work and/or school; however, can function adequately at work and school at least 50% of the time.
9. Severe cramping and pelvic pain, mild relief with NSAID, BCP and narcotic medications. The patient has missed work and/or school due to pelvic pain or complains of reduced effectiveness at work and/or school while symptomatic.
10. Severe cramping and pelvic pain, no relief with NSAID, BCP and narcotic medications. The patient frequently misses work and/or school due to pelvic pain.

monitored with a 10-point pain scale (Table 12-1) experienced improvement in their pain scores. The majority of these patients experienced over a 50% reduction in their pain and relief persistent at 24-month follow-up (Table 12-2). Of the 87 patients followed for at least 6 months (1987 to 1995) in Columbus, Ohio, the majority continued to realize significant improvement in midline pain and dysmenorrhea (Table 12-3). In addition, McDonald and Elliott at the Ohio State University questioned the patients in the multicenter study by Perry and Perez with regard to postoperative pelvic pain, adverse effects and sexual function. This evaluation concluded that presacral neurectomy may be an effective intervention for women suffering from refractory chronic pelvic pain. Most interestingly, these pa-

Table 12-2 *Pain relief following laparoscopic presacral neurectomy*

Time of measurement	N	Mean pain level
Preop	87	7.9 ± 1.7
3 Months	87	2.8 ± 2.2
6 Months	73	2.7 ± 2.1
12 Months	38	2.4 ± 1.9
24 Months	20	2.1 ± 1.4

Table 12-3 *Preoperative and postoperative pain scores*

Pain score	Number of Patients	
	Preoperative	Postoperative
0	—	9
1	—	18
2	—	32
3	—	20
4	—	5
5	—	2
6	8	3
7	11	—
8	22	2
9	17	—
10	29	—

tients reported improvement in sexual sensation, behavior, and function with minimal attending complications from surgery. Laparoscopic PSN seems to augment the beneficial effects of laparoscopic excision of endometriosis, although laparoscopic excision of endometriosis alone may reduce significantly the patient's perception of uterine cramping with the menstrual flow.

CONTRAINDICATIONS

Although there are no specific contraindications, obese patients have more retroperitoneal fatty tissue in the presacral area. This can increase the difficulty of surgery and, rarely, can cause abandonment of the procedure.

Complications

Intraoperative complications related to PSN are rare. Injury to the left common iliac vein is possible because of the variable location of this vascular structure below the aortic bifurcation. The location of the left common iliac vein can be determined before incision of the peritoneum by the presence of the "waterbed sign;" locating it can decrease the chance of injury to this structure.

Long-term complications following PSN are rare. Previous published reports on PSN do not support a view that long-term constipation is a common or predictable result. Malinak, who has extensive experience with presacral neurectomy at laparotomy, has stated in no uncertain terms that "the operation is quite harmless in its effect on the function of the bladder, the bowel, and the uterus."

The left colon acts as a collecting area for stool. It has a different function and innervation than the right and transverse colon. The descending colon and rectosigmoid colon are innervated with parasympathetic (speeds intestinal function) efferent (nerve impulses going toward the bowel) nerve fibers from the pelvic splanchnic nerves. The pelvic splanchnic nerves feed into the inferior hypogastric plexus (also known as the pelvic plexus), and pass on to the left colon. When these fibers fire, the left colon evacuates, resulting in a bowel movement. These parasympathetic stimulatory nerve fibers to the descending colon and rectosigmoid colon do *not* pass through the superior hypogastric plexus and are *not* cut in the performance of a presacral neurectomy. The descending colon and rectosigmoid colon are innervated with sympathetic (slows intestinal function) efferent nerve fibers from four separate plexuses: the inferior mesenteric plexus, the sacral splanchnic nerves, the lumbar splanchnic nerves, and the presacral plexus. Of these, the sympathetic efferent (and some sympathetic afferent) fibers traversing the presacral plexus are severed during a presacral neurectomy. Since the efferent sympathetic fibers which are severed during a presacral neurectomy slow the function of the bowel, it would be impossible to predict constipation as a result of a presacral neurectomy. In fact, one might predict a decrease in constipation following a presacral neurectomy, as has been found (Table 12-4). Since denervation of the uterus is the desired end result of PSN, and since the uterus is known to contract during female orgasm, a decrease of orgasmic potential is a possibility. Perez and Perry found a 12% incidence of lubrication difficulty following presacral neurectomy. Anorgasmia following laparoscopic PSN has been reported by one patient to the Endometriosis Institute of Oregon.

Postoperatively, patients may notice a decreased sensation of bladder fullness, which may be due to interruption of the sympathetic fibers traveling from the bladder superiorly across the presacral space. Urgency is rarely seen. Incontinence or increased susceptibility to urinary infections has not been reported.

Although a subjective decrease in sensation of the first stage of labor has been mentioned as a possible occurrence following PSN, there has never been a case report of a patient entering labor unknowingly following a PSN and delivering precipitously. Nor has there been a case report of a delay of diagnosis of gynecologic cancer following PSN. There is nothing extraordinary in the absence of such reports, since there are many other cues to the onset of labor, and pain is not an early sign of gynecologic cancer.

SUGGESTED READING

Biggerstaff ED, Foster SN. Laparoscopic presacral neurectomy for treatment of midline pelvic pain. *J Am Assoc Gynecol Laparosc* 1994;2:31–5.

Browne OD. A survey of 113 cases of primary dysmenorrhea treated by neurectomy. *Am J Obstet Gynecol* 1949;57:1053–68.

Candiani G, Fedele L, Vercellini P, Bianchi S, DiNola G. Presacral neurectomy for the treatment of pelvic pain associated with endometriosis: a controlled study. *Obstet Gynecol* 1992;167:100–3.

Daniell JF, Kurtz BR, Gurley LD, et al. Laparoscopic presacral neurectomy vs neurotomy: Use of the argon beam coagulator compared to conventional technique. *J Gynecol Surg* 1993;9:169–73.

Freier A. Pelvic neurectomy in gynecology. *Obstet Gynecol* 1965;25:48–55.

Jaboulay M. Le traitement de la neuralgie pelvienne par la paralysie du sympathique sacre. *Lyon Med* 1899;90:102–8.

Lee RB, Sonte K, Magelssen D, Belts RP, Benson WL. Presacral neurectomy for chronic pelvic pain. *Obstet Gynecol* 1986;68:517–21.

Malinak LR. Operative management of pelvic pain. *Clin Obstet Gynecol* 1980;23:191–200.

Meigs JV. Excision of the superior hypogastric plexus (presacral nerve) for primary dysmenorrhea. *Surg Gynecol Obstet* 1939;68:723–32.

Nezhat C, Nezhat F. A simplified method of laparoscopic presacral neurectomy for treatment of central pelvic pain due to endometriosis. *Br J Obstet Gynecol* 1992;99:659–63.

Perez JJ. Laparoscopic presacral neurectomy: results of the first 25 cases. *J Reprod Med* 1990;35:625–30.

Perry CP, Perez J. The role for laparoscopic presacral neurectomy. *J Gynecol Surg* 1993;9:165–8.

Phaneuf LE. Presacral neurectomy in intractable dysmenorrhea. *J Mt Sinai Hosp* 1947;14:553–5.

Polan ML, DeCherney A. Presacral neurectomy for pelvic pain in infertility. *Fertil Steril* 1980;34:557–60.

Redwine DB, Perez JJ. Laparoscopic presacral neurectomy. In: Soderstrom RM, (ed). *Operative Laparoscopy, The Masters' Techniques.* New York: Raven Press, 1993;157–60.

Redwine DB, Perez JJ. Pelvic Pain Syndromes. In: Arregui, Fitzgibbons, Katkhouda, McKernan, Reich (eds). *Principles of Laparoscopic Surgery: Basic and Advanced Techniques.* New York: Springer-Verlag, 1995;545–58.

Tjaden B, Shclaff WD, Kimball, Rock JA. The efficacy of presacral neurectomy for the relief of midline dysmenorrhea. *Obstet Gynecol* 1990; 76:89–91.

Table 12-4 *Average constipation scores—preop vs postop levels among questionnaire responders 1988 to 1991, Endometriosis Institute of Oregon*

Surgical group	Preop score	Postop score
Presacral neurectomy (N = 57)	2.47	1.88
No presacral neurectomy (N = 285)	2.45	1.74

1 = not a problem; 2 = mild; 3 = moderate; 4 = severe; 5 = debilitating.

Operative Laparoscopy, Second Edition
The Masters' Techniques in Gynecologic Surgery
Lippincott–Raven Publishers, Philadelphia © 1998.

13

Laparoscopic Sterilization

Richard M. Soderstrom and Jacques E. Rioux

HISTORY

For women, voluntary sterilization was difficult to obtain until May, 1969. Prior to that date the American College of Obstetricians and Gynecologists (ACOG) required, after approval of both the wife and husband, a three-person committee to review a written request from the patient's physician. Between May, 1969 and October, 1974, the ACOG recognized that most states had no law regarding sterilization and from a legal view the decision could be made between the physician and the patient. They (ACOG) did recommend, however, a consultation from two ''senior'' staff members following voluntary requests. In the 1974 Standards for Obstetric Gynecologic Services the ACOG states, ''If sterilization is requested by the patient and her physician agrees, consultation is not necessary.'' Today, when a medical condition is an indication for sterilization, a consultant skilled in that medical condition is still recommended.

However, by 1970 most medical centers had adopted their own guidelines, similar to those of today. This new freedom of choice made laparoscopic sterilization one of the most common operations performed in the United States by gynecologic surgeons.

During this transformation, one obstacle offered a new challenge to those intrigued by the laparoscope. Previously popular sterilization methods were difficult to use laparoscopically. For instance, the Pomeroy technique, which ties a knuckle of the tube with a plain catgut suture followed by a segmental resection of the devitalized tube, was not possible with laparoscopic techniques without great ingenuity and special instrument design. Unipolar electrocoagulation, a method of seasoned surgeons, seemed to be a suitable alternative approach. Since most sterilization techniques removed about 2 to 3 cm of fallopian tube, it seemed reasonable to coagulate the same amount of tube and if possible remove the coagulated specimen. To prove proper resection, a method to resect an uncoagulated specimen was designed in 1971 and promoted as having a medicolegal advantage, since the ''coagulation first—resect after'' methods frequently left the pathologist with coagulated tissue ''consistent with but not diagnostic of fallopian tube.''

It is no surprise that accidents, presumed to be due to aberrant unipolar electricity, soon became known to those interested in laparoscopy. Two physicians, Rioux and Corson, each working independently, designed bipolar forceps that could circumvent the potential risk of aberrant electrical injury. Rioux's forceps never reached the marketplace because of a bureaucratic logjam within the Canadian patent system. Corson then applied the bipolar principle to an existing forceps, the Frangenheim biopsy scissors. This instrument was difficult to manufacture, and its ability to cut the tube proved to be unnecessary. The Corson forceps (CameronMiller) were next devised, but the manufacturer ceased their production in the late 1970s. As early as 1974, several instrument companies had introduced their models of bipolar forceps; many have been modified as time and experience exposed design defects or bad outcome statistics (i.e., sterilization failures). Richard Kleppinger's bipolar forceps were designed as a system. Working with bioelectrical engineers, Kleppinger married his forceps design to the electrical output characteristics of a generator designed only for bipolar surgery. Today it should be considered the gold standard of bipolar systems.

Mechanical occlusion of the fallopian tube received considerable attention by several investigators. Lay and Yoon, independent of each other, introduced the Silastic rubber ring method used by many today. The Agency for International Development (AID) chose this method for its sterilization training programs in developing countries. In a prospective fashion, Hulka and Clemens created and evaluated a springloaded plastic clip that, with time and redesign, proved effective. Blier of Germany reported great success with a plastic clip that locked in place, but it fell prey

---

Illustrations of the various techniques discussed in this chapter can be found in Appendix 13-A.

to a high failure rate after its introduction in the United States. Filshie from England has developed a clip using a memory characteristic of Silastic rubber to slowly occlude the tube. The Filshie clip was approved in late 1996 by the Food and Drug Administration (FDA).

Though the above methods, as they were designed, discussed, and tested, received great attention during the mid-seventies, little was known of another electrical method—thermocoagulation. An American instrument, manufactured by the Waters Company, coagulates tissue by low-voltage thermal energy, delivered by an apparatus similar to the hot wires of an electric toaster, and severs the tube after coagulation is complete. Semm of Germany designed his "endocoagulator" on the same principle, but without any cutting characteristics. Though the parent companies claim great success with their respective instruments, data through peer review are lacking.

In 1976 the United States Congress enacted the Health Device Act and charged the FDA with the responsibility of control and monitoring of health devices in medicine. Their report on February 26, 1980, in the *Federal Register* classified all instruments designed for laparoscopic sterilization (except unipolar) as class III: approved for sale and use but subject to postmarket surveillance. Unfortunately, the bureaucratic process has delayed the FDA from exercising its option to demand further study by each manufacturer of these devices.

ADVANTAGES/DISADVANTAGES

Laparoscopy for sterilization offers a number of advantages over other sterilization techniques:

- small incisions whose scars are barely visible
- same-day surgery
- no vaginal drainage (i.e., colpotomy)
- no sexual restriction
- lower cost than other approaches
- a panoramic view of the abdominal viscera

The disadvantages of laparoscopic sterilization are few. Though general anesthesia is used by most, regional and local techniques are favored by many, especially in developing countries, where the use of general anesthesia is infrequent. When compared to the minilaparotomy approach to sterilization, laparoscopy requires more training. Vasectomy, which may be preferable for some couples, is less expensive.

CONCEPTS OF ELECTROPHYSICS IMPORTANT TO ELECTROSURGERY

Electrical energy can be harnessed, shaped, and delivered in a variety of ways to accomplish a number of tasks. Equipment used to deliver this energy source must be designed with thought and knowledge about the principles of electricity, or it will not perform as desired. If physicians do not understand the basics of electricity, even the best electrical system, used improperly, will fail. When using electricity for sterilization, two basic objectives must be met: obliteration of the vascular supply to, and complete disruption of, the living tissue. If one of these two objectives is incomplete, tubal patency may persist, which can lead to a sterilization failure.

Electrons are particles of energy that, when passed through living tissue, create heat, intracellular expansion, and cell destruction. When a quantity of electrons passes through tissue (measured in amperes), an *electrical current* is produced. The pressure behind these electrons is measured in volts. As the thermal change develops, water is driven from the cell through expansion and cell disruption. This desiccated tissue then increases the resistance to current flow, which is measured in ohms. An increase in resistance will reduce the current flow unless the current is increased during the electrocoagulation process. Electrical power (measured in watts) is the energy produced. The energy consumed over a period of time is measured in joules. Watts can be expressed as pressure times current, or volts times current, or volts times amperes per second.

Electrosurgery is therefore the art of passing electrons through living tissue with enough force (current) to create heat and tissue disruption. Electrons must be generated (via electrogenerators) and passed through instruments (active electrodes) into the tissue and have an exit pathway (passive electrode) back to their source. For current to flow, this cycle must be complete.

For surgery, *electrogenerators* are machines that produce an alternating current of energy at a frequency that will not stimulate involuntary muscle activity (500,000 to 3 million Hz). An alternating current has a waveform with a positive pole or peak and a negative pole or peak. The measurement from zero polarity to maximum positive or negative polarity is called the peak voltage of the waveform. Peak-to-peak voltage is measured from the positive pole to the negative pole and is twice peak voltage. Bursts of electrical waveforms, interrupted by brief periods (milliseconds) of zero current flow, are used to coagulate tissue; this delivery system is called a damped current. An undamped current without a "rest" period produces a cutting effect. A combination of damped and undamped waveforms is called a blended current.

The amount of heat per square unit of size has a direct relationship to the concentration of electrons within that area and is referred to as current density. Thus the finer the electrode, the more dense is the current. A fine current density (needle electrode) tends to have a cutting effect; a broad current density (ball electrode) leads more to a coagulation effect. With this knowledge, a surgeon can make a damped current (coagulation form) cut if the instrument tip is pointed and an undamped current (cutting form) coagulate if the instrument tip is blunted.

Through all of this discussion about the physics of electricity, we should not forget the return pathway. Ground plates or return electrodes must be part of the circuit to complete the electron's pathway back to the generator. If the return electrode wire is broken, the current will not flow unless an alternate pathway is available. Because of the nuances of electricity, the electrons might find an alternate pathway through an electrocardiogram electrode or through the patient's ring if it is in contact with a piece of grounded metal on the operating table. Because of the current density principle, an inadvertent burn can occur in these locations. Ground plate burns are always due to a loose-fitting ground plate that has created an area of high current density at a point on the surface of the ground plate where it is in contact with the patient's skin.

Moreover, because electrons flow through the path of least resistance, if the tissue resistance as measured in ohms becomes high, the current may cease to flow or search out an alternate pathway (or pathways) with a lower resistance. To complicate the possibilities, if the voltage is increased, the electrons may have more ''push'' to find an alternate pathway. Therefore, one should use the lowest possible voltage necessary to accomplish a given job and be sure that the return or dispersive electrode is in good contact with the patient and broad enough to ''spread out'' the current density far below the level of tissue destruction (heat).

How do you meet these requirements? Reduce the voltage output, select the cutting waveform, and choose an active electrode whose tip design creates the desired current density. However, one point should be remembered. When the voltage is low, the surface tissue to be coagulated must be as dry as possible. For example, if a small bleeding blood vessel is too wet, the electrons may be dispersed through the extravasated blood, and coagulation will be minimal.

How do you eliminate alternate return pathways? Use a generator designed so current can only flow back from the patient through the proper return electrode. Such is the case with low-voltage, high-frequency generators that use a ''floating'' or isolated ground system. Though leakage of electrons makes true isolation impossible, low-voltage isolated units protect against aberrant current flowing through a grounded exit point, such as the cardiac monitor lead or the patient's ring in contact with a metal stirrup. In these circumstances, unless he or she physically touches the patient, even the surgeon is isolated from the circuit. Using this type of equipment can prevent the surgeon from being burned through minute holes in gloves. In fact, one can coagulate tissue barehanded with uninsulated electrodes! Another safety feature of isolated ground systems comes into play when the circuit is not complete: With a broken ground wire, the unit will not activate because the electrons cannot seek an alternate return electrode.

Because laparoscopy is remote control surgery, it is important that unexpected movements of the electrode do not occur. By reducing peak voltage, you reduce the chance of electrons jumping or sparking to nearby structures such as the bowel. An 8000 V pressure can push electrons more than 0.3 cm in room air under certain atmospheric conditions. For electrosurgery sterilization, peak voltage above 600 V is seldom necessary.

These considerations have led the FDA to recommend that for laparoscopic sterilization, low-voltage, high-frequency electrogenerators should not exceed a maximum of 600 V peak voltage or 1200 V peak-to-peak voltage. Experience has shown that the maximum power should be in the range of 100 W. Isolated ground circuitry systems are desirable, as is a fail-safe sentinel system should ineffective or incomplete grounding be present.

Capacitance Effect

In the mid-seventies an electrical problem peculiar to laparoscopy equipment became apparent. It involved a property of electric current called capacitance, which may be defined as the ability to store electrical energy by producing an electrostatic field and releasing energy later. A capacitor is any device that can hold or store electric charge (not current). Physically, a capacitor exists wherever an insulated material separates two conductors that have different potentials.

In laparoscopy, the property of capacitance may explain certain untoward bowel burns. The operating laparoscope, a hollow metal tube, surrounds the active electrode that is placed through the so-called operating channel in the laparoscope. The active electrode is the part of the laparoscope system that grasps the tissue and brings the current to it. Thus there is a tube within a tube, with a difference in electrical potential. When current passes through the active electrode, the laparoscope itself becomes a capacitor. Measurements have shown that from 50% to 70% of the current through the active electrode is induced into the laparoscope wall, and these induced electrons will seek a return pathway.

In 1972, insulated or nonconductive trocar sleeves were introduced to reduce the risk of abdominal wall burns, because laparoscopists were using high-voltage, ground-seeking generators designed for high-energy surgical needs such as in transurethral resections. The standard high-energy spark-gap generator is an example of such equipment. Inadvertent contact of the active electrode with the laparoscope in its trocar sleeve discharges the electrons under high pressure to the metal trocar sleeve and out through the abdominal wall in a small, circumscribed, area, back to the dispersive electrode. This event can occur in either the one-hole or the two-hole technique. Because of the high voltage and wattage then used, enough heat could be generated to cause severe burns of the abdominal wall. This chain of events was compounded with the second-puncture trocar because even less of the surface area of the metal was in contact with the skin, making current density greater.

Now low-voltage generators are used, and this effect is improbable. The pressure behind the electrons in a low-voltage generator is so low that not enough heat is generated to burn. Remember, the surface area of an 11-mm metal trocar in direct contact with the abdominal wall of a patient undergoing laparoscopy probably measures 3 to 4 cm^2 or more. Thus even if an active electrode, in either the one-hole or the two-hole technique, should come into contact with the laparoscope, the energy is dispersed through the metal trocar to the return electrode without tissue damage at the puncture site. When using unipolar electricity through an operating laparoscope, always use a metal trocar sleeve; if a capacitance effect develops, the induced current will leak out through the metal trocar sleeve back to ground without harm. A device has been developed to eliminate any capacitance effect during laparoscopy (See Chapter 3-1).

UNIPOLAR ELECTROCOAGULATION METHODS

Experience has shown that all unipolar electrocoagulation methods are effective and acceptable. The evidence also says that enough tissue must be destroyed to occlude the tubal lumen and obliterate enough of the vascular tree to the coagulated segment to promote atrophy of that segment.

Coagulation Alone

In the United States, electrocoagulation without transection or resection of the fallopian tube has the longest track record of all the methods of female sterilization. When laparoscopic sterilization began its growth, the simple application of unipolar electrical energy to the ischemic portion of the tube seemed logical and efficient. At that time, the high-voltage electrogenerators used for all forms of electrosurgery performed the task in a crisp and rapid fashion — on occasion going far beyond the intended area of destruction. At times, electrical burns to the abdominal wall occurred, which appeared to result from arcing from the active electrode to the metal sheath of the laparoscope, with the energy then discharged into the metal trocar sleeve in contact with the abdominal wall.

Isolated reports of inadvertent bowel injury prompted a similar arcing theory as the cause. With the help of bioengineers and representatives of industry, low-voltage generators became available and proved to be adequate for all of the electrosurgical needs of laparoscopy as performed in the seventies. Though abdominal wall electroinjuries became a rare event, the incidence of bowel injury remained constant. The theory of capacitance (discussed above) introduced a new explanation for bowel injury following laparoscopic sterilization when an operating laparoscope was used to deliver the electrocoagulation energy. In 1980 the FDA health device panel for obstetrics and gynecology endorsed the concept of conductive trocar sleeves greater than 7 mm in diameter. By returning to metal trocar sleeves, any capacitance effect would leak out of the metal trocar sleeve through the abdominal wall back to the return electrode, without generating enough heat in the tissue surrounding the trocar sleeve to create a burn to the abdominal wall. Then, if the bowel should touch the metal laparoscope during the process of electrocoagulation, the capacitance effect induced into the laparoscope sheath would be diverted to the abdominal wall and not to the bowel.

While these struggles to overcome iatrogenic electrocoagulation injuries were going on, large "coagulation alone" studies were published, with impressive outcome statistics. Each author coagulated 2 to 3 cm of the proximal third of each fallopian tube, with a collective failure rate of 0.35%.

In 1981, the CDC published a synopsis of three deaths that occurred following unipolar sterilization. Each patient died of overwhelming sepsis secondary to profound peritonitis following a bowel perforation, found in two of the three patients. Though a perforation was not found in the third patient, the CDC chose to blame an electrical cause of bowel perforation because unipolar electrocoagulation was the sterilization method used. Based on this publication, the American Association of Gynecologic Laparoscopists (AAGL) officially denounced unipolar methods and proclaimed "other methods" as preferable. In 1985, animal studies on the histologic and gross appearance of electrical and traumatic bowel injuries raised serious questions about the veracity of the CDC's conclusions, and the AAGL reversed their position, stating that their statement in 1981 "was no longer valid."

These animal studies showed a clear histologic distinction between electrical injuries and those due to inadvertent trauma. In simple terms, electrical injuries occlude the vascular tree to the injured area; thus the area of injury is avascular and devoid of white blood cell infiltration. In contrast, traumatic injuries are characterized by hypervascularity and extensive white cell infiltration. With this new information a review of many records from cases of assumed bowel burn accidents proved to be traumatic injury confirmed by the histologic findings.

In summary, unipolar electrocoagulation sterilization, and in particular the coagulation-alone method, has stood the test of time and is much safer than once thought. Caution is still important, as with any electrosurgical procedure, when the coagulation-alone method is employed.

Technique

A panoramic view of the operative field is mandatory before the grasping forceps are energized. The distortion and loss of a panoramic field that occurs if the distal lens is too close to the operative area can confuse even the experienced laparoscopist. After the bowel has been displaced from the operative field, the junction of the proximal and middle third of the tube is grasped and elevated away from the pelvic cavity toward the anterior abdominal wall. Once the fimbriae are seen and the proper placement of the grasping forceps confirmed, the active electrode cord is connected to the grasping forceps. If one connects the cord before the tube is secured, accidental activation of the foot pedal may create an electrical burn to a vital organ. In general, 50 W of unipolar power is sufficient to cause complete coagulation of the tissue grasped by the forceps, and a lateral spread of 0.5 to 1.0 cm will be noted. The tube will blanch, swell, and then collapse as electrons are pushed through the tissue on their way to the ground plate.

If 3 cm of tube is not destroyed with one application, more applications will be necessary. Here a principle of unipolar physics is important. Because the electrons return to ground through the path of least resistance, the second (and third if necessary) forceps application should occur *closer* to the uterus. Why? Because after the first application the remaining desiccated tissue has an increased tissue resistance, and the electrons are diverted toward the uterus. In theory, should you move toward the distal end of the tube, the electrons might be driven out of the fimbriae, and if one fimbria tip touches the bowel, electrocoagulation of the bowel can occur.

Some have proposed a word of caution about coagulating the tubouterine junction. They feel that iatrogenic endometriosis, by some called endosalpingosis, will develop, which may lead to fistula formation or increased dysmenorrhea. Others have argued the opposite point of view.

It is wise to move each tube from side to side to confirm adequate coagulation. "Skip areas" in the coagulated area can be recoagulated. A portion of underlying mesosalpinx with its rich supply of blood vessels will be coagulated for at least 0.5 cm.

Coagulation with Transection

This method is practiced by many. However, the failure rate is not improved, and the risk of a tear in the mesosalpinx with subsequent hemorrhage is increased. The advocates of this method argue that they prefer to see the fresh ends of the coagulated tube to assure themselves of a complete coagulation. Unfortunately, only the microscope can answer that question.

Technique

The approach is the same as with the coagulation-alone technique. Once the coagulation process is completed, you can insert *sharp* laparoscope scissors through the operating channel and cut the midportion of the coagulated segment down to the mesosalpinx. If the mesosalpinx has not been coagulated prior to this event, brisk bleeding will occur. Some skilled laparoscopists will gingerly grasp, coagulate, and cut with the laparoscopic scissors, eliminating the use of grasping forceps.

Coagulation and Resection

This method of laparoscopic sterilization is more difficult to master, and the failure rate is not improved. Bleeding from the mesosalpinx is a risk. Several instruments have been used to remove the specimen.

Scissors Technique

With this technique, a wedge resection of the coagulated specimen is performed. The amputated specimen is then grasped and removed through the trocar sleeve with grasping forceps. On occasion, the specimen will fall into the pelvic cavity and be lost. Even when the specimen is removed and given to the pathologist, the histology of the specimen may be so distorted that the pathology report will return with the comment "tissue consistent with but not diagnostic of fallopian tube."

Palmer Drill Technique

The Palmer drill, designed by Raoul Palmer of France, was never meant for tubal sterilization; Palmer designed it for ovarian biopsy. However, since it was one of the first laparoscopic accessories available when laparoscopic sterilization became popular, many chose this tool when they performed sterilization procedures. Once again, the tube must be coagulated first, making pathologic confirmation difficult. The twisting motion of this instrument would frequently twist the tube, and on occasion the mesosalpinx was avulsed. Today most laparoscopists reserve this excellent biopsy instrument for large biopsies of firm masses including the ovary.

Snare Technique

This method uses an operating laparoscope with its grasping forceps and an insulated, self-opening wire snare to coagulate, transect, and resect a tubal specimen adequate for pathologic confirmation. It requires a second trocar puncture. The operating time, however, is equal to that of other methods of laparoscopic sterilization.

Technique. After proper insufflation and introduction of the operating laparoscope, a second 6-mm trocar sleeve with trocar is placed suprapubically in the midline under direct vision. The snare is inserted through the 6-mm trocar sleeve. The surgeon then proceeds through the following steps:

1. Open the snare completely and place it over the middle third of the tube.
2. Thread the tip of the grasping forceps through the open snare. Advance the tip until it touches the tube. The forceps should be spring-loaded to remain closed when

not actively manipulated; a rubber band intertwined between the finger holes will suffice.

3. Grasp the tube. Once the tube is secure, the operator frees his or her hand from the grasper to steady the laparoscope. (The rubber band will maintain the grasping forceps in the closed position.)

4. Slowly withdraw the laparoscope. This ensures a wide view of the operating field and usually will pull a sufficient knuckle of tube (1 to 2 cm) through the open snare wire.

5. Once an adequate specimen has been snared, tighten the snare wire snugly. The resection site should be 2 cm from the uterine cornu.

6. Attach the coagulator cord.

7. Use low-voltage, high-frequency blended coagulation (a setting of 40 W on most models). Apply a steady blended current until blanching extends 5 mm into the mesosalpinx.

8. Close the snare slowly but completely while applying current.

9. Disconnect coagulator cord.

10. Holding the laparoscope trocar sleeve trumpet open, remove the laparoscope and the grasping forceps from the abdomen as a unit. The specimen will be held securely in the jaws of the grasper because of the spring-loaded handle created with the rubber band.

11. Submit the specimen to a pathologist.

12. Inspect the resection site and repeat on the opposite side.

Resection by Biopsy Forceps

A number of biopsy forceps may be used to resect a segment of fallopian tube. Using unipolar energy, each forceps must coagulate the tissue first and then resect the specimen. Unlike the snare method, the pathology report usually reads "coagulated tissue consistent with but not diagnostic of fallopian tube." An increased risk of a mesosalpingeal tear is real. This risk is particularly prevalent if the biopsy forceps are dull. Thus should this method seem reasonable, the instruments should be sharp and the tissue well-coagulated prior to resection.

BIPOLAR ELECTROCOAGULATION METHODS

The principles of bipolar physics play a major role in the bipolar techniques of female sterilization ("Concepts of Electrophysics," above). Though the gross appearance of a tube coagulated by bipolar energy may look, on the surface, the same as it does by unipolar energy, the depth of destruction is seldom the same. Because the characteristic lateral spread of destruction of unipolar energy does not occur with bipolar systems, the tube must be grasped and coagulated more times with the bipolar forceps than with the unipolar forceps. In reality, the success of any electro-coagulation method, unipolar or bipolar, depends upon the length of tube destroyed, not the number of applications. Most authorities feel that a 2-cm segment of coagulated tube is the minimum, and 3-cm is preferable.

By design, bipolar instruments are limited to a power output below 100 W. The voltage output is also low, which creates a narrow range of depth of destruction. The surface of the tube may be well coagulated, but the center may be spared. Bipolar forceps that by design crush the tube may increase their ability to drive the electrons deeper into the tissue. One system, designed by Richard Kleppenger, MD, of West Redding, Pennsylvania, provides a pure cutting (undamped) waveform. His forceps do not crush the tube and are marketed with a warning to the purchaser not to adulterate the card and attach it to another generator. His "bipolar system" has an additional feature worth noting. An Ammeter displays the current flow during the process of electrocoagulation until the current ceases to flow. This technology removes the guesswork when one relies on a visual endpoint. Recently, several companies have introduced similar generators.

As mentioned, the length of tubal destruction is important, not the number of applications. This is important to consider if one chooses a small, thin 3-mm bipolar forceps rather than a larger, broad 5-mm forceps. Remember, the larger the surface of the forceps, the lower the current density, which may require a longer duration of energy to cause deep penetration.

Bipolar forceps should be applied to the isthmic portion of the tube as with the unipolar forcep. When bipolar forceps are placed through the operating channel of an operating laparoscope, the capacitance effect noted with single-puncture unipolar energy is "canceled" by the afferent or return pathway within the forceps.

The tube should be lifted away from the surrounding vital organs after the fimbriae have been located. On occasion, after coagulation is complete, the bipolar forceps may stick to the coagulated tissue. Do not try to pull the forceps free because the mesosalpinx may tear and cause bleeding. In general, a rotation of the forceps in either direction will detach the adherent forceps.

If one chooses to cut the tube or biopsy the coagulated specimen, care should be taken as one approaches the coagulated mesosalpinx. Again, because of the small limit in lateral spread of coagulation with these forceps, the vascular tree beneath the tube may be vulnerable to rupture. Should such an accident occur, the bipolar forceps may not be able to control the bleeding, and unipolar forceps may be needed.

When bipolar sterilization failures occur, in some cases the amount of tubal destruction is incomplete. To reduce this risk at least 2 cm of through-and-through coagulation should be accomplished. Since generators differ in their output characteristics, I recommend you use a nonmodulated (cutting) waveform and field-test your bipolar system (generator and forceps) on a normal fallopian tube; ask your pathologist to analyze the depth of coagulation. Are there "skip areas" within the destroyed segment? Is the endosalpinx coagulated, or is there only "electronic streaking" of the nuclei? Remember, to ensure enough tissue atrophy, tissue must be coagulated to obliterate the vascular tree that supplies the coagulated segment of tube; continuous coagulation of 3 cm of fallopian tube should secure that mission.

THERMAL STERILIZATION

Thermal coagulation, or "true cautery," is available in the United States when one uses one of two instruments. The Waters instrument is a wire hook heated much like an electric toaster wire, the hook being sheathed in a heat-resistant plastic tube. The hook is extended beyond the sheath and hooked under the fallopian tube. The hook is then withdrawn into the protective sheath, the wire is heated, thermal cautery occurs, and the tube is severed by the wire hook when thermal damage is complete. A ground plate is not necessary, but the tube should be elevated away from surrounding structures because the protective sheath can become hot. The amount of tissue destruction after using the Waters instrument is less than 1 cm.

The second instrument, by Semm, looks like a grasping forceps but is coated in Teflon. Again, the instrument is heated (about 100°C), and direct cautery occurs. The area of damage is limited to the width of the forceps, so many applications are required to coagulate 2 to 3 cm of tube. Most of the experience with the Waters instrument has been concentrated in only a few states, and experience with Semm's thermal forceps has come from Europe. Neither advocate has presented controlled or convincing studies that this approach to female sterilization has an acceptable failure rate.

MECHANICAL METHODS

Band Method

Using a Silastic rubber band or ring, Inbae Yoon successfully occluded the fallopian tube in the early 1970s. He adapted this technology to the operating laparoscope and to the two-puncture technique. It has become a popular method for both laparoscopic and nonlaparoscopic approaches to sterilization.

The applicator is more complex than the instruments used for the electrical methods of sterilization. The applicator has two concentric cylinders with a grasping forceps within the inner cylinder, which grasps and elevates a segment of fallopian tube. By means of a "ring loader," the Silastic rubber ring is stretched over the distal end of the inner cylinder, and the outer cylinder retracted up the inner cylinder shaft about 5 mm.

The handle of this applicator allows the surgeon to extend the grasping forceps beyond the inner cylinder, grasp the fallopian tube, and draw a knuckle of tube inside the inner cylinder. Once the knuckle of tube is secure within the inner cylinder, the handle of the applicator is squeezed slowly against the outer cylinder, causing this cylinder to push or fire the ring onto the secured tubal segment or loop. The applicator is designed to draw into the inner cylinder a loop of tube measuring 2.5 cm before the band is fired.

The area to grasp is the junction of the proximal and middle third of each tube. If one attempts to fire the ring on the proximal segment next to the uterus, the grasping forceps may sever the tube because of increased tension, secondary to lack of tubal mobility; should the tube separate before the band is fired, bleeding may be brisk. Conversely, if the distal third of the tube is grasped, the diameter of the tube will be too large for the inner cylinder, a problem that can lead to bleeding or only partial occlusion of the tube.

Because the ring applicator is a mechanical device with several moving parts, the proper care and maintenance of this instrument should be understood by the operating room personnel and surgeon. If the applicator is not correctly disassembled, cleaned, and reassembled, the instrument may freeze or misfire the ring. Imagine the frustration if the ring fires onto the grasping tongs before the knuckle of tube is drawn into the inner cylinder. Should that happen, it is possible to "milk" the ring off the grasping forcep onto the tube, but a wiser decision would be to insert another secondary trocar sleeve through which scissors can be passed to cut the Silastic band. This accident can also occur if the ring is improperly applied onto the inner cylinder.

If the ring is not stretched more than 6 mm, it has an elastic memory of 100%; a stretch beyond 6 mm may render the elastic memory ineffective, and tubal occlusion may not occur. Some feel the success of this device is its ability to continue to compress tissue after it has been applied to the tube, unlike permanent suture; silk has not performed well when used for postpartum sterilization (i.e., Madlener technique).

The grasping tongs are thin and delicate in their construction. If the handle is squeezed shut in a brisk fashion, the tongs may transect the tube. When this occurs, a click can be heard as the two handles snap together during the squeezing process. Should bleeding occur, a skilled laparoscopist usually can apply a band to each tubal stump to control the bleeding and occlude the tube. Electrocoagulation may be necessary in some cases.

By mistake, rings have been applied to surrounding structures, such as the round ligament and bowel. For this reason, a wide, panoramic view of the operating field should be obtained before the ring is applied. If the bowel is "banded" and this accident noted, operating scissors can cut the band, and the patient should be closely followed. A band that is lost or dropped into the abdominal cavity is of no concern and may be left behind.

Because of the acute tissue necrosis that follows band application, postoperative discomfort can be a problem. Many laparoscopists apply sterile anesthetic jelly or solu-

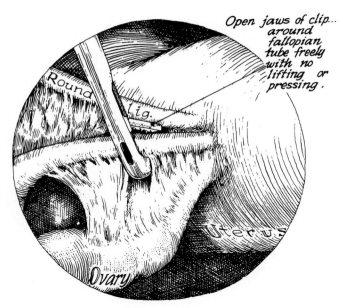

Figure 13-1 Grasping the tube. (Reprinted with permission from Hulka JF. *Textbook of Laparoscopy.* Philadelphia: WB Saunders, 1985.)

tion on the tube when they perform ring sterilization. This helps in some patients, but many will require intramuscular or intravenous narcotics to control their discomfort in the first few hours after surgery.

Unlike electrical methods, especially unipolar methods, tissue destruction and atrophy are confined to the knuckle of tube involved in the initial procedure. Later, should a patient request a reversal operation, the chances for tubal restoration are better than following electrocoagulation techniques.

Clip Sterilization

Tantalum clips used for vascular occlusion have been used for tubal occlusion, but the failure rate is high because the clip binds over the muscular tube and occlusion is incomplete. Even multiple tantalum clip application has a high failure rate unless the vascular tree to a segment of tube is occluded and that segment dies.

Blier, from Germany, reported success with a hinged plastic clip that snap-locked in place over the tube. When introduced in the United States, it is alleged that a change in manufacturing methods weakened the hinge, and a high failure rate became evident.

At this time, only one clip is available in the United States, but another clip, the Filshie Clip, has received FDA approval and should be available soon. The clip in current use is the Hulka-Clemens clip, made of 3-mm-wide Lexan plastic jaws hinged by a small metal spring that opens the jaws for application. Once the jaws are applied over the tube, a U-shaped gold-plated steel spring is pushed over

and down the length of the jaws to hold them closed under constant pressure. In some patients it may take several days for this spring to squeeze the tube to complete occlusion. This latter fact protects the tube from an abrupt transection, which could lead to bleeding or allow the clip to fall away from the tube.

Clip Application

An operating laparoscope designed for clip application is available, although the clip can be applied with the use of a second-puncture applicator. The clip, once secured in the applicator, can be used as grasping forceps to lift and hold the tube securely. Caution should be exercised during this portion of the procedure to prevent accidental firing of the gold spring, thus prematurely securing the clip. After placing the clip into the applicator, the clip should be opened and closed with the upper ram before placing the applicator into the abdomen. This function check reduces the risk of malfunction and prevents accidental jamming of the clip.

The clip should be applied at a 90° angle to the isthmic portion of the fallopian tube, about 2 to 3 cm from the cornu (Figure 13-1). Application further out on the tube may render the clip ineffective due to the increased volume of tissue held between the jaws of the closed clip (Figure 13-2). Care should be taken to ensure that the clip is completely across the oviduct. Proper placement is easier to confirm in the two-incision technique because the applicator can be rotated from side to side, which improves the angle of view

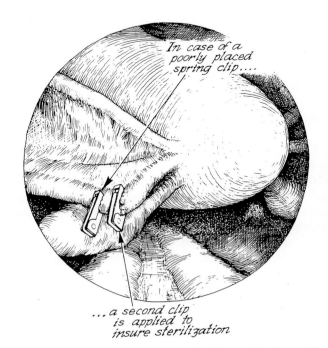

Figure 13-2 Correct and incorrect clip applications. (Reprinted with permission from Hulka JF. *Textbook of Laparoscopy.* Philadelphia: WB Saunders, 1985.)

(Figure 13-3). With the operating laparoscope, the angle of view is restricted; this limitation can be overcome with practice.

Once the clip is in proper position, the upper (outer) ram closes the jaw when the handle of the applicator is slowly squeezed (Figure 13-4). Once the jaws are closed, the middle (inner) ram pushes the gold spring over the clip to hold the clip in place on the tube. Once the clip is applied, the handle of the applicator is opened, retracting the two rams and permitting the clip and the tube to fall free of the applicator (Figure 13-5). Experienced surgeons achieve success rates equal to those of other laparoscopic sterilization methods, but practice is necessary to learn the proper mechanics of the applicator and clip application. Always inspect the placement of the clip after it has been released from the applicator. If one finds the clip has been applied improperly (on an angle or not surrounding the tube), a second clip can be applied.

Complications unique to spring clip sterilization operations result from mechanical difficulties. Should the clip be dislodged and dropped into the abdomen, it can be removed using an operating laparoscope with a grasper and lifted through the laparoscope trocar sleeve. The trumpet valve should be held open to prevent accidental trapping of the clip as the laparoscope, grasper, and clip are removed together. If an operating laparoscope is not available, place a grasper (placed through a secondary trocar sleeve), grasp the clip, and push the clip into the abdominal end of the laparoscope trocar sleeve. During this maneuver, withdraw the laparoscope up the trocar sleeve in advance of the clip.

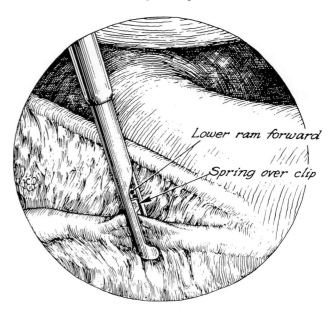

Figure 13-4 Closing the clip. (Reprinted with permission from Hulka JF. *Textbook of Laparoscopy.* Philadelphia: WB Saunders, 1985).

Thus, in simultaneous maneuver, the clip is pushed through the trocar sleeve with visual guidance as the laparoscope is withdrawn from its trocar sleeve. On occasion, a minilap incision may be necessary. If so, the laparoscope should be left in place, the minilap incision made as small as possible, and a sturdy instrument, such as a long Kocher clamp,

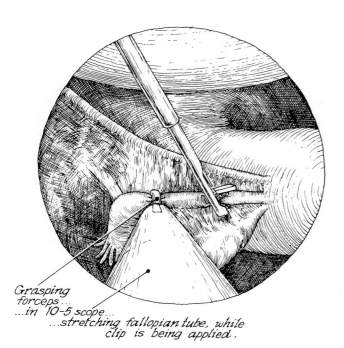

Figure 13-3 Stretching the tube with grasping forceps in an operating channel. (Reprinted with permission from Hulka JF. *Textbook of Laparoscopy.* Philadelphia: WB Saunders, 1985.)

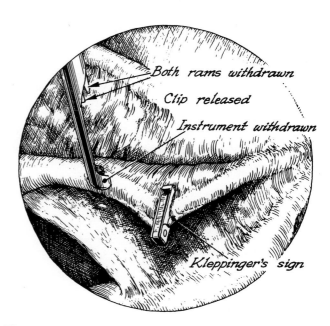

Figure 13-5 Correct application of clip. (Reprinted with permission from Hulka JF. *Textbook of Laparoscopy.* Philadelphia: WB Saunders, 1985.)

passed through the incision. The operator can use the laparoscope to watch the clamp grasp the clip and withdraw it from the abdomen.

STERILIZATION FAILURES

Unfortunately for patient and physician, sterilization failures occur. Each technique has inherent problems, and Mother Nature has a remarkable propensity to reconstitute the integrity of the normal fallopian tube. Statistical reports on the success and/or failure of techniques are usually flawed because of anecdotal experience, retrospective review, and short-term follow-up. Too frequently, different techniques are modified by the individual surgeon, who in essence invents another method without the luxury of adequate statistics. The following comments are summarized from reports in the literature, anecdotal experiences of others, and the personal experience of the two authors.

By 1996, the world's first prospective study of all female sterilization techniques was completed. Over 14 years with a ten-year follow-up period, over 10,000 cases of sterilization procedures were analyzed by the Centers for Disease Control (CDC). All of the methods were found to have a higher risk of failure than previously stated from retrospective studies. All of the laparoscopic methods had sufficient numbers of patients to claim statistical validity. Of the nine study centers, six were teaching institutions, which may influence the higher than expected failure rate. Of particular concern was the finding of a one-in-twenty failure rate in patients under the age of twenty-eight who had a bipolar method. A failure frequently resulted in an ectopic pregnancy, a life-threatening event. Table 13-1 reveals the risk of each method resulting in a failure.

Thus, of the laparoscopic procedures described, unipolar electrocoagulation without transection has boasted the lowest failure rate of all of the laparoscopic techniques to date. When unipolar failures occur, a fistula is always the culprit. The presumed risks of unipolar electrocoagulation, as previously mentioned, moved the laparoscopist to other techniques presumed to be safer.

Prior to the CDC prospective study, problems with bipolar failure have become apparent in the literature. Incompatible equipment and inadequate coagulation appear to play a major role in these disturbing reports. Bipolar techniques that coagulate less than 2 cm of tube and in which the energy delivered to the tube is below 20 to 25 W of power appear to have an unacceptable failure rate. A cutting waveform is preferred, with the power setting at 24 to 35 W.

When bipolar failures are examined, a healthy endosalpinx is usually found, with scarred muscular tissue consistent with incomplete electrocoagulation, suggesting that the visual endpoint of electrocoagulation is not sufficient information to declare the tube coagulated. The use of an Ammeter or optical meter as provided by the Richard Wolf Company would appear to reduce the risk of incomplete coagulation.

Failures associated with a Hulka clip frequently follow misplacement of the clip, either too distally on the tube or at oblique angles to the axis of the tube, or misapplication to other structures. When mechanical devices in medicine are used, occasional flaws in the individual device may render the operation unsuccessful.

When ring failures occur, in general, they are secondary to spontaneous reanastomosis. In these cases, once the loop contained above the applied clip has atrophied, the tube does not separate, as is the usual case, and spontaneous reanastomosis occurs. In such cases, the ring is frequently found perched on top of the anastomosis or adjacent to the anastomosis on the mesosalpinx.

At this point, a word about the management of failed tubal sterilization is appropriate. Too often, the repeat procedure is performed by another physician who may or may not have a keen knowledge of the technique previously employed. At the second sterilization procedure, it is the duty of the surgeon to approach this matter in a scientific fashion. The description of the anatomy should be clear, and when possible photographs or video film taken of the operative site. At either the operating table or in the pathology laboratory, the tube suspected of patency should be instilled with chromotubation to identify the exact point of failure. If necessary, multiple microscopic slides of the area in question should be obtained for close scrutiny by a trained and informed pathologist. The use of a Mallory Trichome stain will help to identify tissue previously destroyed by electrical energy. To say casually "The tube looked normal to me" serves no one well.

SUGGESTED READING

Hulka JF, ed. *Textbook of Laparoscopy*. Orlando, FL: Grune & Stratton, 1985.

Peterson HB, Xia Z, Hughes JM, Wilcox LS, Tylor LR, Trussell J. The risk of pregnancy after tubal sterilization: findings from the U.S. collaborative review of sterilization. *Am J Obstet Gynecol* 1996; 174: 1161–70.

Phillips JM, ed. *Endoscopic Female Sterilization*. Downey, IL: American Association of Gynecologic Laparoscopists, 1983.

Phillips JM, ed. *Laparoscopy*. Baltimore, MD: Williams & Wilkins, 1977.

Table 13-1 *Relative risk of failure by method*

Postpartum partial salpingectomy	1.0
Unipolar	1.5
Spring clip	2.3
Bipolar	3.7
Silicone band	3.9

APPENDIX 13-A

Female Sterilization: Advantages, Disadvantages, and Special Equipment

UNIPOLAR STERILIZATION (Figures 13-A.1, 13-A.2, 13-A.3)

Advantages

1. Complete coagulation of the tissue is guaranteed by the nature of the electrophysics involved.
2. Any insulated forceps that can grasp the tube can be used.
3. The mesosalpinx and the vascular tree are coagulated.
4. This method has the lowest reported sterilization failure rate.

Disadvantages

1. Extensive electrical coagulation may occur.
2. Reanastomosis may be impossible.
3. Aberrant electrical pathways are possible (the use of low-voltage generators eliminates this risk).
4. Ground plate burns are possible.
5. Touching vital organs by accident may cause severe damage.
6. Capacitance occurs when using an operating laparoscope.

Special Equipment

1. Low-voltage generator (isolated ground circuitry is desirable).

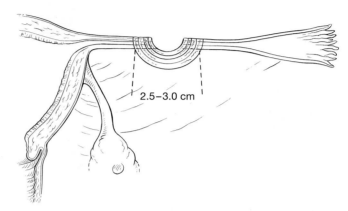

Figure 13-A.2 Coagulation and cutting, unipolar.

2. Grasping forceps (insulated).
3. Ground plate.

SNARE STERILIZATION METHOD (Figures 13-A.4 and 13-A.5)

Advantages

1. It produces adequate and uniform coagulation low-voltage, high-frequency coagulators).

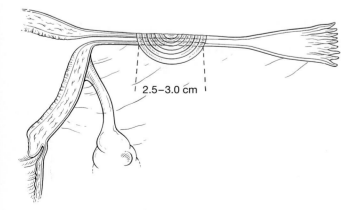

Figure 13-A.1 Coagulation only, unipolar.

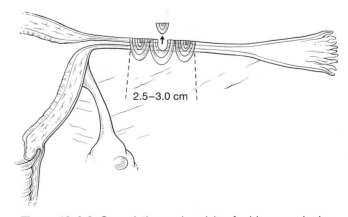

Figure 13-A.3 Coagulation and excision for biopsy, unipolar.

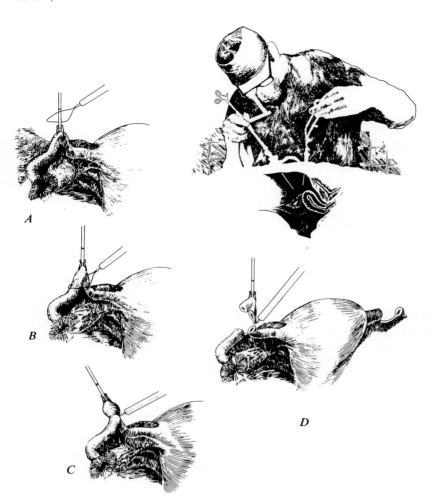

A

B

C

D

Figure 13-A.4 The Soderstrom-Smith technique of midtubal resection. **A.** A grasping forceps, introduced through the operating laparoscope, is guided through an open snare that has been introduced through the suprapubic trocar sleeve, to grasp the middle segment of the fallopian tube. **B.** The forceps, grasping the tube segment, are pulled back through the open snare. **C.** The snare is tightened to constrict the tube segment just before electrocoagulation is applied. **D.** Once the tube blanches white, low-voltage, high-frequency cutting current is applied, and the tube segment is resected. The resected tube segment is removed with the grasping forceps and the laparoscope through the umbilical trocar sleeve.

2. It guarantees adequate transection.
3. It guarantees adequate resection.
4. It is the only method yet described that removes a normal (uncoagulated) specimen for pathologic confirmation.
5. It exposes the abdominal viscera to a small active electrode, thus reducing the risk of visceral burn.

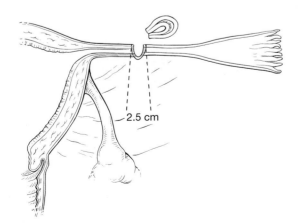

Figure 13-A.5 Unipolar coagulation with excision, Soderstrom method.

2.5 cm

Disadvantages

1. It is a two-hole technique (debatable).
2. An operating laparoscope must be available.
3. The technique is more complicated to learn; it should be reserved for the skilled laparoscopist.
4. It is more difficult to teach than other methods.

BIPOLAR STERILIZATION (Figure 13-A.6)

Advantages

1. The ground plate is eliminated.
2. There is better control over electron spread.
3. Reanastomosis is usually possible.
4. Aberrant pathways are not possible.
5. Touching vital organs by accident will, in general, cause little harm.
6. Capacitance cannot occur.

Disadvantages

1. Because of the electrophysics involved, the extent of coagulation is limited and may be incomplete.

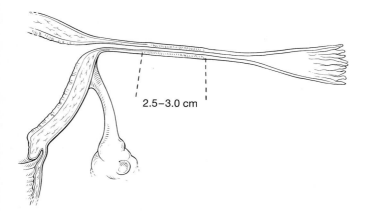

Figure 13-A.6 Coagulation only, bipolar.

2. Some forceps may not be compatible with all generators.
3. Higher failure rates than unipolar and silastic band methods, especially in younger women.

Special Equipment

1. Bipolar generator.
2. Bipolar forceps.

THERMAL STERILIZATION (Figures 13-A.7 and 13-A.8)

Advantages

1. A ground plate is not required.
2. No aberrant pathways are possible.
3. The burn is discrete.
4. Reanastomosis is usually possible.

Disadvantages

1. Tissue destruction may be insufficient to impede spontaneous reanastomosis (Waters instrument).

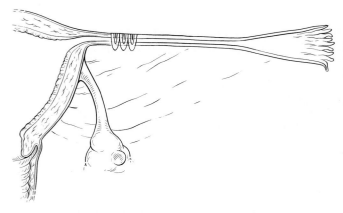

Figure 13-A.8 Thermocoagulation.

2. Failure rates are unknown.
3. Double-puncture technique is required (debatable).

Special Equipment

1. Twelve-volt generator and compatible forceps or hook.

BAND STERILIZATION (Figure 13-A.9)

Advantages

1. The technique is nonelectrical.
2. It secures and destroys 2.5 cm of tube.
3. The applicator is programmed to secure an adequate amount of tube.
4. It has had wide use.
5. Reanastomosis is usually possible.

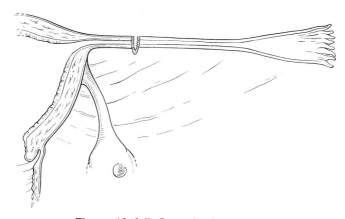

Figure 13-A.7 Cauterization section.

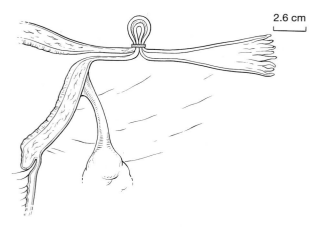

Figure 13-A.9 Falopering.

Disadvantages

1. Applicator tongs may sever the tube and cause bleeding.
2. The band may "milk" itself off the tube, especially "fat" tubes.
3. Tubes bound down with adhesions may preclude band application.
4. Short-term postoperative pain is often experienced.
5. The band may aggravate subclinical salpingitis.

Special Equipment

1. Band applicator.
2. Cone-shaped device to stretch band onto the applicator.

HULKA-CLEMENS CLIP STERILIZATION (Figure 13-A.10)

Advantages

1. Only 5 mm of tube is destroyed; reanastomosis is always possible.
2. The technique is nonelectrical.
3. The clip received extensive premarket testing and appraisal.
4. Less postoperative pain is experienced than with the band method.

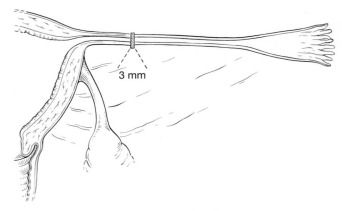

Figure 13-A.10 The Hulka clip.

Disadvantages

1. It requires more training than the band method (debatable).

Special Equipment

1. Clips.
2. Clip applicator.

Operative Laparoscopy, Second Edition
The Masters' Techniques in Gynecologic Surgery
Lippincott–Raven Publishers, Philadelphia © 1998.

14

Nongynecologic Uses

Alan B. Gazzaniga, Kim James Charney, Theodore Coutsoftides, Brian A. Palafox, and Jeffrey M. Johnsrud

The number and variety of laparoscopic procedures done by general surgeons has broadened dramatically since 1987, when Mauret in France introduced laparoscopic cholecystectomy. Laparoscopic cholecystectomy was then introduced in the United States by Reddick in 1989 and, because of his effort, it is now the treatment of choice for almost all gallbladder diseases. Laparoscopic cholecystectomy has become a landmark in the development of surgery and can be compared to such surgical milestones as the introduction of vascular surgery and organ transplant. In this chapter we will discuss laparoscopic techniques in the treatment of gallbladder disease, abdominal trauma, appendicitis, hiatus hernia, colon disease, and inguinal hernia.

LAPAROSCOPIC CHOLECYSTECTOMY

Laparoscopic cholecystectomy should be considered in every patient who has the indication for cholecystectomy. During the initial introduction of laparoscopic cholecystectomy, it was felt that patients with acute cholecystitis, previous upper abdominal surgery, morbid obesity, intraabdominal sepsis with septicemia, and common bile duct obstruction with jaundice should not be treated by laparoscopic cholecystectomy. With time and experience, however, many of these "absolute contraindications" have fallen by the wayside. The advantages of laparoscopic cholecystectomy were outlined by Reddick et al (1989). In that study, the patients had less morbidity, required less analgesia, had fewer side effects, faster recovery, and were able to return to work earlier than patients who received the conventional treatment for cholecystectomy. The cost of laparoscopic cholecystectomy in our institution is about one-half the cost of cholecystectomy. Laparoscopic procedures have caused a fundamental alteration in the management of gallstones and cholecystitis. Laparoscopic cholecystectomy is here to stay and is the treatment of choice for gallbladder lithiasis. Newer tech-

niques, adherence to sound surgical principles, and advancements in instrumentation, have made the surgery safe. Laparoscopic common bile duct exploration is evolving and will be applied increasingly by the majority of laparoscopic surgeons.

Technique

The patient is positioned on the operating table, which may be rotated to facilitate the procedure. Patients undergoing cholecystectomy should receive some form of deep venous thrombosis prophylaxis. In our institution, patients routinely have intermittent pneumatic compression devices placed on their lower extremities. Most surgeons administer preoperative antibiotics. Following induction of general endotracheal anesthesia, the patient initially is placed in the Trendelenburg position to allow the intraperitoneal contents to shift cephalad out of the pelvis. The entire abdomen is prepared and draped. A 1-cm incision is made in the lower half of the umbilical skin, and the umbilical fascia is grasped with two hemostats or towel clips and elevated. At this point, a Veress needle is introduced with a light touch so that one can feel the entry into the peritoneal cavity. There are disposable Veress needles that allow the surgeon to see that the blunt obturator has moved forward when the needle passes through the fascial and peritoneal barrier. The open or Hasson technique is used when there has been previous surgery or adhesions may be expected, or if there are difficulties with percutaneous insertion. A drop of saline in the open end of the needle will be sucked in on elevation of the hemostats and help to establish that the needle is in the peritoneal cavity. Usually the abdomen is distended to 11 to 15 mmHg. Lower pressures are recommended for patients with significant pulmonary or cardiac compromise. CO_2 is insufflated (usually 1 L to start), and the abdomen is carefully percussed to be sure the CO_2 is entering the peritoneal cavity and not subcutaneous tissue. Once it is ascertained that the CO_2 is intraperitoneal, more rapid insufflation can occur, up to 3 to 4 L. At this point, the insufflators will allow continuous pressure at a certain level. Under ordinary circumstances, intraabdominal pressure of 15 to 20 mmHg is well-tolerated, but, in the presence of hypotension or shock, this pressure can lead to a further fall in blood pressure and cardiac output (Toomasian et al, 1978).

Following introduction of the needle, a 10/11-mm cannula is introduced into the umbilical incision, followed by the laparoscope. Various types of laparoscopes are available, and familiarity with their use is mandatory. Some prefer a 30°-angle scope, though I find it more difficult to use. Before the camera is attached, the lenses are inspected for any water vapor or foreign material that might obscure the video picture. With most video cameras, a white balance is necessary to be sure that the picture is absolutely clear. Another 10/11-mm cannula is introduced near the midline, approximately two to three finger breadths below the costal margin. It is important that this cannula be below the inferior aspect of the liver, so one does not have to work around the liver to gain access to the gallbladder. An additional 5-mm cannula is placed at an extreme lateral to allow instruments to rotate the gallbladder, and another one between the other two cannula ports (Figure 14-1). Most right-handed surgeons prefer to stand on the right-hand side of the table. However, if the surgeon is left-handed, the assistant can stand on the right-hand side of the table and handle the laparoscope and the lateral cannula, while the left-handed surgeon can manage the two medial upper abdominal cannula sites.

Once in place, and after the entire peritoneal cavity has been explored with the laparoscope, the cholecystectomy can begin. The patient is now placed in reverse Trendelenburg to allow the stomach, colon, and duodenum to fall away from the gallbladder. It is best to have the assistant grasp the gallbladder near the fundus and rotate it cephalad. The surgeon then can grasp the gallbladder near the neck and begin the dissection in the triangle between the gallbladder, cystic duct, and cystic artery. Once this triangle has been opened and care taken to be sure the cystic duct is indeed the cystic duct, a clip applicator is passed through the 10/11-mm cannula and a clip applied at the junction between the gallbladder and cystic duct. The best way to prevent common duct injury is to grasp the gallbladder as described and straighten out the gallbladder so that the cystic duct is perpendicular to the common duct during dissection.

Once the cystic duct/gallbladder junction has been occluded with a clip, a transverse incision is made in the cystic duct with scissors and a catheter is introduced (Figure 14-2). I have found a balloon-type catheter introduced through a small needle to be the most effective. After the cholangiogram, the cystic duct catheter is removed and the duct clipped, three times, if possible, before complete tran-

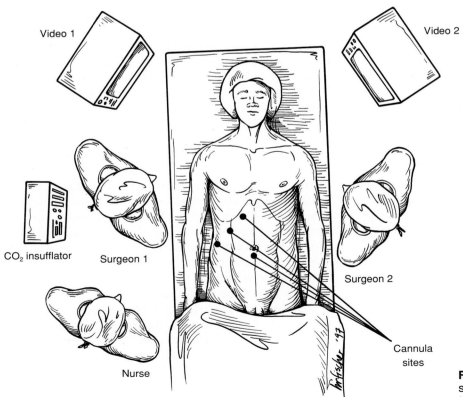

Video 1

Video 2

CO_2 insufflator

Surgeon 1

Surgeon 2

Nurse

Cannula sites

Figure 14-1 The primary surgeon can stand on either side of table and work effectively with the assistant.

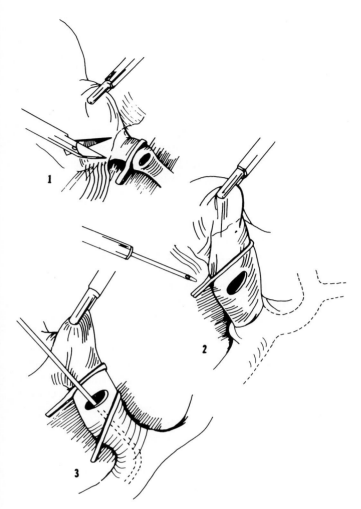

Figure 14-2 Normal cystic duct cholangiogram.

liver bed is identified and coagulated. The gallbladder is grasped by the 10-mm grasping forceps and can be brought out either through the umbilical cannula site or through the upper midline abdominal cannula site. I prefer the midline cannula site, since it does not require moving the camera. The gallbladder is brought to the epigastric 10/11 cannula site and the cannula removed. The gallbladder is then grasped with clamps and opened. If the gallbladder should rupture on removal, it is easier to remove the stones from the upper abdomen than it is from the bowel, when rupture occurs at the umbilical site.

Once the gallbladder is brought to the abdominal wall and has been decompressed, it may be difficult to remove all the gallstones. This can prevent delivering the gallbladder through the cannula site. Dilating the fascia with a Péan clamp is useful and works in most cases. Sometimes this is not satisfactory, particularly in an obese patient with large stones. It may be necessary to crush the stones in the sack, but this must be done carefully with video assistance so that perforation and spillage does not occur. Although some experimental evidence suggests that free gallstones are usually isolated by the omentum, it has been our experience that if stones are left behind in the peritoneal cavity they cause an inflammatory reaction and can produce adhesions. Bile leakage from perforation of the gallbladder can occur during laparoscopic cholecystectomy. In small amounts, whether infected or not, this appears to be relatively harmless. However, in combination with gallstone loss, this can significantly increase the risk of postoperative adhesions and intraabdominal abscesses.

After the stones are removed from the gallbladder, the gallbladder is pulled through the abdominal wall. The 10/11 cannula then is reintroduced and the upper abdominal area inspected. It is easier to aspirate blood and bile over the right lobe of the liver by introducing the suction irrigator to that area. As long as the tip is under fluid, the pneumoperitoneum will not be lost and one can irrigate thoroughly. It is important to remove all bloody material and clots, to reduce morbidity. It is not recommended that you suction near clips, since they can be aspirated off the cystic artery or duct, making reclipping very difficult.

Once the gallbladder bed, cystic duct area, and cystic artery area have been thoroughly irrigated and inspected, the insufflation is released and the 10/11 cannulas removed. Surgeons are not unanimous about whether or not the fascia at the 10/11 cannula site needs to be closed. Most surgeons, however, feel that closure of fascia may offer some advantage in preventing herniation, and whenever possible I close it with absorbable sutures. The skin is closed with 3-0 absorbable suture and a dressing is applied.

COMPLICATIONS

Intraoperative complications in our experience and that of others have included 1. pneumothorax, 2. bowel injury

section. At this point, the cystic artery is usually identified; it may branch into an anterior and posterior branch. Occluding the cystic artery with a clip will ensure minimal problems when removing the gallbladder. If present, it is imperative that the posterior branch of the cystic artery be identified, since troublesome bleeding can occur if it is transected during the cholecystectomy.

Once the cystic artery has been clipped and divided, the gallbladder can be removed in an antegrade fashion using electrocoagulation. There was initial enthusiasm for a cutting and coagulating laser, but its advantages over electrosurgery are questionable. Lasers (1) are expensive, (2) create safety hazards in the operating room, (3) are more cumbersome to use, and (4) offer no distinct advantage over standard electrosurgery. The use of the electrode scissors and/or J hook has made the removal of the gallbladder safe and usually bloodless. With electrical instruments, the gallbladder can be rapidly mobilized and dissected from its bed in a fashion similar to that of traditional open cholecystectomy. As the gallbladder is removed, any bleeding from the from active electrode or laser burns, 3. cholangiographic findings that demand formal traditional surgical intervention, 4. bleeding from the gallbladder itself, or inability to grasp the gallbladder because of the thickened wall to allow mobilization and dissection, and 5. bile leakage that may result from several injuries. These include the classic injury related to missed identification of anatomy, leading to a number of variants of injury: 1. Partial or total interruption of the common bile duct, 2. Missed accessory duct from the gallbladder bed and 3. Cystic duct stump leakage caused by displacement or removal of the clip or necrosis of the cystic duct during ligation.

A pneumothorax can be seen by viewing the pneumoperitoneum above the liver and looking at the diaphragm as the lung expands. Under ordinary circumstances, the lung will depress the diaphragm when the patient is ventilated. However, a loss of this excursion and a billowing down of the hemidiaphragm indicates a pneumothorax. The cause for this is unknown but is probably related to a connection in the diaphragm with subsequent leakage of CO_2 into the chest. In any case, if pneumothorax is identified, a tube thoracostomy must be placed right away. It can be suspected under general anesthesia when there is a fall in oxygen saturation and a rise in CO_2 retention.

Bleeding, if seen to fill the monitor screen, requires rapid laparotomy. In most cases, however, this does not occur and, with experience, bleeding can be controlled with clips and cautery in the usual fashion. If there is excessive bleeding from the liver bed and there is continued oozing at the conclusion of the procedure, then a closed drainage system must be used.

The presence of common duct stones at the time of cholangiography does not necessarily mean open cholecystectomy is indicated. If the stones are small and located in the distal common duct with the dye flowing around them, they probably can be left in place and removed later by endoscopic retrograde cholangiopancreatography (ERCP). If, however, the dye flows very slowly around the stone, indicating the stone is nearly occlusive or occlusive in the mid-common duct, immediate removal of the stone or stones is necessary, by laparoscopic or open exploration technique. If a stone is retained in the common duct and it is nearly occlusive, it may become totally occlusive postoperatively, raise proximal common duct pressure and lead to cystic duct perforation.

We have had two common bile duct injuries in our series, and when they occurred, immediate laparotomy was undertaken and the duct repaired either with direct anastomosis or a Roux-en-Y of jejunum.

Postoperatively, the patient usually complains of shoulder pain if complete removal of the pneumoperitoneum was not accomplished. There is usually mild abdominal pain, and we always infiltrate the incisions with local anesthesia to alleviate the initial discomfort. Most patients get along with light Demerol analgesia, and 90% of patients go home within 24 hours. On occasion, small fevers occur, related to atelectasis, but they do not require vigorous intervention and will resolve within 48 hours.

Comment

Laparoscopic cholecystectomy has become an established procedure in a short period of time. It offers a tremendous advantage over traditional cholecystectomy; the patient's discomfort is reduced, and ability to return to work is accelerated. Traditional cholecystectomy and laparoscopic cholecystectomy have the same intraperitoneal tissue dissections. It is the abdominal incision that is different, and it is the size of the incision that produces the morbidity. The elimination of large, painful, abdominal incisions, with the attendant effects on colon and pulmonary function, has made laparoscopic cholecystectomy a desirable and necessary part of the general surgeon's armamentarium.

The training of general surgeons to do laparoscopic cholecystectomy has occurred over a rapid period of time with tremendous success. The use of videotapes, animal laboratories, etc., has allowed this procedure to go from hospital to hospital, state to state, throughout the country. Various hospitals have set up standards for appropriate training in this procedure. When one considers the number of operative procedures performed, it is clear that the technique is accepted and is safe throughout the country.

However, despite this glowing presentation, there remain many problems with laparoscopic cholecystectomy. There continue to be technical errors in terms of complete visualization of the cystic duct, injury to the common duct, bleeding, etc. The question of what to do when cholangiography reveals the presence of stones in the common duct has not been fully resolved. If at all possible, the common duct stone should be recognized prior to laparoscopic cholecystectomy. This will prepare the surgeon for transcystic duct exploration, or even for laparoscopic common bile duct exploration. While these techniques are in evolution, surgeons will have to become familiar with them to be able to give complete intraoperative and postoperative endoscopic management of common bile duct stones. Currently, when common duct stones are encountered on cholangiogram, ERCP continues to be the most favored approach for dealing with them.

During our first 150 laparoscopic cholecystectomy procedures, twelve patients had conversion to open laparotomy. Since that time, we have done over 1500 laparoscopic cholecystectomies and only a small number had to be converted to open cholecystectomy. The most common reason for this has been acute cholecystitis or complicated common duct stones.

LAPAROSCOPY FOR ABDOMINAL TRAUMA

In 1976, we introduced laparoscopy in the management of both blunt and penetrating injuries to the abdomen (Gazzaniga et al, 1976). At that time, the standard laparoscope was used without video camera. We were able to evaluate a large number of patients and become adept at predicting which patients did or did not need laparotomy. Our interest in emergency laparoscopy waned because of introduction of computerized tomography (CT) scanning and a better interpretation of peritoneal lavage fluid. With the introduction of laparoscopic cholecystectomy, interest was rekindled in laparoscopy for blunt trauma. For example, Berci et al (1991) introduced laparoscopy at the bedside, either in the intensive care unit or in the emergency department. They used a 4-mm miniature laparoscope, which is approximately the same diameter of a lavage catheter, allowing easier, faster, and safer entry into the peritoneal cavity. In trauma patients, their indications for emergency laparoscopy included an obscure clinical picture and physical signs with impaired level of consciousness, stab or blunt abdominal trauma, unexplained hypotension and equivocal signs of physical examination of the conscious patient. Since their reintroduction of laparoscopy for blunt trauma, there have been many authors who have supported laparoscopy in trauma (Smith, Sosa, Poole).

I continue to prefer laparoscopy in the operating room and use it for the same general indications outlined above. It is particularly useful in patients who have stab or gunshot wounds of the abdomen, in which peritoneal penetration cannot be ascertained, or when other surgical procedures are necessary, such as drainage of a subdural hematoma, when there is not time to evaluate the abdomen by CT scanning.

Procedure

The abdomen is prepared and draped and a 1-cm incision is made in the midline above the umbilicus. The Veress needle is introduced in the same fashion as previously described. After CO_2 insufflation and placement of a 10/11 cannula, the laparoscope is introduced into the peritoneal cavity. Inspection usually begins by looking at the liver for any fractures. Frequently, liver lacerations are seen, but are not bleeding, and surgery is not indicated. The patient is then turned 30° with the right side down, and the omentum is teased away from the spleen via forceps introduced through a second left upper quadrant 5-mm cannula. This gives an excellent view of the left upper quadrant. In my experience there has never been a ruptured spleen when blood was not present in the left upper quadrant. In almost all cases where blood and omentum are present, the spleen is ruptured. There have not been any reports of splenectomy for trauma through the laparoscope, but splenorrhaphy has been done (Smith, et al).

With the patient supine, a panoramic view of the peritoneal cavity can be accomplished by withdrawing the scope to the umbilicus and looking directly downward into the peritoneal cavity. The lateral gutters can be visualized and inspected for spilled abdominal contents. The small bowel can be run by using another cannula and grasping forceps to pull the bowel, while looking for any hidden hematomas or collection of bile-stained fluid. In patients with a fractured pelvis, a view of the pelvis will often show a hematoma in the midline and laterally. This hematoma can be quite extensive and can be the source of the so-called "positive tap." The lavage catheter does not enter into the peritoneal cavity, but remains in the hematoma, giving a false positive result.

In the presence of penetrating injury, the penetrating site can be identified. On a number of occasions, although there was abdominal fluid and muscle injury, the object did not penetrate the peritoneum and laparotomy was not necessary.

Comment

In most cases, the diagnosis of intraabdominal injury is made by standard techniques, including clinical assessment, radiologic studies, and laboratory tests. However, diagnostic laparoscopy can prove helpful. If the laparoscopic examination was negative or minimal injury was found, no patient in our series and the series by Berci required subsequent exploratory laparotomy. In those patients with positive laparoscopy, where minimal to moderate hemoperitoneum was identified, the injury was usually minimal. In Berci's series, only one patient who had laparoscopy, but not laparotomy, subsequently went to laparotomy. Whenever severe hemoperitoneum was identified, laparoscopy in all cases revealed injuries that would not have resolved without surgical intervention. Recent reports by other authors have agreed with this approach (Poole et al, Pommer et al, Sosa et al). The advantages continue to include a rapid diagnosis with minimal risk. Extensive use reduces the number of unnecessary laparotomies and subsequent morbidity. It is generally agreed that there is a reduction of complication rate when laparoscopy is used in preference to routine laparotomy in trauma patients. This leads to reduced hospital stay and, ultimately, to lower cost.

LAPAROSCOPIC COLECTOMY

Colorectal surgery using the laparoscope was a natural progression, following the development of laparoscopic cholecystectomy. In this publication, I have documented that this procedure can be carried out without an untoward number of complications in both benign and malignant colorectal disease. Laparoscopic colectomy is more complicated and requires a larger learning experience than does laparoscopic cholecystectomy. It is estimated that it takes between 30 and 50 procedures (Wishner et al, Senagore AJ et al), to feel comfortable. This is due in part to the more complex nature of the procedure and also the variation in anatomy from patient to patient. During this learning curve period, the conversion to open laparotomy may be as high as 25% (Wishner et al). The latter is due to either obscure anatomy, large lesions, and/or complications. Most authors feel that converting to an open procedure, both in the learning phase and any time that patient safety and outcome appear to be compromised, is good judgment and not failure.

The indications for laparoscopic colectomy are the same as for open surgery. There is a question at this time as to whether using the laparoscope in malignant colorectal disease is justified, in view of the absence of data showing that cure rates are not comprised. Relative contraindications include extreme obesity and history of previous abdominal procedures (Guillou). Preoperative evaluation and bowel preparation is the same for both open and laparoscopic colectomy. Procedures can be done completely with the laparoscope, or assisted with the laparoscope. The latter procedure requires a larger incision, because, often, parts of the procedure, such as division of bowel and anastomosis, are done extracorporeally (Bernstein et al).

Procedure

The patient is placed supine on the operating table and the abdomen is prepped widely, from the nipples to the upper thigh. Pneumoperitoneum is established as described before, with the Veress needle or the open or Hasson technique, depending on whether the patient has had previous surgery. Once pneumoperitoneum is established, a 10/12-mm cannula is inserted via a small infraumbilical incision, and the operative laparoscope is inserted via this cannula. If the surgeon deems that the procedure can be done safely, then secondary 10/12-mm cannulas are inserted in the right lower quadrant, left upper quadrant and left lower quadrant. Occasionally it is necessary to insert an additional cannula in the right upper quadrant. If this is needed, then we insert the cannula in a location that will be used to make the abdominal incision to remove the specimen (Figure 14-3). The colon is grasped with atraumatic instruments (Babcocks or gallbladder clamps), inserted from the left side and retracted medially. During this part of the dissection, the patient is placed in the left lateral position with the head up. Using the electrocautery scissors or the harmonic scalpel, the peritoneum of the right gutter is divided and the colon retracted medially. Care is taken not to damage the ureter that is usually exposed during the dissection, or the duodenum, which should always be visualized. Attachments of the hepatic flexure to the liver and gallbladder are carefully dissected and the most lateral part of the gastrocolic omentum is carefully divided until the lesser sac is entered. The gastrocolic omentum is taken with the specimen in malignant cases, or lifted off the colon in benign disease.

At this point, the colon is well-mobilized but one needs to mobilize the distal small intestine as it is attached to the pelvic brim on the right side. Dissection here is fraught with some difficulty, because the ureter and iliac vessels may be lying close to the brim. Having mobilized the distal ileum, right colon, and proximal transverse colon, one can proceed in one of two ways.

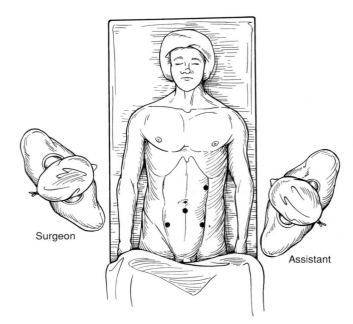

Figure 14-3 Laparoscopic colectomy port sites.

Intracorporeal: The mesentery of the distal small intestine, the ileocolic vessels, the right colon vessels, and the right branch of the middle colic vessels are divided in order to resect the specimen. A true right colic artery arising from the superior mesenteric artery is frequently absent. This can be accomplished by using the harmonic scalpel or the electrocautery scissors for small vessels or peritoneum and the use of vascular endo GIA or endoloops for the major vessels which usually have to be skeletonized prior to division. Once the blood supply is severed the bowel itself is transected using endo GIA and an anastomosis can be performed intracorporeally or extracorporeally using staples. The specimen is removed via a small right upper abdominal incision that is placed closer to the midline rather than the flank. This same incision is used to perform the extracorporeal anastomosis and close the mesenteric defect.

Extracorporeal: Once the colon is mobilized a 3 to 4-inch right upper abdominal incision is made, closer to the midline than the flank, and the colon is delivered through this incision. If the mobilization has been adequate, the mesentery also is delivered easily via this incision and can be serially clamped and divided. By making the incision in this position, one is looking down to the origin of the ileocolic and right colic vessels. An extracorporeal anastomosis is made, using the intestinal stapler, the mesenteric opening is closed in a routine fashion, and the bowel is returned to the abdominal cavity.

LEFT COLECTOMY, SIGMOID RESECTION AND LOW ANTERIOR RESECTIONS

The patient is placed in a modified lithotomy position, using adjustable low-profile stirrups. Positioning and securing the patient safely to the operating table are extremely important; during the dissection the patient will need to be placed in various positions. The rectum is irrigated with diluted Betadine solution and the rectal tube is left in place to help with decompression. The abdomen and perineum are prepped and draped in a standard fashion. Pneumoperitoneum is established in a routine fashion, a 10/12-mm cannula is inserted via a small supraumbilical incision, and the operative laparoscope is inserted. Following this, 3 to 4 additional cannulas are inserted in the right lower quadrant, left lower quadrant, right paraumbilical region, and left upper quadrant. The positions and sizes of the cannulas will vary, depending on the anatomy and configuration of the colon. In all of these procedures, it is necessary to mobilize the splenic flexure fully. Exposure is facilitated by having the patient in the head-up position, with rotation of the table to the right. To begin, the colonic flexure is grasped with instruments inserted via the right lower quadrant and right paraumbilical cannulas. The peritoneum is divided with the electrocautery scissors or harmonic scalpel. Staples or the harmonic knife are needed to control the bleeding from the attachments to the left upper quadrant. Once the flexure is mobilized, the patient is taken out of the head-up position and the peritoneum is divided along the left gutter (the ureter is always identified). The patient is now placed in the head-down position, to facilitate the dissection of the peritoneum in the pelvis. If a low anterior resection is contemplated, the lateral stalks are divided, using clips to the level of the levators. Once the stalks are divided on the left side, the stalks on the right side are divided, if a low anterior resection is contemplated. If not, the dissection is halted at the peritoneal reflection for left colectomy or sigmoid resection. When doing an anterior resection, the medial exposure of the sigmoid and rectum is augmented by placing the patient head-down. The inferior mesenteric artery and vein are identified by pulling the colon and mesentery laterally and dividing them with the endovascular GIA. The rectum is grasped or pushed anterior, away from the sacrum, and the mesentery is serially divided again, using either clips or the stapler, until the wall of the rectum is clearly seen. We try to use the cautery as little as possible for dissection, as there could potentially be thermal injury to the sympathetic and parasympathetic plexus. The rectum is transected by using a 60-mm endo-GIA inserted through the right lower quadrant cannula, or, on occasion, another cannula is inserted in the suprapubic region. These cannulas are usually larger, in order to accommodate the larger endo-GIA. Alternatively, the same can be accomplished by using the 30-mm endo-GIA, except that more cartridges are needed.

Having mobilized the colon and transected the bowel in its distal part, a small left lower quadrant transverse incision is made, and the colon is delivered through this. The proximal point of transection is chosen, a pursestring is applied, and the colon transected. A 29-mm intraluminal stapling device is used. The head is inserted in the proximal colon and the shaft is grasped with a grasp specially designed to facilitate "docking" for the anastomosis. The proximal colon is returned to the abdominal cavity, the left lower quadrant incision is closed in layers, and pneumoperitoneum is reestablished. An anastomosis is now effected under direct vision by inserting the anvil part of the stapler transanally to complete an end-to-end anastomosis. Saline is then inserted in the pelvis, air insufflated in the rectum, and the integrity of the anastomosis is tested. For very low anterior resection or for coloanal anastomosis, an alternate technique can be used. After complete mobilization is carried out, the rectum is transected approximately 6 to 8 cm above the levators. The distal segment is everted transanally and the proximal segment is delivered perineally, via the everted anus. Points of transection are chosen and an end-to-end anastomosis is fashioned, using the intraluminal stapling device, or done by hand.

ABDOMINOPERINEAL RESECTION

The dissection is carried out in much the same way as in a low anterior resection except that this is carried inferiorly to the levators and the rectum is separated anteriorly from the vagina or the prostate seminal vesicles, depending on the case. The colon is transected at the junction of the sigmoid descending colon and a colostomy is established at the previously marked site. Usually, the left lower quadrant cannula is inserted at the same site as the colostomy, obviating need for another incision. Once the colostomy is constructed, the perineal dissection, which is the same as that in an open technique, is completed.

Comment

A number of articles show a percentage of complications in laparoscopic surgery similar to those of procedures done in an open fashion. Some reports even show fewer complications; however, these reports may be those of highly selective groups (Ballantyne). In a large review from the Laparoscopic Bowel Surgery Registry, intraoperative complications were the same as from open operative complications (Ortega et al). This conclusion was challenged in an editorial following the article, stating that the study may have been flawed because the results were reported voluntarily and with this methodology, the problem may be understated (Abscarin). However, certain complications, such as vascular injury, are specific to laparoscopic surgery and can be avoided using the open technique to establish pneumoperitoneum (Geers et al).

Earlier reports of tumor implantation at the cannula site have been bothersome and reported in the literature with sufficient frequency (Wexner et al). The question as to whether laparoscopic colectomy is adequate cancer surgery is still unanswered. Although reports have shown that the distal margin and number of lymph nodes harvested are comparable with those from the open procedure, no studies have been done to show whether the circumferential dissection is as adequate as the open procedure (Guillou, Vignati et al, Ballantyne). There appears to be a higher incidence of local recurrence, and occasionally the wrong segment of colon removed, because of inadequate preoperative marking (Vignati et al, Nelson et al). Reports to date do not show any significant differences in survival (Franklin et al) but longer follow-up and prospective studies will be needed to answer this question (Nelson et al). At this point, it appears that a considerable number of physicians are reluctant to use this technique for large malignant lesions of the colon, while some physicians use this in highly selected patients (Zucker et al). It is clear that patients who have a laparoscopic colectomy have a shorter hospital stay and costs are less than for comparable surgery done in the standard fashion. Laparoscopic techniques in colorectal surgery are gaining popularity and are being done more frequently. The indications for the procedure are the same as for open technique, but the controversy still exists regarding this procedure in patients with cancer.

ACUTE APPENDICITIS

Semm (1984) was the first to describe the treatment of acute appendicitis by laparoscopy. Since that time, there has been steadily increasing interest in the use of the laparoscope for appendectomy. The advantages of laparoscopic appendectomy are an incision of reduced size, accelerated convalescence, and rapid return to work. Even retrocecal appendix and other variations of anatomy do not prevent laparoscopic appendectomy. With expanded use of the laparoscope for colonic resection, laparoscopic appendectomy has become more popular, although most surgeons still hesitate to use it routinely.

Procedure

A Foley catheter is placed in the urinary bladder. The Veress needle is introduced in a similar fashion to that described before and a 10/11-mm cannula is introduced below the umbilicus. Once inspection is made and the diagnosis is confirmed, the patient is placed in Trendelenburg and turned to a left 30° position, to allow the bowel to fall away and expose the appendix. A second 5-mm cannula is placed in the left lower quadrant. A third 10/11 cannula is placed in the right upper quadrant in the anterior axillary line. Depending on the location and the skill of the examiner, these cannulas can be reversed, with the 10/11 mm cannula being in the left lower quadrant and the 5-mm cannula in the right upper quadrant (Figure 14-4). Either way, the appendix is grasped with forceps and the mesoappendix is taken down, using an endoscopic automatic stapler. When the mesoappendix is divided and the appendix is isolated, it can be closed either with an Endoloop or by endoscopic stapling. I prefer to do endoscopic stapling and to bring the appendix

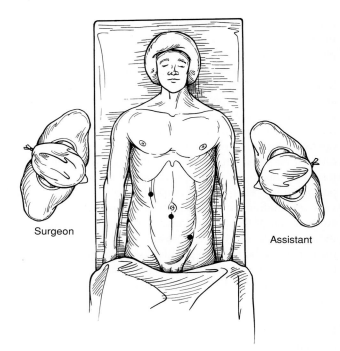

Figure 14-4 Appendectomy port sites.

out through the 10/11-mm cannula site. Before retraction, the appendix can be placed in a sterile bag, if necessary. After the appendix is removed, the peritoneal cavity is irrigated thoroughly and inspected for bleeders. Postoperatively, the patient can be discharged the first day after surgery. Antibiotics should be used whenever appropriate.

Comment

Laparoscopic appendectomy is appealing and has become widely used. It permits minimal invasion, avoiding the associated problems of a right lower quadrant incision. This will be appealing to female patients who are concerned about scars or athletes who do not want their abdominal musculature interrupted. Furthermore, elective prophylactic appendectomy can be considered in patients who are planning to travel through remote areas where surgical assistance may not be readily available, e.g., scientists wintering in Antarctica or astronauts in space. In some cases, appendectomy may be difficult through the laparoscope, but, with experience, these anatomic and instrument limitations have been overcome.

LAPAROSCOPIC FUNDOPLICATION

The first "Nissen fundoplication" was described in 1936, for an esophageal ulcer penetrating the pericardium. Sixteen years later, Nissen noted that the patient did not have esophagitis and later used this technique to treat esophageal reflux. This operative procedure has improved over the years and currently over 20,000 patients a year have Nissen fundoplication done through the laparoscope.

The physiology for reflux has been well described in the last decade. The anatomy of the area is shown in Figure 14-5. The major factors are: 1) the need to maintain a high pressure zone in the distal esophagus, 2) the sphincter function is best when it resides in the abdomen, and 3) the esophageal sphincter is too flaccid for long periods of time, or too short. The observation of associated hiatus hernia with gastroesophageal reflux (GER) is documented in large series in the United States. In groups of patients that have severe GER, 75% have hiatal hernias. However, less than 10% of the population have a hiatal hernia. The indications for surgery include esophagitis that does not respond to medical therapy, bleeding, obstruction and Barrett's mucosal changes, which is considered a premalignant lesion.

Procedure

An orogastric tube is placed to decompress the stomach after induction of general endotracheal anesthesia. The patient is positioned in a modified lithotomy, with elbows protected to minimize compression of the ulnar nerve. The hips should be located over the break in the table, and the patient's legs should be well-padded. It is important to secure the patient to the table, so that when the table is placed in the reverse Trendelenburg position, the patient will not slide. This is accomplished by using sheets tied to the table and looped around the patient's legs, securing the free ends of the sheet to the table. Great care is taken not to compromise circulation or place undue stress on the hips.

The surgeon positions himself between the legs, the assistant on the patient's left side and the scrub nurse on the patient's right side (Figure 14-6). The assistant controls the camera. The scrub nurse holds the liver retractor unless a table attachment is available. Insufflation of the abdominal cavity is done as previously described at the umbilicus. A 10/12-mm cannula is inserted between the xyphoid process and the umbilicus. If the entry site is too distal, the length of the laparoscope will not reach the esophageal hiatus, limiting visualization of the posterior aspect of the hiatus.

The right subcostal (5-mm) cannula is positioned to allow access to the left lobe of the liver, so it can be elevated without interference of the round ligament. Once placed, there is little reason for this retractor to be manipulated. The more laterally the cannula is placed the less likely it is that it will interfere with the other cannulas.

The left subcostal 10/12-mm cannula is placed in such a position that a grasper, ultrasonic scalpel, coagulator, and automatic suturing device, can be used. Placement depends on the location of the spleen relative to the stomach in order to optimize and control the short gastric vessels. The last two cannulas (5-mm) are placed to the right and left of the midline above the level of the viewing port. They do not need to be symmetrically placed, the position being determined by the intra-abdominal anatomy. Depending on the

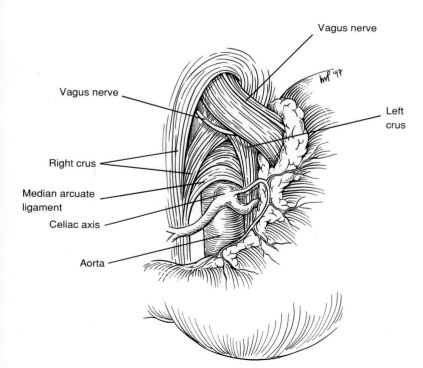

Figure 14-5 Exposed anatomy for Nissen fundoplication.

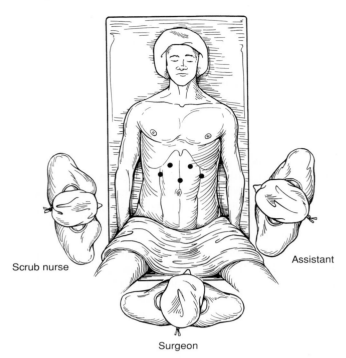

Figure 14-6 Laparoscopic Nissen fundoplication. Three 5mm ports and two 10/12 mm ports are inserted. Notice the 10/12 mm port for the camera is in the midline superior to the umbilicus. The second 10/12 mm port is placed lateral and below the costal arch.

Scrub nurse

Assistant

Surgeon

skill of the surgeon and his assistant, there is no assigned operator of a given cannula, though the assistant is assigned to control the camera.

After placing the cannulas, abdominal exploration is done to see whether the patient is still a candidate for laparoscopic repair. Contraindications include a short esophagus, occult malignancy, stomach adherent to the spleen, and difficulty in identifying the anatomy at the gastroesophageal junction. The table is placed in the reverse Trendelenburg position. Using atraumatic graspers, the stomach is pulled inferiorly and laterally to expose the gastroesophageal junction. The fat pad and peritoneum surrounding the hiatus should be inspected to locate the anterior vagus nerve, which is to be avoided. The vagal branch of the gallbladder and/or an aberrant left hepatic artery must not be divided. This maneuver will expose the right crus of the diaphragm. The proximal stomach is then retracted to the patient's right and dissection is continued to visualize the left crus. When the hiatus is adequately mobilized, inspection of the area behind the esophagus should assure that the posterior vagus nerve has not been separated from the esophagus. At this point, the orogastric tube is removed. The esophagus must not be grasped or traumatized in any way. Manipulation of the esophagus should be done by grasping gastric mucosa. Under direct vision, the esophagus is encircled, passing the instrument from the right to the

left, taking care not to go posterior to the crura, entering the left chest, which will cause a pneumothorax. The "C"-shaped cable retractor is then passed behind the esophagus under direct vision. This retractor has the advantage over a Penrose drain. It is relatively atraumatic and tissue manipulation is more direct. The esophageal window posteriorly is enlarged by gentle blunt dissection to free the areolar tissue and enlarge the space for the wrap. This also will ensure that the posterior vagus nerve is in continuity with the esophagus. The posterior free space should be about 5 cm long. To ensure there is enough redundant stomach for a tension-free wrap, the short gastrics are divided.

The instrumentation for division of the short gastrics is dependent on the surgeon's confidence in achieving hemostasis. Endoscopic suture ligation with the automatic suturing device, "free hand" suturing, endo-clipping, use of an Endoloop or the harmonic scalpel, are methods that work equally well (Figure 14-7A). A combination of modalities can be utilized to ensure hemostasis. I have a bias against using clips on the gastric side of the short gastrics, because they can be dislodged with manipulation of the stomach while creating the wrap. Dual clips should be used on the splenic side. Recently, I have been using the harmonic scalpel in the slow coagulation mode, and have had good hemostasis. It is important that when dividing the short gastric, enough counteraction is utilized to identify the individual vessels, dissect them out and then use whatever modality is decided upon for hemostasis. Ligation of the short gastrics can be started from the proximal stomach, working distally until about 10 cm of greater curve is freed. If the proximal portion is obscured, then an arbitrary opening is made about mid-spleen, and the dissection carried cephalad. The wrap can be fashioned after hemostasis has been checked. If the stomach demonstrates no tension (not retracting) after the grasper is released, then no more dissection of the short gastrics needs to be done. It is better to err on the side of too much stomach being freed. During this traction test, the 60°F dilator has not been placed, so one must take that into account.

Closure of the crura is done to prevent slippage of the repair into the chest, which may cause it to fail. The crura should be closed in patients with large hiatal hernias. The cable retractor lifts the esophagus to the left and anterior, exposing the right and left crura. Simple interrupted sutures, using the automatic endosuturing device or free-hand suturing with 0 or 2-0 nonabsorbable braided suture, is best. Intra- or extracorporeal knots can be fashioned. The crura is closed loosely until a 10-mm blunt dissecting forceps can be passed along the esophagus without a bougie in place. Again, care is necessary to prevent occluding the posterior vagus nerve in the approximation.

The wrap is the most important part of the procedure and must be tension-free. Great care must be taken in the orientation of the wrap so proximal stomach is attached to fundus and not to the body of the stomach. The latter can cause a two-compartment stomach, precipitating dysphagia,

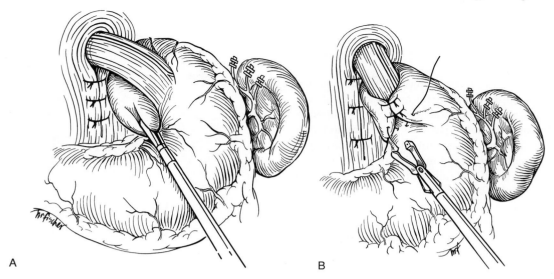

Figure 14-7 Automatic suturing device as used in fundoplication. **A.** A switch of the toggle lever passes the needle smoothly through the tissue for easy, accurate placement. **B.** Jaws return to a closed, neutral position for added safety from inadvertent needle punctures.

bloating, and volvulus. The stomach is passed from the patient's left to the right and proper orientation is noted by identifying the short gastrics. An atraumatic forceps is used to grasp the stomach as it is advanced under direct vision. When enough stomach has been pulled through and the proper orientation confirmed, a 60°F dilator is passed by the anesthesiologist. It is important to watch the dilator exit the hiatus and pass into the stomach. If the stomach is under excess tension it will fall away rapidly when released and more short gastrics need to be taken down.

Once the appropriate orientation is verified, the wrap can be secured, using interrupted mattress or simple 2-0 braided nonabsorbable sutures. The automatic sewing device or free-hand intracorporeal sewing techniques are equally reliable. The first stitch is taken from the stomach through the esophagus, avoiding the anterior vagus nerve, and then through the stomach of the opposite side. It is important to take individual bites for optimal placement of sutures. This process is repeated until a 1.5-2-cm wrap is completed (Figure 14-7B). The wrap is formed around the esophagus and not around the proximal stomach. An additional one or two sutures can be used to anchor the proximal portion of the wrap to the hiatus.

A tension-free fundoplication should be supple when manipulated after the bougie is removed. The hiatus, splenic bed and lesser curve areas are then irrigated with warm saline. All the vascular ligation sites are checked. Local anesthetic is used in the cannula sites to ease postoperative pain.

Comment

In my experience with more than 50 laparoscopic fundoplications, I have had two major complications. During placement of a 60°F dilator, the dilator perforated the distal esophagus when passed. This was repaired primarily and a Nissen fundoplication was placed over the repair to buttress the area further. Postoperatively, the patient did well and did not have a leak. The second complication occurred four days after an uneventful fundoplication. On the patient's second day after discharge, he had a period of violent and repetitive vomiting. He was readmitted and laparotomy showed breakdown of the crura with ischemic perforation of the stomach. The ischemic area was resected and a repeat fundoplication completed. The left chest was drained and the patient made a slow but uneventful recovery.

Other complications include damage to structures at the time of fundoplication; these include injury to the vagus nerve and spleen. Beyond these technical considerations, complications such as the "gas bloat" syndrome occur in about 5% of patients. Esophageal reflux with esophagitis, and the potential for subsequent development of a cancer, is a serious clinical problem. Laparoscopic Nissen fundoplication has made this procedure more acceptable, with excellent and comparable results to open laparotomy repair. As more and more patients are identified with esophageal reflux and mucosal changes, this operation will become more commonplace.

LAPAROSCOPIC INGUINAL HERNIA

Experience with laparoscopic herniorrhaphy has broadened over the past several years, as more surgeons become familiar with the technique. A number of reports, documenting more than 500 repairs, have appeared in the literature. In these reports, a variety of approaches and techniques have been evaluated. Presently, however, two exposures are favored by most surgeons and both use non-absorbable prosthetic material (Polypropylene) and a multiple firing stapling device.

Even as the procedure becomes more standardized, the debate over its place in hernia repair continues. While the rationale for its use lies in the potential for less postoperative pain and shorter disability periods, there remain larger questions about increased cost, unknown long-term outcomes, added complications and mandatory use of general anesthesia. Time is needed before a firm conclusion on its usefulness can be drawn. It has become clear, however, that the surgeon who does the occasional laparoscopic hernia repair is not adept nor can he or she perform this operation as well as someone who is doing the procedure more often.

Technique

There are two generally accepted approaches to laparoscopic hernia repair, with the actual floor repair done the same way in both cases. There is the Transabdominal Preperitoneal Prosthetic Repair, the favored approach because it is technically easier. The pure Intraperitoneal Inlay Prosthesis approach has generally been abandoned, with its only indication for use in small, indirect, hernias.

The patient is placed supine on the operating table, and following induction of general endotracheal anesthesia, the entire abdomen is prepped and draped. The patient is placed in the Trendelenburg position and CO_2 insufflation is carried out at the umbilicus, as previously described. During the Transabdominal Peritoneal Repair a 10/11 cannula is placed at the umbilicus. Two additional 10/11 cannulas are placed for instrument and mesh access. These are in the left and right mid-quadrants at about the same level as the umbilicus cannula (Figure 14-8). After inspection, the pelvic peritoneum is incised above the hernia defect and the area is exposed. An indirect sac can either be inverted and excised with cautery or just incised from the peritoneum and left in place in the inguinal canal.

The preperitoneal fat is then swept away to expose the anatomy in preparation for mesh placement. A large piece (10 × 12 cm) of polypropylene mesh is used and generally is most readily held in position with endostaples. The mesh should extend from the pubic tubercle along the ileopubic tract and Cooper's ligament inferiorly, and beyond the internal ring laterally, with a slit cut in the mesh for the cord structures. Superiorly, the mesh should be attached along the transversus abdominis arch. After fixation of the mesh, the peritoneum should be brought over to cover the repair.

The Preperitoneal Approach is similar in its attachment of the mesh but differs in that the abdominal cavity is not entered. Rather, a preperitoneal space is created with CO_2 insufflation, to perform the repair. This repair is more tedious in the dissection and more time-consuming, because of the smaller working area and the difficulty of remaining outside of the abdominal cavity.

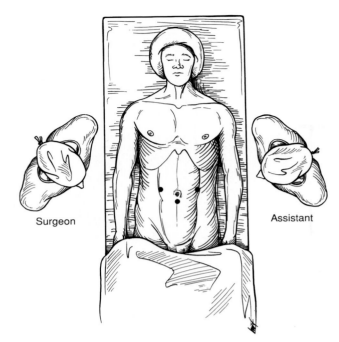

Figure 14-8 Laparoscopic hernia port sites.

Comment

The general use of the laparoscopic hernia repair remains unclear although interest continues in modifying and perfecting it. There seem to be definite indications for the laparoscopic approach in the case of bilateral inguinal hernias. Patients who have had laparoscopic hernia repair seem to recover more rapidly and have a shorter disability period following surgery. When compared to standard open repair, the incidents and types of complications appear to be similar. Early recurrence rates are slightly higher and as yet no long-term recurrence rates are available.

The future use of laparoscopic herniorrhaphy would seem to depend on the factors of cost, long-term recurrence rates, complications, and the need for additional training and expertise over that of standard open repair.

SUGGESTED READINGS

Cholecystectomy

Barton JR, Russell RCG, Hatfield ARW. Management of bile leaks after laparoscopic cholecystectomy. *Br J Surg* 1995;82:980–4.

Deans GT, Wilson MS, Brough WA. The ability of laparoscopic clips to withstand high intraluminal pressure. *Arch Surg* 1995;103:439–41.

Deziel DJ, Millikan KW, Economou SG, et al. Complications of laparoscopic cholecystectomy: a national survey of 4,292 hospitals and an analysis of 77,604 cases. *Am J Surg* 1993;165:9–14.

Duensing TA, Williams RA, Collins JC, Wilson SE. Managing choledocholithiasis in the laparoscopic era. *Am J Surg* 1995;170:619–23.

Liu CL, et al. Combined laparoscopic and endoscopic approach in patients with cholelithiasis and choledocholithiasis. *Surgery* 1996;119:534–7.

McGinn FP, et al. Randomized trial of laparoscopic cholecystectomy and mini-cholecystectomy. *Br J Surg* 1995;82:1374–7.

Miller RE, Kimmelstiel FM, Winkler WP. Management of common bile duct stones in the era of laparoscopic cholecystectomy. *Am J Surg* 1995;169:273–6.

Mouret P. From the first laparoscopic cholecystectomy to the frontiers of laparoscopic surgery: the prospective futures. *Dig Surg* 1991;8:124.

Peters JH, et al. Reasons for conversion from laparoscopic to open cholecystectomy in an urban teaching hospital. *Am J Surg* 1994;168:555–9.

Phillips EH, et al. Bile duct stones in the laparoscopic era: Is preoperative sphincterotomy necessary? *Arch Surg* 1995;130:880–6.

Reddick EJ, Olsen DO. Laparoscopic cholecystectomy: a comparison with mini-lap cholecystectomy. *Surg Endosc* 1989;3:131–3.

Reddick ES, Olsen DO, Daniell JF, et al. Laparoscopic laser cholecystectomy. *Laser Med Surg News* 989;7:38–41.

Reddick EJ, Olsen D, Spawi A, Baird D, et al. Safe performance of difficult laparoscopic cholecystectomies. *Am J Surg* 1991;161:377–81.

Rieger R, et al. Selective use of ERCP in patients undergoing laparoscopic cholecystectomy. *World J Surg* 1994;18:900–5.

Schol FPG, Go PMNYH, Gouma DJ. Outcome of 49 repairs of bile duct injuries after laparoscopic cholecystectomy. *World J Surg* 1995;19:753–7.

Toomasian JM, Glavinovich G, Johnson MN, Gazzaniga AB. Hemodynamic changes following pneumoperitoneum and graded hemorrhage in the dog. *Surg Forum* 1978;29:32–3.

Welch N, et al. Gallstones in the peritoneal cavity: a clinical and experimental study. *Surg Laparosc Endosc* 1991;87–97.

Trauma

Berci G, Sachein SM, Paz-Partlow M. Emergency laparoscopy. *Am J Surg* 1991;161:332–5.

Carey JE, Koo R, Miller R, Stein M. Laparoscopy and thoracoscopy in evaluation of abdominal trauma. *Am Surg* 1995;61:92–5.

Gazzaniga AB, Stanton WW, Bartlett RH. Laparoscopy in the diagnosis of blunt and penetrating injuries to the abdomen. *Am J Surg* 1976;131:315–8.

Pommer S, Lange J. The value of laparoscopy in diagnosis and therapy of the traumatized abdomen. Klinik fur Chirurgie, Katonsspital, St. Gallen, Schweiz. *Wien Kline Wochenschr* 1995;107:49–53.

Poole GV, Thomae KR, Hauser CJ. Laparoscopy in trauma. *Surg Clin N Am* 1996;76:547–56.

Rashiah KK, Crowe PJ. Laparoscopic repair of a traumatic diaphragmatic hernia. *J Laparoendosc Surg* 1995;5:405–7.

Smith RS, Fry WR, Morabito DJ, Koehler RH, Organ CH Jr. Therapeutic laparoscopy in trauma. *Am J Surg* 1995;170:632–9.

Sosa JL, Arrillaga A, Puente I, Sleeman D, Ginzburg E, Martin L. Laparoscopy in 121 consecutive patients with abdominal gunshot wounds. *J Trauma* 1995;39:501–6.

Laparoscopic Colectomy

Abscarin N. Invited editorial *Dis Colon Rectum* 1995;38:685–6.

Ballantyne GH. Laparoscopic assisted colorectal surgery: review of results in 752 patients. *Gastroenterologist* 1995;3:75–89.

Bernstein MA, et al. Is complete laparoscopic colectomy superior to laparoscopic assisted colectomy? *Am Surg* 1996;62:507–11.

Darzi et al. Stapled laparoscopic rectopexy for rectal prolapse. *Surg Endosc* 1995;9:301–3.

Franklin ME, et al. Prospective evaluation of laparoscopic colon resection for adenocarcinoma: a multicenter study. *Surg Endosc* 1995;9:811–6.

Garcia-Ruiz A, et al. Right colonic arterial anatomy: implications for laparoscopic surgery. *Dis Colon Rectum* 1996;62:507–11.

Geers J, et al. Major vascular injury as a complication of laparoscopic surgery: a report of three cases and review of the literature. *Am J Surg* 1996;62:377–9.

Guillou P. Laparoscopic surgery for diseases of the colon and rectum-quo vadis? *Surg Endosc* 1994;8:669–71.

Liberman MA, et al. Laparoscopic colectomy vs. traditional colectomy for diverticulitis. *Surg Endosc* 1996;10:15–8.

Nelson H, et al. Proposed phase III trial comparing laparoscopic assisted colectomy with open colectomy for colon cancer. *Monogr Natl Cancer Inst* 1995;19:51–6.

Ortega A, et al. Laparoscopic bowel surgery registry: preliminary results. *Dis Colon Rectum* 1995;38:681–6.

Senagore AJ, et al. What is the learning curve for laparoscopic colectomy? *Am J Surg* 1995;61:681–5.

Tucker JG, et al. Laparoscopic assisted bowel surgery. *Surg Endosc* 1995;9:297–300.

Vignati P, et al. Endoscopic localization of colon cancers. *Surg Endosc* 1994;8:1085–7.

Wishner JD, et al. Laparoscopic assisted colectomy. *Surg Endosc* 1995;9:1179–83.

Zucker KA, et al. Laparoscopic assisted colon resection. *Surg Endosc* 1994;8:12–8.

Appendectomy

Pier A, Gotz F, Bacher L. Laparoscopic appendectomy in 625 cases: from innovation to routine. *Surg Laparosc Endosc* 1991;1:8–13.

Semen K. Operationshehur fin endoskopiche abdominal chirurgie. *Stuttgart: Schattauer* 1984.

Nissen Fundoplication

Collet D, Cadiere GB, et al. Conversions and complications of laparoscopic treatment of gastroesophageal reflux disease. *Am J Surg* 1995;169:622–6.

DeMeester TR, Johnson LF, Joseph GJ, et al. Patterns of gastroesophageal reflux in health and disease. *Ann Surgery* 1976;184:459–70.

Ellis H. The Nissen fundoplication. *Ann of Thoracic Surg* 1992;54:1231–5.

Garcelon JC, O'Leary JP. Vignettes in medical history: Dr. Rudolph Nissen—The man and his other contributions. *Am Surgeon* 1995;61:468–9.

Hinder RA, Filipi CJ, Wetscher G, et al. Laparoscopic Nissen Fundoplication is an effective treatment for gastroesophageal reflux disease. *Ann Surg* 1994;22:472–83.

Hunter JG, Soper NJ. New approaches to the management of gastroesophageal reflux. *Problems in General Surgery* 1996;13:1–114.

Jamieson GG, Watson DI, Britten-Jones R, et al. Laparoscopic Nissen fundoplication. *Ann Surg* 1994;220:137–45.

Kahrilas PJ. Gastroesophageal reflux disease: review. *JAMA* 1996;276:983–8.

Pope CE. Acid reflux disorders. *New Engl J Med* 1995;335:656–60.

Raiser F, Hinder RA, Kraus MA, et al. Pitfalls in the surgical management of gastroesophageal reflux disease. *Contemporary Surg* 1996;49:189–94.

Inguinal Hernia

Nyhus L, Condon R. *Hernia.* 4th Edition. Philadelphia: JB Lippincott, 1995;253–61.

Ramshaw Bruce, et al. Technical considerations of the different approaches to laparoscopic herniorrhaphy: an analysis of 500 cases. *Am Surg* 1996;61:69–75.

Vogt D, et al. The past, present and future of laparoscopic hernia repair. *Int Surg* 1994;79:280–5.

Operative Laparoscopy, Second Edition
The Masters' Techniques in Gynecologic Surgery
Lippincott–Raven Publishers, Philadelphia © 1998.

15

Laparoscopic Repair of Hiatal Hernia and Gastroesophageal Reflux

Ralph W. Aye, Daniel R. Marcus, and Lucius D. Hill

Gastroesophageal reflux is the most common disorder of the upper gastrointestinal tract, affecting at least one-third of Americans on a regular basis and accounting for a significant portion of health care costs. Nevertheless, prior to the advent of the laparoscopic approach, surgical correction of reflux was often considered a last resort, with only 3000 antireflux procedures performed in the United States in 1990. The adaptation of minimally invasive surgical techniques to antireflux surgery has ushered in a new era in management, with much greater acceptance of surgical repair by patients and referring physicians. In 1995, approximately 30,000 antireflux procedures were done nationally, the majority being performed laparoscopically. This increased demand, driven partly by the lay public, places increased responsibility on the surgeon to screen and select surgical candidates carefully, and to pay the utmost attention to surgical technique in a field which has often been fraught with suboptimal results.

Minimal preoperative workup includes a careful history and physical, with special attention to differential etiologies such as coronary disease, esophageal spasm or other motility disorders, cholelithiasis, peptic ulcer, or functional bowel disorders; flexible upper endoscopy; and esophageal motility studies in a competent lab. A 24-hour pH study is highly recommended, especially if there is any question about the diagnosis or the source of symptomatology, because correction of reflux in a patient whose symptoms are from another source will result in misery for both patient and physician.

Contraindications to the laparoscopic approach include the surgeon's lack of qualifications to perform, or the patient's inability to tolerate, an open repair, and inadequate planning, equipment, or proctoring. These procedures can be quite demanding of judgment and technical expertise; active proctoring for at least the first 10 cases is recommended. Relative contraindications include massive obesity, previous upper abdominal surgery, or giant hiatal hernia, until the surgeon has gained enough expertise with straightforward cases. Reoperative GE junction surgery can be extraordinarily difficult, and should only be attempted laparoscopically after strong consideration.

The three most commonly performed laparoscopic antireflux procedures are the Hill, Nissen, and Toupet repairs. Repair of the often-associated hiatal hernia is one component of the procedure, aside from the very rare true paraesophageal hernia without associated reflux; even in these cases, an antireflux procedure should perhaps be added.

GENERAL CONSIDERATIONS

No special preoperative preparation is required, aside from thorough discussion with the patient about indications, alternatives, and expected postoperative course. A low dorsal lithotomy position is used, taking care to protect the lower legs and utilizing a sequential compression device to prevent venous stasis. As a dilator is generally used to calibrate the repair, we prefer to endoscope the patient prior to prepping and draping, to rule out any previously unrecognized pathology and to pass a guide-wire over which a hollow-core dilator can be safely passed later, when needed. For the Hill repair, a specially modified nasogastric tube with a manometric side port 12 cm from the tip (Island Scientific, Bainbridge Island, WA), is passed at this time as well, and hooked to the manometric machine or to the anesthesiologist's CVP monitor. Several position combinations for surgeon, assistant, and camera operator are possible, but we prefer either having the surgeon between the patient's legs, with assistant on the patient's left and camera operator on the right, or having the surgeon on the patient's left, with the assistant on the right and camera operator between the legs. The scrub nurse is on the patient's left with a Mayo stand near the patient's left knee.

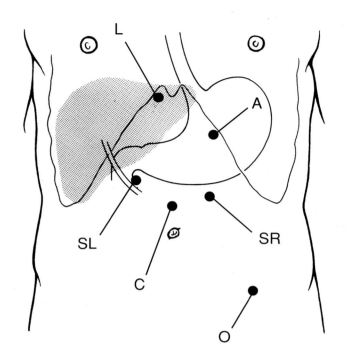

Figure 15-1 One common trocar placement scheme. Sr = surgeon's right-hand work port; sl = surgeon's left-hand work port; c = camera port; a = assistant port; l = port for liver retractor; o = optional port for babcock retractor.

Five ports are used. In the past, all ports were 10 mm, but with improvements in 5 mm liver retractors, Babcock clamps, and angled telescopes, it has been possible to substitute 5 mm ports at most locations. One common port location is illustrated (Figure 15-1). It is important that the reducer system used for the surgeon's right hand and the assistant port be of good quality to prevent excess loss of pneumoperitoneum during extracorporeal tying, and the only three brands we have found acceptable to date are Applied Medical, Ethicon, and U.S. Surgical. Sutures used for repair are of 0-Ethibond. We use a multipack with two different colors to help avoid crossing or confusing sutures.

Initial Dissection

With trocars in place and the left lobe of the liver lifted with a fan retractor secured with a self-retaining system to prevent motion and the potential for liver laceration, dissection begins over the caudate lobe, dividing the "clear zone" of the gastrohepatic ligament, clipping or cauterizing the artery accompanying the hepatic branch of the vagus nerve. Alternatively, the harmonic scalpel has been found to be a very helpful instrument in the laparoscopic dissection of the GE junction. Dividing the gastrohepatic ligament

consistently leads the surgeon to the right crus, which is just posterior to the upper limit of the gastrohepatic ligament. Care must be taken to avoid the inferior vena cava, which has been mistaken for the right crus by some, with predictably disastrous results. The anterior aspect of the gastroesophageal junction is dissected out from patient's right to left, coming down onto the anterior aspect of the left crus, and taking care not to injure the anterior vagus nerve or to disrupt the fibroareolar tissue overlying the anterior aspect of the GE junction, referred to as the *anterior phrenoesophageal bundle* (Figure 15-2). Next, attention returns to the right crus, with dissection continuing inferiorly along its border, down to, but not into, the region of the celiac axis. Entry into this relatively avascular space behind the esophagus, with blunt dissection posterior to the esophagus, permits exposure of the left crus and its confluence with the right, the confluence representing the most superior and visible aspect of the *preaortic fascia*.

Laparoscopic Hill Repair

The Hill repair is considered by some to be more difficult to learn to do correctly, but once accomplished, surgeon and patient are rewarded with a repair that has been extensively tested over time, is more anatomically true to normal, less prone to slippage and other undesirable complications, and easily modified to accommodate motility disorders. Intraoperative manometry is an important part of the procedure, a fact which causes many to throw up their hands in discouragement, but this is easily performed using a readily available and inexpensive modified nasogastric tube hooked to the CVP monitor available in almost any operating room.

Once the retro-esophageal space has been opened with blunt dissection, the left crus is followed superiorly and the window behind the esophagus is completed, exposing the

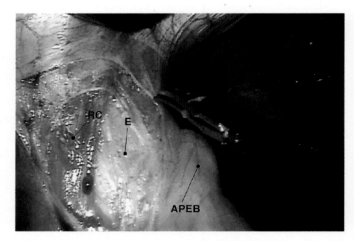

Figure 15-2 Anterior dissection of the GE junction. Rc = right crus; e = esophagus; apeb = anterior phrenoesophageal bundle.

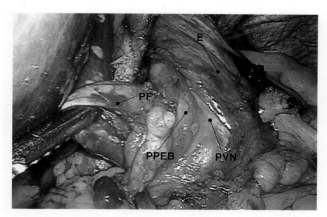

Figure 15-3 Exposure of the posterior phrenoesophageal bundle. Pf = posterior fundus; ppeb = posterior phrenoesophageal bundle; pvn = posterior vagus nerve; e = esophagus.

posterior aspect of the fundus. This is most easily accomplished by working high on the left crus, between it and the esophagus. This window is enlarged inferiorly, by dividing the posterior gastric arterial branch arising from the left crus, and by separating the fibroareolar tissue which overlies the posterior fundus. The left gastric artery lies at the lowermost extent of this dissection, and must be kept in mind. It is important to free the posterior fundus sufficiently to allow it to be easily brought midline to the preaortic fascia, without tension. In the course of dissecting inferiorly, the inferior-most aspect of the preaortic fascia is also defined, marked at the lowermost end by the celiac axis, which is avoided. We do not dissect out the median arcuate ligament for the laparoscopic Hill repair, using instead the inferior aspect of the preaortic fascia for the repair stitches. Identification of the anterior vagus nerve by downward traction on the anterior phrenoesophageal bundle, and the posterior vagus nerve by retracting the anterior phrenoesophageal bundle to the patient's left, complete the dissection. Identification of the posterior vagus nerve is a critical step in locating the posterior phrenoesophageal bundle, which lies immediately posterior and to the right of the posterior vagus nerve, and is an important component of the Hill repair (Figure 15-3).

Following dissection, the hiatus is closed posteriorly using interrupted suture, tied extracorporeally. The same suture is used throughout, a heavy gauge nonabsorbable (0-Ethibond). Usually two sutures are enough for closure, but more may be needed if the hiatus is large. It is important to close the hiatus securely, but not too tightly, thus avoiding a difficult-to-manage source of dysphagia. If further sutures would create an unacceptable posterior ridge effect over which the esophagus must stretch, it may be necessary to complete closure of a large hiatus anteriorly after the rest of the repair has been completed.

Next the posterior aspect of the fundus is anchored to the left aspect of the preaortic fascia. This is not an essential feature of the basic Hill repair, and is best omitted during the early learning curve, but adds further reinforcement to the repair, taking stress off the repair sutures in the event of trauma. It also elevates the posterior bundle, making subsequent repair sutures easier to place. Two or three sutures are placed in the posterior fundus several cm posterior to the posterior phrenoesophageal bundle, and then through the left aspect of the preaortic fascia and left crus. Great care must be taken not to penetrate too deeply, as the aorta lies immediately beneath.

At this point, the repair sutures for the Hill repair are placed, but not tied, allowing for adjustment of tension following initial manometric pull-through. The first and second sutures are placed through the surgeon's right work port, the third and fourth through the assistant port. With some attention to angle of entry, crossing of these sutures is rare. We alternate the color of the sutures to help keep them separate. Exact location of placement is important, and has often been illustrated or described incorrectly. The first suture, working from lowermost to uppermost (in contrast to the order for open repair), is passed through the anterior bundle immediately to the patient's left of the anterior vagus nerve, and almost parallel to the nerve, in an inferior to superior direction, taking care to place the suture sufficiently inferior and deep to penetrate the seromuscular layer of the stomach (Figure 15-4). The same suture is then passed through the posterior bundle, as inferior as possible without risking injury to the left gastric artery, with point of entry being just posterior to the posterior vagus nerve, and again being sure to take part of the seromuscular layer of the stomach. This suturing is oriented in an anterior to posterior direction, and is facilitated by cocking the needle backward to get deep penetration, and by having the assistant grasp and pull the tissue between the two bundles anteriorly and to the left for better exposure (Figure 15-5). This same suture is then passed through the preaortic fascia

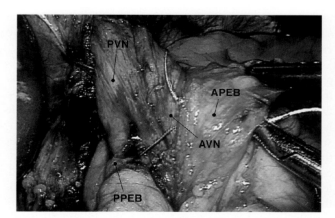

Figure 15-4 Placement of second repair suture through anterior phrenoesophageal bundle. Ppeb = posterior phrenoesophageal bundle; pvn = posterior vagus nerve; avn = anterior vagus nerve; apeb = anterior phrenoesophageal bundle.

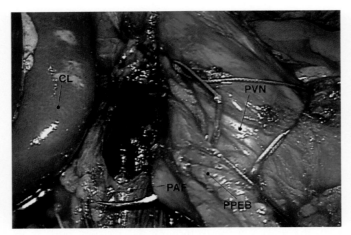

Figure 15-5 Placement of third repair suture through posterior phrenoesophageal bundle. Cl = caudate lobe; paf = preaortic fascia; ppeb = posterior phrenoesophageal bundle; pvn = posterior vagus nerve.

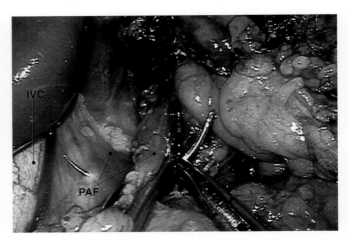

Figure 15-6 Placement of first repair suture through the preaortic fascia. Note that the preaortic fascia is being lifted up away from the aorta as suture is placed; note also the location of the vena cava. Ivc = inferior vena cava; paf = preaortic fascia.

from patient's left to right, as inferior as possible while avoiding the celiac artery, and elevating the fascia off the aorta with a Babcock clamp so that a secure suture can be placed (Figure 15-6). As the needle is pulled back out of the trocar, it should be obvious that care must be taken to avoid sawing through tissue by pulling through in increments or placing an instrument against the suture to deflect stress from the tissue. After the suture is placed, the ends are clamped together externally with a hemostat.

The second, third, and fourth repair sutures are placed in a similar fashion, advancing laterally up the anterior bundle and superiorly up the posterior bundle, 2 to 3 mm each time. Final LESP is determined partly by how tightly the sutures are tied, and partly by how far up and lateral on the bundles the third and fourth sutures are placed. Thus, if the distance between sutures is too great, the repair will be too tight, even with the sutures tied loosely. Conversely, inadequate distance between sutures as they pass through the bundles will result in a repair that is too loose, despite tying the sutures securely. Judgment of placement comes with experience.

After all sutures have been placed, a 36 French dilator is passed over the guidewire alongside the modified nasogastric tube and positioned across the GE junction. The top two (third and fourth) sutures are now tied with a single half-hitch and clamped, the top being clamped by an instrument through the surgeon's left-hand port, and the other through the right-hand port. These two sutures are the greatest determinants of final LESP. The dilator is removed, leaving the guidewire in place, and a manometric pull-through is taken (Figure 15-7). The high-pressure zone is usually located somewhere between the 45 and 50 marks on the manometric tube. A first pull-through helps locate the high-pressure zone, and a second is then done more slowly for greater accuracy. Using the anesthesiologist's

CVP monitor, there can be some delay in pressure rise, and pulling through too rapidly will miss the peak pressure. Ideal pressure is 35 mmHg, ±5, using this particular system, which reads a bit lower than standard manometry lab equipment. Based on the reading obtained, the sutures can be tightened or loosened and another pull-through taken before tying sutures permanently, or the dilator can be passed again and all sutures tied completely (Figure 15-8). A final pull-through is taken. At this point, if the repair appears too tight, it can still be loosened somewhat by pulling laterally on the anterior bundle with a Babcock clamp, and sometimes by dividing thin bands of tissue, which cross the GE junction just above the anterior bundle. If the repair

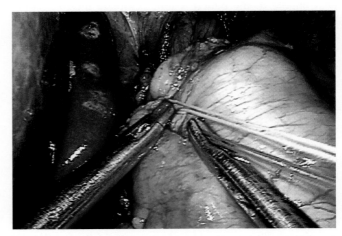

Figure 15-7 Clamping of top two repair sutures during initial manometric reading. A single half-hitch has been tied in each suture prior to clamping and can be easily readjusted if necessary.

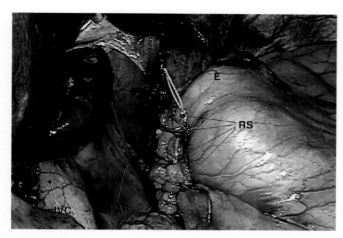

Figure 15-8 Final configuration of the completed Hill repair. Note the firm anchoring of the repair to the preaortic fascia, and the reestablishment of the angle of His and intraabdominal esophagus. lvc = inferior vena cava; paf = preaortic fascia; e = esophagus; rs = repair sutures.

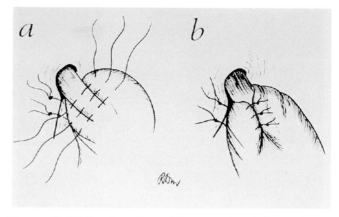

Figure 15-10 Configuration of the completed Nissen fundoplication. Not shown is posterior fixation of fundus to crura and preaortic fascia.

still seems too loose, the anterior bundle can be pulled down further to the preaortic fascia, using additional interrupted sutures.

Finally, as additional reinforcement of the repair, and to accentuate the newly recreated valve and to prevent paraesophageal hernia, a series of 3 or 4 sutures are placed between the fundus and the rim of the hiatus. The most important of these, from the standpoint of accentuating the configuration of the valve, is the suture placed between fundus and the right aspect of the hiatus.

Nissen Repair

The Nissen repair is the most commonly performed and probably the most easily learned antireflux operation world-wide. When performed correctly, it is highly competent, but as such it carries some risk of dysphagia and gas-bloat syndrome, and is not appropriate for patients with significant motility aberrations in the body of the esophagus. For both the Nissen and Toupet repairs, the short gastric vessels are divided prior to developing the retroesophageal space. This is important to ease tension on the fundoplication, and has been shown to result in a lower incidence of dysphagia postoperatively. The linear coagulation shear/harmonic scalpel is a useful instrument for this step, but surgical clips can also be used. Division begins with the short gastric vessel at the midportion of the greater curve, proceeding cephalad from there until the fundus is free (Figure 15-9). Following this, the retroesophageal space can be developed as described above to allow the fundus to be brought around the back of the esophagus. Dissection is not as inferior for the Nissen and Toupet repairs as it is for the Hill, focusing more on freeing the fundus for fundoplication. At its completion, it should be possible to bring the fundus behind the

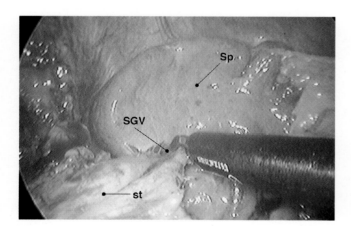

Figure 15-9 Division of short gastric vessels. Sp = spleen; st = stomach; SGV = short gastric vein.

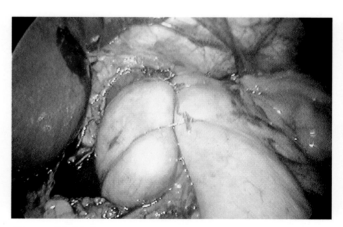

Figure 15-11 Laparoscopic view of the completed Nissen.

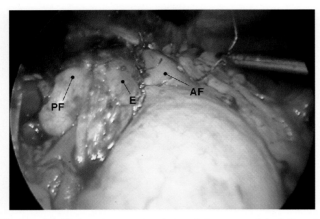

Figure 15-12 Laparoscopic view of the completed Toupet procedure. Af = anterior fundus; e = esophagus; pf = posterior fundus.

esophagus with a Babcock clamp, at the level of the GE junction, without tension.

The repair is performed by first closing the hiatus posterior to the esophagus, generally using two sutures and tying extracorporeally. With the fundus pulled around behind the esophagus, the posterior aspect of the fundus overlying the crural repair is then sutured, with interrupted suture, to the crura with 2 to 3 sutures, to create a posterior fixation. Next a fundocrural stitch is placed from the apex of the left wrap to the left crural apex on the left side of the esophagus. With a 56 French dilator in place, (46 to 48 French if passed alongside the modified nasogastric tube), the wrap is then completed by placing 2 to 3 sutures from the left wrap into the anterior wall of the esophagus, taking care to avoid the anterior vagus nerve, and then into the right wrap, bringing the two edges of the wrap together and tying intracorporeally, thus completing the 360° wrap (Figures 15-10 and 15-11).

Toupet Repair

The Toupet repair has gained more popularity as a result of recent studies favorably comparing it with the Nissen, and with the advent of laparoscopic repair as an alternative to the Nissen in patients with abnormal motility in the esophageal body, because it is only a partial fundoplication and hence potentially less obstructing. The repair is similar to a Nissen, except that following the posterior fixation stitches a 270° wrap is created by suturing the left and right wraps to either side of the esophagus along either side of the anterior vagus nerve, taking care to avoid and protect the nerve. Three sutures on each side are utilized, tying intracorporeally to minimize trauma to the esophagus (Figure 15-12).

FINAL CONSIDERATIONS

At the end of the procedure, the completed repair is viewed endoscopically, both antegrade and retroflexed. While this is not an absolutely necessary part of the procedure, we have found it to be enormously helpful as a teaching tool, to assess the configuration of the newly recreated gastroesophageal valve and to seek refinements in suture placement. It is also useful to assess evidence of obstruction caused by an overly tight repair. It is hard to stress sufficiently how we feel the quality of our performance of the repair has been improved by the timely feedback this simple inspection provides.

The nasogastric tube can be removed at the completion of the procedure. The patient is encouraged to begin clear liquids without ice or carbonation and to progress to full liquids or pureed foods, generally being discharged the day following surgery. The patient is cautioned that some dysphagia for solids is not uncommon during the first few weeks following surgery and that the condition will improve with time. Normal activity usually resumes within 7 to 14 days postop. Follow-up esophageal manometry and 24-hour pH studies at 6 months are encouraged, both as a baseline data point for the patient and to provide feedback to the surgeon for adjustments in technique.

SUGGESTED READING

Hill LD, Aye RW, Ramel S. Antireflux surgery: a surgeon's look. In: McCallum RW, Mittal RK, guest eds. *Gastroenterology Clinics of North America* Vol 19, 3 Philadelphia: W. B. Saunders, 1990;745–75.

Hill LD, Snopkowski P. The Hill repair. In: Sabiston DC, Spencer FC (eds.). *Surgery of the Chest, Sixth Edition*. Philadelphia: W. B. Saunders, 1995;1039–52.

Low DE, Anderson PP, Ilves R. Fifteen-to-twenty year results after the Hill antireflux operation. *J Thor CV Surg* 1989;98:444–50.

Rossetti ME, Liebermann-Meffert D. Nissen antireflux operation. In: Nyhus LM, Baker RJ, eds. *Mastery of Surgery*. Boston: Little, Brown, 1992:504–16.

Operative Laparoscopy, Second Edition
The Masters' Techniques in Gynecologic Surgery
Lippincott–Raven Publishers, Philadelphia © 1998.

16

Laparoscopically Assisted Vaginal Hysterectomy

16-1   Laparoscopically Assisted Vaginal Hysterectomy

Marshall L. Smith, Jr.

Traditionally when the decision is made between the patient and her gynecological surgeon to proceed to hysterectomy, one of the next decisions is whether to approach the removal of the uterus abdominally or vaginally. Some of the factors that influence this decision are the patient's pelvic and vaginal anatomy, as well as any specific pelvic pathology. Because of the reduced morbidity and patient's recovery time from the vaginal approach, it is usually recommended by most gynecologists as the preferred access. Over the last several years, techniques have been developed to allow the gynecological surgeon the ability to convert to the vaginal approach the cases that usually would have required an abdominal one. Thus is the goal of the laparoscopically assisted vaginal hysterectomy, simply converting the abdominal to the vaginal approach. This conversion then allows the patient the reduced morbidity and recovery time of the vaginal hysterectomy.

When my patient and I have decided that a hysterectomy is the indicated procedure, my first choice is always to perform it vaginally, if possible. If I believe I can perform the hysterectomy vaginally then no discussion of laparoscopy need be initiated. If I do not believe I can easily remove the uterus vaginally, my next decision concerns whether I can perform enough dissection laparoscopically to remove the uterus vaginally. In the first several years of performing these procedures there were very few conditions under which I would not attempt an LAVH. However, at this point, I find myself becoming more conservative (or perhaps only wiser). One thought process I always complete involves trying to estimate how long it will take me to perform the procedure laparoscopically. We have all heard about the gynecologist performing a prolonged LAVH, requiring hours and hours to complete the procedure (foreveroscopy). Certainly the patient does not benefit from a prolonged operative time and anesthesia, not to mention the increased operating room costs. My rule of thumb is that I will proceed if I think I will only increase the length of the procedure by 50% or less, by performing an LAVH. I feel any laparoscopic procedure which more than doubles the time of the abdominal approach should probably be reconsidered.

There are also other contraindications to my initiating a hysterectomy laparoscopically. The first is certainly any condition in which laparoscopy itself is contraindicated. I have had several cases in which previous operative reports have indicated there is essentially no free space in the abdominal cavity; that is, the bowel is completely encased in adhesions, resulting essentially in an obliteration of the peritoneal cavity. Certainly this case would lend itself much better to an exploratory laparotomy and an abdominal hysterectomy. Another situation in which I proceed cautiously in regard to an LAVH is when there is a very large uterus that extends laterally. This is often seen with fibroids, and if the fibroids extend well laterally to the pelvic walls, I become very cautious. I have found that it is very difficult to dissect around the fibroids laterally and yet be able to gain access to the uterine vessels laparoscopically in these patients. Certainly uterine size or fibroids are not a contraindication either to the vaginal or the laparoscopic approach, but care should be taken when there is significant lateral extension. Thus, the ideal candidate for me to consider for an LAVH procedure is a patient with minimal uterine descent or vaginal access and perhaps with the presence of bowel or adnexal adhesions and/or endometriosis.

In the preoperative discussion with the patient I tell her that there is always the possibility that the procedure cannot be completed vaginally. In addition I tell her that if any type of emergency arises, there is the possibility that it might need to be addressed through an open incision. The patient is always aware that she may awaken from anesthesia with an abdominal incision. However, as this would be the situation if we did not attempt a laparoscopic approach initially, most patients readily accept this contingency.

INITIAL INTRAOPERATIVE STEPS

After the patient is placed under general anesthesia (I do not use regional anesthesia for extensive laparoscopic

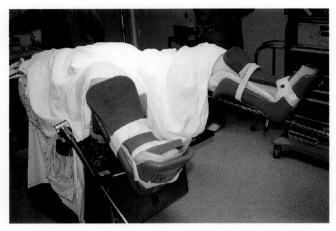

Figure 16-1.1 Patient's legs in Allen stirrups for LAVH. Note the padding, the support for the foot and lower leg, and the ability to elevate or lower the stirrups, under sterile drapes, for either the laparoscopic or vaginal portion.

work), I position the patient's legs myself, using the adjustable Allen type stirrups (Figure 16-1.1). These have the advantage of cushioning and supporting the patient's feet and lower legs and can easily be converted from the abdominal to the vaginal approach intraoperatively, even while the patient is draped. I carefully place the legs in the stirrups and pad them well with some type of foam rubber padding. I then elevate and lower the legs into both the abdominal and vaginal positions before the patient is prepped. In this way, I can observe the legs in each position to ensure there are no undue stretching or positional problems. If the patient has given me any history of back pain or nerve problems of the lower extremities, I will position the legs in both positions prior to initiation of anesthesia. This way the patient can assure me while she is awake that there is no undue stress or discomfort in either position. The last thing I do is to assist in tucking the patient's arms at her sides. With the deep Trendelenburg position that is often required, having the patient's arms extended on arm boards will prevent the surgeon from standing comfortably at the patient's side. There have been many brachial plexus injuries reported from hyperextension of the upper extremity, and this usually occurs when the arm board is raised above 90° from the body under the drape as the surgeon is trying to obtain more room or become more comfortable.

After the abdominal and vaginal prep are performed, a Foley catheter is placed. Next a weighted speculum is placed and traction is placed on the cervix with a single-toothed tenaculum. At this point I stop and make a very important assessment of the uterus. I decide how much of the dissection is going to be performed laparoscopically and how much can be performed easily vaginally. This decision is made by judging the size of the uterus, descent of the uterus, the vaginal access, and the pathology of that particular patient. I strongly believe every good gynecological

surgeon is much more time-efficient in securing pedicles with a vaginal clamp than they are securing them laparoscopically. Thus, my goal is to do the minimal amount laparoscopically to ensure that this becomes an easy vaginal hysterectomy. For instance, if I am having trouble even visualizing the uterosacral ligaments and the uterus is still very high, I make the decision to take the uterine vessels laparoscopically and essentially to carry the dissection down to the uterosacral ligaments. If, on the other hand, I do have some vaginal access, I may remove the adhesions and endometriosis and take only the ovarian pedicles laparoscopically. Once this decision is made, I place a uterine manipulator (e.g., Valtchev Uterine Mobilizer) for movement of the uterus during the procedure, as I have found that it is much more helpful than a simple tenaculum. I no longer place a sponge under the anterior vaginal mucosa, as I have found the technique described below to be more time-efficient and hemostatic. After insertion of the uterine manipulator, the legs are lowered and the laparoscopic portion begins.

LAPAROSCOPIC DISSECTION OF THE UTERUS

I use three trocar insertions for the laparoscopic part of the procedure. I place a 10-mm trocar through the umbilicus for the laparoscope and two lateral 5-mm trocars for the instrumentation (Figure 16-1.2). I utilize the short 5-mm trocars with some type of spiral grooves to keep them in place, and these are placed lateral to the inferior epigastric vessels. Obviously, care has to be taken with the insertion of the lateral trocars, as the large iliac vessels lie under their insertion site, and the bowel is usually closer to the abdominal wall than with a midline insertion.

All bowel adhesions are removed as necessary. Both ovaries are mobilized in the event they are adherent to the lateral pelvic wall, and any endometriosis or endometrial im-

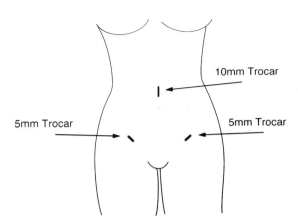

Figure 16-1.2 Trocar placement for LAVH. The 5-mm trocars are placed laterally to the inferior epigastric vessels, but great care should be exercised when inserting them.

plants that will not be removed with the specimen are excised. Often a small portion of the peritoneal reflection of the sigmoid at the pelvic brim has to be incised and the sigmoid mobilized in order to access the left infundibulo-pelvic (IP) ligament. If the ovaries are to be removed, I take each IP ligament, using a bipolar coagulation device. I no longer use staplers for the pedicles, due to the cost factor and to the need for larger trocars for insertion. I do occasionally use sutures or free ties on the pedicles if I am worried about the proximity of the ureter or other heat-sensitive structures (e.g., bowel), but my preference is bipolar desiccation of the vessels.

I always insist that the bipolar unit be tested prior to initiation of the procedure. We have all been in situations where bleeding is encountered, the bipolar coagulation instrument is requested, and it does not work for any of a myriad of reasons. A small sponge soaked with saline and placed between the blades will result in a hissing sound when the unit is activated, and I insist that this be done prior to beginning any procedure. If there is a defect in the unit (which at least in my hospital is not uncommon) then it can be corrected before the procedure has begun, not later, with everyone frantically running around, while watching the patient bleed on the monitor screen.

Approximately two centimeters of each IP pedicle is desiccated and the vessels transected. The round ligament is also coagulated with the bipolar current and transected. Usually the step which is the most time-consuming at this point is that of switching instruments back and forth through the trocar ports. Thus, I coagulate all structures that I can before removing the bipolar unit. For instance, I coagulate both the round ligament and the IP ligament before I remove the bipolar unit and insert the scissors. If the ovaries are being left in situ, then the coagulation and transection are taken down the utero-ovarian ligaments. This is actually the more time-consuming step (compared to the removal of the adnexa) as there is much more vasculature in this region. An error I try to avoid is coagulating and cutting too close to the uterus. If the transections of the utero-ovarian ligament are made too proximal to the uterus it usually results in bleeding that becomes cumbersome to control. Once I have transected the ligaments and entered the broad ligament, I usually skeletonize the peritoneum. The posterior peritoneum can usually be taken down to the uterosacral ligaments, and the anterior peritoneum taken over to include the bladder dissection.

The peritoneum over the anterior lower uterine segment (bladder flap) is one of the few areas in an LAVH where I use unipolar current. There are often small vessels in the bladder flap, and underlying tissue, which can be easily controlled with the unipolar current on the scissors, as the cut is made across the anterior peritoneum above the lower anterior uterine surface. Usually this area is well away from any bowel and the unipolar current can be utilized more safely. Once the bladder is mobilized and taken down, the underlying tissue over the lower uterus and cervix is in-

cised, again using unipolar current. In this way, the bladder is reflected down until the endopelvic fascia overlying the lower uterine segment and cervix is visualized. Once this is done, the uterine vessels are addressed.

The uterine vessels are skeletonized until they can be visualized and are then desiccated, utilizing bipolar current. In doing this, care is taken to stay high up on the uterus, exactly as one would do when placing uterine clamps, providing a safety margin for avoiding the ureter. My approach is to desiccate the vessels on one side and then move to the other side to desiccate the contralateral vessels, prior to transecting either side. It is often difficult to completely desiccate all the vasculature of the ascending uterine plexus, and can require several steps to complete this part of the procedure. Skeletonization of these vessels removes the peritoneum and prevents it from acting as a heat sink, when I am trying to desiccate these vessels. In addition, even after the uterine vessels have been totally transected and released laterally, there can still be several areas of bleeding encountered, as further dissection is carried down the lateral uterine segment to the uterosacral ligaments. Usually, the ascending uterine artery branches several times in this location and there is often a plexus of vessels on the lateral aspect of the uterus. There are branches of the ascending vaginal arcade here, and you must be aware of them, as they can bleed quite profusely. Once the dissection is carried down to a region just above the uterosacral ligaments, I make my final laparoscopic maneuver. I will take the unipolar cautery and cut transversely low across the anterior cervix (Figure 16-1.3). This dissection is carried down through all of the endopelvic fascia into the cervix itself. This eliminates any difficulty in ''getting in'' anteriorly on the vaginal dissection. When the anterior bladder peritoneum has been incised and the endopelvic fascia over the anterior cervix here has been completely transected, enter-

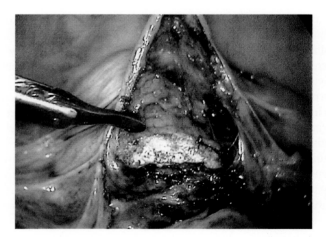

Figure 16-1.3 Transverse incision in the endopelvic fascia overlying the anterior lower uterine segment. When this incision is made deeply with the unipolar current, then the anterior colpotomy is greatly facilitated when dissecting vaginally.

ing the anterior cul-de-sac from below becomes very simple. You cannot miss this opening as you dissect up from the vagina.

At this point, the procedure is converted to the vaginal approach. In the past I would have performed the posterior colpotomy laparoscopically, but I have come to feel it is much more time-efficient to perform it vaginally. In addition, when the posterior colpotomy incision is made laparoscopically, the angle of dissection is such that inevitably a centimeter or two of vagina is taken with the uterus. By performing the colpotomy vaginally, one can ensure that the maximum vaginal length is maintained. However, it is always prudent to make a quick inspection of the posterior cul-de-sac laparoscopically to ensure it is clear before going on to the vaginal portion of the procedure.

VAGINAL APPROACH

At this point, a traditional vaginal hysterectomy is performed. As mentioned above, the anterior cul-de-sac is usually much easier to enter because of the laparoscopic dissection over the cervix, and the posterior cul-de-sac has already been inspected to be sure it is clear. And when dissecting from below up the lateral aspects of the uterus, remember the laparoscopic incisions above lie laterally in the broad ligament, away from the uterine vasculature. When operating laparoscopically, we tend to make these incisions more lateral so as to avoid the ascending branch of the uterine artery. Conversely, we all keep the vaginal dissection very close to the uterus, or medially, so as to avoid the ureter. Thus, two parallel incisions are often made in the broad ligament, and it is not uncommon when dissecting from below to have difficulty finding the upper incision. Be certain to look for it more laterally.

Once the uterus is removed I place my angle sutures for support and close the vagina with interrupted figure-of-eight sutures. I do not close the peritoneum separately, but I often include the peritoneum with the figure-of-eight sutures, especially along the posterior cuff. Then attention is directed again laparoscopically. The patient's legs are lowered again and my assistant and I change gloves. The patient is again placed in Trendelenburg position and the pelvis is irrigated. I am often amazed at how much debris and blood clots remain in the pelvis, even when the vaginal hysterectomy has seemed to be dry and hemostatic. After the pelvis is irrigated thoroughly, all pedicles and vessels are carefully inspected for hemostasis. If any bleeders are encountered, I usually utilize bipolar current to control them. If a pedicle or vessel is oozing and I am uncomfortable with the proximity of the ureter or other structures,

than a simple Endoloop can be placed. However, most of the time the pelvis is dry and only an occasional bleeder along the cuff or posterior bladder wall is seen; this can be easily controlled with the bipolar current used very superficially. Once the pelvis has been irrigated well, I leave a small amount of irrigation in the pelvis. This is to reduce the amount of residual pneumoperitoneum so as to prevent shoulder discomfort. A single suture is placed in the fascia of the umbilicus and the skin of the trocar incisions is closed with a subcuticular stitch.

POSTOPERATIVE CARE

I usually admit the patient for a 24-hour observation stay and discharge her early the next morning. Occasionally, she may go home the same afternoon, but most choose to stay the full 24 hours. I limit her activity for approximately one week and then have her return to full activity at her own rate, but I do recommend pelvic rest for six weeks so as to allow healing of the vaginal cuff. Usually she is feeling well within only a few days, and afterward the most common complaint is that of a lack of energy and stamina. In fact, the problem I have had more often is patients not realizing they have had major surgery inside their abdomens because of the small incisions outside; hence, they will often try to do too much too soon. However, seeing a patient originally destined for an abdominal incision be discharged within 24 hours and be able to return to work within a couple of weeks certainly should inspire the gynecologist to devote the additional amount of time required to learn and perform this procedure.

All the surgical modalities are modifying their procedures towards the minimally invasive approach, and the overall direction of medicine certainly seems to be toward outpatient procedures. The laparoscopically assisted vaginal hysterectomy provides the gynecologist with the armamentarium to allow patients improved morbidity and recovery time, as well as to stay competitive in the transition toward treatment in the outpatient setting as we move into the years of change ahead for medicine and surgery.

SUGGESTED READING

Garry R. Various approaches to laparoscopic hysterectomy. *Curr Opin in Obstet Gynecol* 1994;6:215–22.

Liu CY. Laparoscopic hysterectomy: a review of 72 cases. *J Reprod Med* 1992;37:351.

Ou, Chau-Su, Beadle E, Presthus J, Smith M. A Multicenter Review of 839 Laparoscopic-Assisted Vaginal Hysterectomies. *J Am Assoc Gynecol Laparoscop* 1994;1:417–22.

Reich H, De Caprio J, McGlynn F. Laparoscopic hysterectomy. *J Gynecol Surg* 1989;5:213–16.

Smith ML Jr., Reich H. Laparoscopic hysterectomy. In: *The Video Encyclopedia of Endoscopic Surgery for the Gynecologist*. Shirk, G. (ed). St. Louis, Missouri; Medical Video Productions, 1994.

Operative Laparoscopy, Second Edition
The Masters' Techniques in Gynecologic Surgery
Lippincott–Raven Publishers, Philadelphia © 1998.

16-2 Laparoscopically Assisted Vaginal Hysterectomy (LAVH)

Delbert Alan Johns

Since first reported by Harry Reich in 1989, laparoscopically assisted vaginal hysterectomy (LAVH) has grown from a mere curiosity to a widely utilized but often controversial procedure. The most recent debate has centered on indications for LAVH and the techniques necessary to make this procedure both safe and cost-effective.

Since every gynecologist applies different criteria for approaching a hysterectomy vaginally or abdominally, absolute indications for LAVH are extremely difficult (if not impossible) to determine. In my surgical practice, LAVH is indicated in the following circumstances:

1. The patient with endometriosis undergoing hysterectomy for pain.
2. The patient who would, in *my* hands, require an abdominal approach. Most often this is a patient with "limited vaginal access" to the cervix, uterus or adnexa.
3. The patient with suspected (but undocumented) pelvic pathology, including endometriosis and adhesive disease.

Other indications for LAVH depend totally on the gynecologist's skill and experience in vaginal surgery and operative laparoscopy.

Several authors have reported LAVH to be a very expensive procedure, often eclipsing abdominal hysterectomy in total hospital cost. All of these authors, however, used disposable laparoscopic equipment, and most recommend endoscopic stapling devices. My experience has been quite different. By utilizing *only* reusable laparoscopic equipment, electrosurgery, and simple suturing techniques, LAVH (*in our hands*) is consistently associated with operating room costs slightly more than vaginal hysterectomy, but considerably less than abdominal hysterectomy. Although the cost of LAVH is only one consideration in evaluating its efficacy, it also offers the benefits of vaginal surgery to patients who would otherwise require laparotomy. Cost, recovery time, complications, and patient comfort must all be considered in evaluating this procedure.

The gynecologist skilled in vaginal surgery and operative laparoscopy, using reusable laparoscopic equipment and electrosurgery, can provide for the majority of their patients the unquestioned benefits of vaginal surgery without increasing the cost beyond that of abdominal hysterectomy. With this in mind, the techniques I use for LAVH will be reviewed.

PREOPERATIVE EVALUATION

The patient undergoing LAVH *must* be made aware of those complications (unique to laparoscopy) which do not occur during vaginal or abdominal hysterectomy. The possibility of trocar injuries to major vessels or bowel must be discussed with every patient prior to her surgery. Although these complications are rare, the potential cannot be ignored. The patient should understand that laparoscopy adds additional risks to those associated with abdominal or vaginal hysterectomy, but these risks are offset by the benefits of the laparoscopic approach in her particular situation.

Those patients able to undergo simple vaginal hysterectomy (with or without BSO) should not have a trocar inserted without a good clinical indication. There is no proven benefit of LAVH over simple vaginal hysterectomy. Use of the laparoscope simply adds cost, operating time, and risk.

In every case, the indications for using the laparoscope to complete the hysterectomy should be explained to the patient and carefully documented. Every patient should be aware that laparotomy may be required at *any* time. This might be necessary to evaluate and handle complications, treat newly discovered pathology, or complete the hysterectomy. Although these situations are unusual, the patient should never be surprised by this occurrence.

PATIENT POSITIONING AND OPERATIVE PREPARATION

Before the patient is transported to the operating room, *all* laparoscopic equipment is assembled and checked. CO_2 tanks are filled; electrosurgical equipment (including generators) are tested; light sources, television monitors, and cameras are checked. The worst possible time to discover malfunctioning equipment is *after* the patient is under anesthesia.

After the patient is anesthetized, her legs are positioned in fully adjustable stirrups supporting the knees and calves. The legs should be placed in a relatively low position with the femur parallel to the abdominal wall. This allows a full range of motion for instruments placed through the suprapubic sleeves.

I first perform a pelvic exam under anesthesia. This exam determines how much of the procedure must be done laparoscopically to ensure vaginal removal of the uterus and/ or ovaries. I evaluate the mobility of the uterus and cervix, the amount of ''space'' available for operating, and look for any abnormalities not previously identified.

Since I operate from the left side of the operating table, the patient's left arm is tucked at her side. This prevents her outstretched arm from limiting my ''maneuvering area'' and avoids any tendency to lean on the arm during the procedure.

A simple, straight, reusable uterine manipulator is then placed through the cervix to the uterine fundus. With practice, this can be accomplished without the physician sitting or using a vaginal speculum. I simply place my fingers into the vagina and identify the cervix. The cervix is grasped with a single-toothed tenaculum just over the tips of my fingers. While applying traction to the cervix, I am able to direct the manipulator through the cervical os and into the uterine cavity. Direct visualization of the cervix is unnecessary and considerable time is saved.

The bladder is emptied with a simple, red rubber catheter. I prefer *not* to leave an indwelling Foley catheter, since the Foley bulb can be mistaken for intraabdominal pathology. Since most LAVHs can be completed in two hours or less, the patient will rarely require intraoperative catheterization.

The sites of the umbilical incision and the two suprapubic 5-mm incisions are injected with 0.5% Marcaine. This significantly decreases postoperative discomfort in the incisions.

The lower fold of the umbilicus is grasped and elevated with Allis clamps. A 1.5- to 2-cm incision is made transversely *inside* this fold of tissue. When healed, this incision is almost invisible, hidden inside the umbilicus.

The primary intraumbilical trocar should *always* be inserted with the patient flat. If the operating table is tilted in any direction while the primary trocar is being inserted, the proper angle is required to avoid major vessels which may be less obvious.

In the majority of cases, I prefer a direct trocar insertion technique, without prior insufflation. The abdominal wall is grasped with my left hand a few cm beneath the umbilicus and elevated, and the tip of the reusable trocar spike is placed through the umbilical incision to the fascia. While holding up the abdominal wall with my left hand, I aim the trocar spike toward the hollow of the pelvis with my right hand. I carefully advance and rotate the trocar very slowly through the abdominal wall. I believe a slow, twisting, motion of the trocar allows a more controlled entry into the peritoneal cavity. By using this slow, twisting, motion I am better able to feel the trocar advance through the layers of the abdominal wall and estimate when it has penetrated into the peritoneal cavity.

As soon as the trocar is felt to be through the peritoneum, I insert the laparoscope to make certain that the placement is appropriate. If the sleeve is in an intraabdominal position, CO_2 insufflation is begun.

If I am concerned about intraabdominal adhesions at the umbilicus, I prefer to insert the first trocar in the left subcostal position. The Veress needle is inserted beneath the last rib on the left in the mid-clavicular line. Three liters of carbon dioxide is instilled in the abdominal cavity and a 5-mm trocar is inserted. A 5-mm laparoscope or hysteroscope is then used to find an appropriate area for placement of the 10-mm primary trocar.

Virtually all reusable 10-mm trocars have a trumpet valve or other device (usually spring-loaded), which seals the trocar sleeve when the laparoscope is removed. All of these devices produce friction on the laparoscope as it moves up and down through the sleeve. This often results in the trocar sleeve sliding out of the umbilical incision, a maddening and frustrating problem which always seems to happen in the midst of a difficult case.

To avoid this frustration, I disassemble the 10-mm trocar sleeve and remove any spring or other device that forces this valve closed or pushes against the laparoscope. Now, the only friction on the laparoscope comes from the gasket sealing the end of the trocar sleeve. As a result, rarely (if ever) do umbilical trocar sleeves slide out of the abdominal wall during my cases.

Once the abdomen is inflated, the patient is placed in steep Trendelenburg position and a quick visual inspection of the abdominal cavity undertaken. The uterus is identified and the optimum placement of the two suprapubic trocar sleeves determined (medial or lateral to the inferior epigastric artery). Since placement medial to the epigastric vessels minimizes risk of injury to the iliac vessel, I prefer this anatomic area when it will provide adequate access to the pelvis.

The inferior epigastric arteries are identified as they course just beneath the peritoneum. The appropriate insertion point is determined by pressing on the anterior abdominal wall, while visualizing the epigastric vessels laparoscopically. An incision is made, and a threaded 5-mm secondary trocar is inserted. These trocars should have no gaskets, insufflation ports or valves. These devices interfere with tissue removal, complicate insertion and removal of sutures and needles, and (because of friction on the instrument) make manipulation of instruments less precise and more difficult.

Two blunt irrigation/dissection probes are used to manipulate the small and large bowel out of the pelvis. I thoroughly examine the entire abdominal cavity, including the appendix, terminal ileum, and upper abdomen, and record the findings on videotape. Only *after* thorough inspection of the upper abdomen do I begin to evaluate the pelvic cavity.

The pelvic cavity is then carefully examined and the findings recorded. Only now do I begin to determine those laparoscopic procedures that will be necessary to complete the operation vaginally.

If the patient is undergoing hysterectomy for pelvic pain, dyspareunia or dysmenorrhea, and she has *significant* endometriosis (particularly endometriotic nodules), these implants *must* be removed along with the uterus or ovaries. If the disease is deeply invasive, overlays ureter or bowel, or invades into the rectovaginal septum, its removal requires very careful and precise dissection. Because of its predictability and precision, I prefer the CO_2 laser in these circumstances. In addition, when used through the operating channel of a single puncture laparoscope, the CO_2 laser is a "third hand," allowing the other two ports to be used for traction, counter-traction, and dissection. In these cases, the 10-mm umbilical trocar is removed and an operating laparoscope coupled to the CO_2 laser is inserted.

You should be operating with the best video equipment available. I prefer a 3-chip video camera coupled with a digital video enhancer, high resolution monitor, and matched light source. Since the surgeon *totally* relies on a video image for information, it should always, absolutely, positively, be the highest quality available. A less than optimal video image compromises the surgeon's abilities, and can lead to complications that would otherwise be avoidable. If funds are to be expended for laparoscopic equipment, they should first be spent on a quality video system. All other equipment is of secondary concern.

Additionally, I prefer scissors, bipolar instruments, graspers, and dissectors through which irrigation fluid can be forced. This allows me to irrigate the operative field, clearing blood and debris from the object of my attention. Otherwise, one is required to work in an operative field covered with blood and clots.

If bowel or adnexal adhesions are the only impediment to vaginal hysterectomy, they are lysed with (reusable) operating scissors until vaginal hysterectomy can be accomplished. If endometriosis is identified, *all* endometriotic implants and nodules are either excised or destroyed,

depending on their depth of penetration. This may require dissection in and around major vessels, ureter, bowel or the rectovaginal septum.

After endometriosis, pelvic adhesive disease, and any other pelvic pathology has been treated, I begin the process of freeing adnexal structures in preparation for vaginal hysterectomy. Techniques for LAVH with and without BSO will be covered.

LAVH WITH BSO

The *right* round ligament is secured with grasping forceps through the *left* suprapubic sleeve. It is pulled medially, desiccated with bipolar electrosurgery through the right suprapubic sleeve, and transected with monopolar electrosurgery or scissors.

Next, the *right* tube and ovary are grasped through the *left* suprapubic sleeve and pulled medially. This stretches the peritoneum medial to the iliac vessels. The peritoneum is opened with scissors or unipolar electrosurgery, allowing access to the retroperitoneal space. This peritoneal incision is extended caudad to the round ligament stump and cephalad to the level of the infundibulopelvic ligament (Figure 16-2.1). As the tube and ovary are pulled medially, the retroperitoneal space is carefully dissected with a blunt irrigation/dissection probe through the right suprapubic sleeve until the medial leaf of the broad ligament is found. If not otherwise obvious, the ureters should also be easily identifiable in the retroperitoneal space.

With continued medial traction on the right tube and ovary, the peritoneum overlaying the "infundibulopelvic ligament" is incised and the ovarian vessels identified. The ovarian artery and vein should now be isolated and skeletonized. For optimum desiccation and minimal lateral thermal spread, a 2 to 3-cm length of these vessels should be skeletonized.

With continuing medial traction on the right tube and ovary, the ovarian artery and vein are grasped with unipolar or bipolar electrosurgical instruments, desiccated and coaptated (Figure 16-2.2). The process of bipolar electrosurgical desiccation should be monitored with an in-line ammeter. A non-electrolyte solution (Glycine) is passed through the electrosurgical instruments during desiccation of the infundibulopelvic ligaments. This cools the surrounding tissue and minimizes lateral thermal injury. In addition, the tips of the metal instrument are cooled and are less likely to adhere. You should refer to the chapter on electrosurgery for further information on monopolar and bipolar desiccation and coaptation techniques.

Once thoroughly desiccated, the infundibulopelvic ligament is transected with operating scissors. Should the coaptation be incomplete, these vessels will bleed, but this is easily controlled with a pre-tied laparoscopic "loop" suture (which should be readily available during *every* case). This retroperitoneal approach ensures more complete and pre-

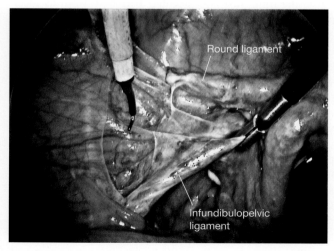

Figure 16-2.1 The peritoneum overlying the retroperitoneal space between the round ligament and the infundibulopelvic ligament has been opened, allowing access to the retroperitoneal space.

dictable coaptation of the ovarian vessel and vein and also reduces the risk of ureteral injury.

The ovary and tube are again grasped and pulled medially, stretching the posterior leaf of the broad ligament. While visualizing the ureter, the remaining peritoneum is opened to the level of the uterine artery. Using the same technique (but bringing instruments through the opposite side), the left tube and ovary are freed to the uterine artery.

This same retroperitoneal approach is used if either ovary is densely adherent to the pelvic sidewall. Rather than trying to dissect the ovary off the sidewall peritoneum, the ovary *and* peritoneum are removed en bloc by dissecting the peritoneal sidewall from retroperitoneal structures medially (with the ovary still attached). This minimizes the risk of ureteral injury and decreases the possibility that you will later be faced with an ovarian remnant.

Next, using the uterine manipulator, the uterus is pushed cephalad, stretching the peritoneum overlaying the vesicouterine fold. My assistant maintains the uterus in this position while I grasp and elevate the anterior cul-de-sac peritoneum. This allows me to accurately identify the junction between the dome of the bladder and the lower uterine segment. The peritoneum is incised at this level with unipolar electrosurgery or scissors, and the incision is extended laterally to the round ligament stumps.

While pushing the uterus cephalad, the edge of the bladder is grasped and elevated. Using scissors and/or an irrigation/dissection probe, the bladder is carefully dissected away from the lower uterine segment (Figure 16-2.3). Completion of this step makes transvaginal entry into the anterior cul-de-sac *very* simple, thereby decreasing the risk of bladder injury. I closely inspect the posterior cul-de-sac to make certain that a transvaginal colpotomy will be simple and associated with minimal risk of rectal injury.

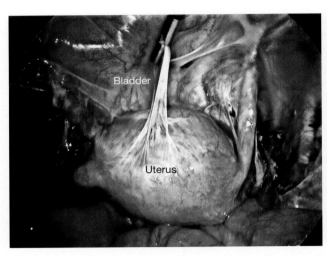

Figure 16-2.3 The uterus is pushed cephalad, the peritoneum elevated, and the bladder dissected from the lower uterine segment.

At this point, the adnexal structures are freed to the level of the uterine artery, the bladder is dissected from the lower uterine segment, all implants of endometriosis are excised or coagulated, and all clinically significant adhesions are lysed. In most cases, the patient is now ready to be repositioned for vaginal hysterectomy.

LAVH WITHOUT BSO

A slightly different technique is used when the ovaries are to be retained. The right round ligament is grasped through the left suprapubic sleeve approximately 1 cm from the cornu, pulled medially, desiccated approximately 2 to 3 cm from its insertion into the uterus, and transected. Similarly, the right tube is desiccated 1 to 2 cm from its insertion into the uterus and transected.

The utero-ovarian ligament and a portion of the broad ligament remain attached to the uterus. Unfortunately, this broad ligament segment contains numerous large veins which can be difficult to control by electrosurgical coaptation. To avoid bleeding from these vessels, I prefer to isolate this segment of the broad ligament and control it with sutures rather than electrosurgery.

The right round ligament is grasped through the left suprapubic sleeve and the uterus pulled medially. The right utero-ovarian ligament is desiccated and transected. Using an irrigation/dissection probe through the right suprapubic sleeve, the medial leaf of the broad ligament is identified through the defect created by transection of the round ligament. The medial leaf of the broad ligament is opened, creating a "window" through which sutures can be passed, encircling the remaining attachment of the broad ligament to the uterus. A second suture is passed through and around the pedicle to prevent back bleeding. The sutures are se-

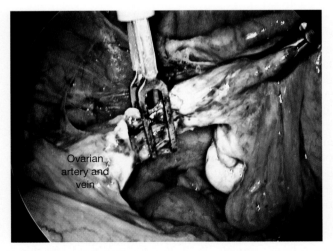

Figure 16-2.2 The ovarian artery and vein have been dissected and isolated, the medial leaf of the broad ligament opened, and bipolar desiccation of the ovarian artery and vein has begun. (Bipolar forceps manufactured by Karl Storz Co.).

cured around this remaining attachment with an endoscopic knot-pusher, and the broad ligament is transected. If the veins in this area are relatively small, this connection is desiccated with unipolar or bipolar electrosurgery and transected.

After repositioning the graspers and electrosurgical instruments, the same procedure is carried out, detaching the left round ligament, utero-ovarian ligament and broad ligament from the uterus. Endoscopic stapling instruments can also be used to detach adnexal structures from the uterus, but the added cost is prohibitive and not adequately offset by any decrease in operating time.

Both adnexa are carefully inspected for bleeding from the proximal portion of the transected vessels. If bleeding is encountered it is controlled with sutures or electrosurgery. Additionally, both adnexal structures are examined for ''rotational mobility.'' If it appears that either adnexa might be at risk for torsion, the transected utero-ovarian ligament and tubal segment are sutured to the round ligament stump.

The bladder is dissected from the lower uterine segment as previously described. In most cases, the uterus is now ready for transvaginal removal.

THE UTERINE ARTERY

Because of its proximity to the ureter, the uterine artery poses unique problems for the laparoscopic surgeon. Most gynecologists are capable of controlling the uterine artery during vaginal hysterectomy, but few develop the skills necessary to isolate and control the uterine artery laparoscopically. In reality, it is very rarely necessary to control the uterine artery laparoscopically. In the majority of cases, this can be done much more quickly and safely during the vaginal portion of the LAVH.

If, from the preoperative and intraoperative evaluation, I feel that the uterine artery must be taken laparoscopically, I use the following approach: The obliterated umbilical artery (umbilical ligament) is followed down the abdominal wall into the retroperitoneal space which has been previously opened. At the point where the umbilical ligament nears the ureter, the uterine artery can be identified where it crosses over the ureter.

Since the uterine artery branches several times prior to reaching the uterus, I prefer to isolate and ligate it *prior* to its crossing the ureter. Once I identify the uterine artery after it branches from the hypogastric artery, I dissect and isolate a 2 to 3 cm segment of this vessel. Proximal and distal sutures are passed around this segment and it is ligated and transected (Figure 16-2.4).

COLPOTOMY

In the very rare circumstance when the entire uterus must be removed laparoscopically, only the cardinal and utero-

sacral ligament complexes remain after the uterine artery is taken. To enter the vagina anterior to the cervix, I press the uterus cephalad, elevate the bladder and anterior vagina, and enter the anterior cul-de-sac just above the cervix with unipolar electrosurgery.

The cervix is then amputated from the apex of the vagina, cardinal ligaments, and uterosacral ligaments with unipolar electrosurgery. A moistened sponge placed in the vagina maintains pneumoperitoneum during this time. The uterus is then removed intact through the vagina or morcellated and removed through a suprapubic sleeve. The vaginal cuff is closed laparoscopically.

REPOSITIONING AND VAGINAL HYSTERECTOMY

It is imperative that the patient be properly repositioned on the operating table for the vaginal portion of the operation. Every difficult vaginal hysterectomy requires the patient's legs to be positioned vertically and somewhat lateral, giving the surgical assistants enough room to provide adequate exposure. If the patient is not properly positioned, even the simplest vaginal hysterectomy can become extremely difficult and potentially dangerous.

When I am finished with the laparoscopic portion of the LAVH, the operating room nurses rotate the patient's legs vertically and the feet and ankles slightly outward. A sterile drape is placed over the abdomen, the legs and perineum are covered with standard perineal drapes. The laparoscope and trocar sleeves are left in place.

Since the laparoscopic portion of the operation is performed with the patient in a deep lithotomy position, she may shift forward on the operating table. If this occurs, adequate retraction can be virtually impossible. Correcting the problem at this time may avoid a lot of frustration during

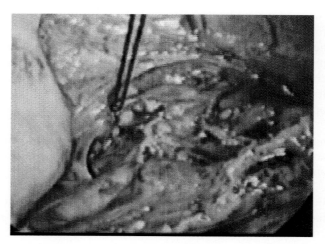

Figure 16-2.4 The uterine artery has been isolated and ligated prior to the point it crosses over the ureter.

the case. Once the patient is properly repositioned, I begin the vaginal portion of the LAVH.

The cervix is grasped and the remaining attachments of the cardinal and uterosacral ligaments are controlled and transected as with any vaginal hysterectomy. If not taken with the cardinal ligament, the uterine artery remains the only attachment and can be easily ligated and transected. The uterus (with or without ovaries) is removed. Morcellation or fragmentation may be required to remove a larger uterus, but no blood is lost since the entire vascular supply of the uterus has been interrupted. The vaginal cuff is then closed by standard methods.

The patient's legs are rotated downward and she is repositioned as she was at the beginning of the laparoscopic procedure. The abdomen is reinflated, and irrigating probes reinserted through the suprapubic sleeves. The abdominal cavity is cleansed of all blood clots and debris. During this time, bleeding points are commonly identified. These are controlled with electrosurgery or sutures, depending on the location and severity of the bleeding.

The entire abdominal cavity and operative field is once again irrigated and inspected. All irrigating fluid is aspirated. While maintaining the patient in Trendelenburg position, instruments are removed from the suprapubic sleeves and 1 to 2 liters of isotonic saline solution or Ringer's lactate is introduced into the abdomen through the umbilical sleeve insufflation port. As it fills the upper abdomen, the fluid forces the carbon dioxide out of the abdomen through the suprapubic ports, minimizing postoperative shoulder pain. Trocar sleeves are removed and the incisions are closed. Fascial closure is mandatory in all incisions larger than 5 mm.

POSTOPERATIVE CARE

Postoperative care of the patient having undergone LAVH is identical to that for vaginal hysterectomy. The patient's bladder is emptied prior to leaving the operating room and 3 to 4 hours after admission to the recovery room. She then undergoes intermittent catheterization, as needed, until dismissal. LAVH patients rarely require more than 2 catheterizations before regaining bladder control. Only if the patient underwent a procedure for incontinence is an indwelling Foley catheter used postoperatively.

The patients are given injectable analgesics every 3 to 4 hours for a maximum of three doses. Oral fluids are encouraged as soon as the patient is awake and alert, and oral analgesics are begun very shortly thereafter.

By 8 hours after surgery, these patients are able to take liquids and oral analgesics, and most are voiding spontaneously. The intravenous line is removed between 4 and 6 hours after surgery. Remember, the patient is unlikely to become dehydrated since she has 1000 to 1500 cc of isotonic fluid in her abdomen when she leaves the operating suite; therefore, continuous intravenous fluids are unnecessary.

By the morning after surgery, the patient is on the diet of her choice, taking oral analgesics, is voiding spontaneously, and has no intravenous line. In our experience, approximately 80% of these patients can be dismissed *within* 24 hours of their procedure. Those patients undergoing prolonged procedures (particularly those with AFS Stage 3 or 4 endometriosis) may require hospital stays up to 48 hours.

After dismissal, LAVH patients are allowed to gradually resume their normal activities as soon as their pain is controlled with non-narcotic analgesics. This usually occurs within 7 to 14 days. Many are able to return to work in 2 weeks.

CONCLUSIONS

Although some authors have concluded that LAVH is considerably more expensive than its abdominal counterpart, there is ample evidence to indicate that this is primarily due to use of disposable laparoscopic instruments and stapling devices. These have been shown to significantly increase the cost of these procedures without any demonstrable off-setting benefit.

The gynecologic surgeon who has skill and experience in the techniques of vaginal hysterectomy as well as operative laparoscopy can perform most, if not all, hysterectomies for benign disease via the vaginal route.

Operative laparoscopy is simply a valuable adjunct to vaginal hysterectomy.

These three simple rules apply:

1. Always use reusable laparoscopic instruments, electrosurgery, and sutures.
2. Perform only those laparoscopic procedures necessary to complete the hysterectomy vaginally.
3. If it can be done vaginally, *do not* put a laparoscope in.

When these rules are followed, the cost of LAVH will be below that of TAH, complications will be minimized, and abdominal hysterectomy will be relegated to its proper place.

This accomplishes two major goals: Overall medical costs associated with hysterectomy are reduced, thereby increasing our "cost-effectiveness." More importantly, however, most of our patients will benefit from the lower complication rate and shorter, more pleasant recovery associated with vaginal surgery.

SUGGESTED READING

Boike GM, Elfstrand EP, DelPriore G, Schumock D, Holley HS, Lurain JR. Laparoscopically assisted vaginal hysterectomy in a university hospital: report of 82 cases and comparison with abdominal and vaginal hysterectomy. *Am J Obstet Gynecol* 1993;168:1690–701.

Johns DA. Laparoscopically assisted vaginal hysterectomy (LAVH). *J Reprod Med* 1994;39(6):424–8.

Johns DA. Laparoscopically assisted vaginal hysterectomy: electrosurgical techniques. In: Diamond MP, Daniell JF, Jones HW III, eds. Hysterectomy. Boston: Blackwell Science, 1996:45–58.

Johns DA. *Laparoscopic Hysterectomy and Pelvic Floor Reconstruction.* In: Liu, CY, ed. Laparoscopically Assisted Vaginal Hysterectomy. Boston: Blackwell Science, 1996:149–67.

Kovac RS, Christie SJ, Bindbeutel GA. Abdominal versus vaginal hysterectomy: a statistical model for determining physician decision making and patient outcome. *Med Decis Making* 1991;11:19–28.

Kovac RS, Pignotti BJ, Bindbeutel GA. Hysterectomy: a comparative statistical study of abdominal vs. vaginal approaches. *Missouri Med* 1988;85:312–6.

Reich H, DeCaprio J, McGlynn F. Laparoscopic hysterectomy. *J Gynecol Surg* 1989;5:213–6.

Reich H, McGlynn F, Sekel L. Total laparoscopic hysterectomy. *Gynecol Endosc* 1993;2:59–63.

The Medical and Economic Impact of Laparoscopically Assisted Vaginal Hysterectomy in a Large Metropolitan Not-For-Profit Hospital. *J Ob Gynecol* 1995;172(6):1709–15.

Operative Laparoscopy, Second Edition
The Masters' Techniques in Gynecologic Surgery
Lippincott–Raven Publishers, Philadelphia © 1998.

16-3   Laparoscopic Supracervical Hysterectomy

Thomas L. Lyons

Laparoscopic supracervical hysterectomy (LSH) was originally proposed by the present author in 1990 as a method of increasing conversion of the relatively high morbidity procedure total abdominal hysterectomy (TAH) to a less morbid procedure for the patient. Of course this was the original goal of the laparoscopically assisted vaginal hysterectomy (LAVH), which then and now seems not to have been met in most reviews. Originally, the indications for LSH were somewhat limited, excluding all patients with any cervical disease, pelvic prolapse, gynecologic malignancies, etc. However, in our hands virtually any patient with indications for hysterectomy (excepting invasive carcinoma of the cervix and cancer of the endometrium) may currently be considered an LSH candidate. This fact has allowed the author to develop several "pearls" of technique which can assist gynecologic surgeons in the performance of LSH on a wide variety of patients with varying diagnoses, physiognomies, and idiosyncrasies, and make this procedure an easy, safe alternative for most patients.

TECHNIQUE

Pearl 1. *Basic surgical techniques and rules should always be followed. Exposure, traction and countertraction, meticulous hemostasis, anatomic analysis, and adherence to tried and true surgical techniques, will help the operator's chances of completing the task at hand successfully.*

The patient's consent is obtained with full documentation and discussion of the risks and potential benefits of conservation of the cervix. This discussion includes recommendations for continued cytologic surveillance and, as with all proposed laparoscopic procedures, the possibility of laparotomy. Our consent form now specifically includes direct language on bowel or urinary tract damage in addition to the risks of bleeding, infection, anesthesia, etc. Bowel preparation (Golitely prep, Braintree Laboratories, Braintree, MA) is used very liberally in any patient with suspicion of significant adhesive disease or endometriosis and routine MetroGel (Curatek Pharmaceuticals, Elk Grove, IL) vaginal insertion is prescribed the evening prior to surgery. If bowel prep is not indicated, a Fleet phosphosoda enema is used at bedtime the night prior to the procedure.

Pearl 2. *The surgeon is wise to supervise or participate in patient positioning and to document this or have it documented in the patient's chart. Patients may have medical problems which necessitate this surveillance or there may be an idiosyncrasy specific to the case which will require a change in position.*

The patient is positioned in the modified dorsal lithotomy position, Allen Stirrups (Allen Medical) as shown in Figure 16-3.1. The distribution of equipment may vary surgeon to surgeon, but the primary surgeon should always have the insufflator, and therefore the intraabdominal pressure readout, immediately in view. Basic equipment needs include camera/lightsource (best if produced by the same manufacturer), bipolar forceps, suction/irrigation (33-cm length is preferred), a cutting device (we prefer the Contact Nd:YAG laser through the operating channel of the laparoscope or the Harmonic Scalpel but CO_2 laser or monopolar cutters may be used), and various means of vessel occlusion (clips, ligatures, or traditional sutures). Stapling devices or hybrid devices such as coagulator/cutters have not proved to facilitate the procedure in our hands.

Pearl 3. *A good uterine manipulator can be a significant benefit in this as well as other laparoscopic procedures. I recommend either the Pelosi or the Valchev manipulator, due to their singular abilities to create the necessary traction and exposure for gynecologic endoscopy.*

Pearl 4. *Trocar placement is critical to the performance of the procedure. The trocars must be placed high enough in the abdomen to see well around the uterus and adnexal structures. The lateral trocars must be wide enough to exert good lateral traction on the fundus.*

Open laparoscopy is performed, as this site (the subumbilical site) is used for tissue removal at the termination of the case. Also, open laparoscopy may be the entry of choice in patients with suspected adhesive disease or with large intraabdominal masses. This author has performed the procedure on patients who have had up to 17 prior laparotomies and up to a 32-week size fibroid uterus. Trocar placement is illustrated in Figure 16-3.2. Note the upper abdominal placement in patients with larger uteri and the lateral placement (well lateral to the rectus musculature). Five-mm trocars are used laterally unless a larger trocar is dictated by the situation. For example, if adhesive disease requires placement of the operating laparoscope in a lateral port for access to adhesiolysis, larger ports may be necessary in these sites. It is important to note that trocar distribution is related to pathology, not simply placed in a rote fashion in the same way for each case. Generally, four trocars are used, which enable the surgeon to triangulate the pathology, but variations of this may be necessary to accomplish the

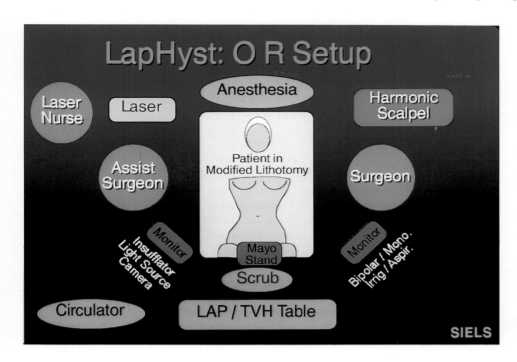

Figure 16-3.1 The operating room setup is graphically demonstrated.

desired task. A second 10-11 trocar is helpful, as this site can be used to pass curved needles for suturing and clips or stapling devices may be used through this portal, while the laparoscope is being used through the other 10-mm port. **Pearl 5.** *Always perform an exploration prior to initiating the procedure. This may facilitate or change the actual procedure to be performed.*

Exploratory laparoscopy is performed, pathology is identified, and adhesiolysis is accomplished as necessary at the onset of the case. After careful identification of the ureters at the pelvic brim, the infundibulopelvic ligaments are desiccated with a bipolar cautery, divided with the Nd:YAG laser scalpel or scissors and can be ligated using Endoloop (Ethicon Endo Surgery, Cincinatti, OH) of O-PDS.

Pearl 6. *Control back-bleeding by bipolar desiccation of the round ligament, tube, and utero-ovarian pedicle on the specimen side prior to division of any pedicles.*

Back-bleeding is carefully controlled with bipolar cautery. We find that the BI-Coag curved dissector/grasper (Everest Medical, Minneapolis, MN) is a highly useful instrument to be used in this procedure as it reduces the number of instrument changes necessary to complete the dissection. If any pedicles are not able to be freed, careful lateral sidewall dissection and ureterolysis is first performed, then ligatures are passed and extracorporeal knotting techniques may be used to ligate these pedicles. Sidewall dissection is best performed by entering the avascular space lateral to the fallopian tube and above the round ligament while proceeding down into the pelvis. The ureter is located within the peritoneal leaf, medial and inferior to the hypogastric vasculature. The round ligament is desiccated

and divided in similar fashion. The uterovesicle fold is dissected using the Nd:YAG laser scalpel, harmonic scalpel, or scissors and blunt and sharp dissection of the bladder flap is carefully accomplished. An endoscopic kittner (Ethicon Endo Surgery, Inc., Cincinatti, OH) may be employed in this blunt dissection as this is atraumatic and may decrease the tendency for bladder injury. It is imperative that this portion of the procedure be carefully carried out because this opens the uterine vessel fossa for dissection of the uterine vasculature. It is of further importance to note that aqua dissection in this area may be a difficult or impossible technique to use, due to dense adherence of the bladder flap in cases of prior cesarean section. Also, the distortion of the anatomy which is incumbent with aqua dissection can make identification of vital sutures, i.e. the uterine arteries and the ureter, very difficult and, therefore, division and dissection/ligation of these structures may be more difficult if aqua dissection is used extensively. The LCS (Ultracision, Inc., Providence, RI) device can be used to coagulate and divide the larger vascular pedicles of the IP and utero-ovarian ligament, if the operator desires.

Pearl 7. *Dissection of the posterior leaf of the broad ligament allows the ureter to splay laterally and with good countertraction on the uterine fundus, facilitates skeletonization of the uterine vessels, and maximizes the distance between the ureter and the vasculature.*

The posterior leaf of the broad ligament is dissected carefully, allowing the ureter to splay laterally. This posterior leaf dissection allows the surgeon, along with good countertraction on the uterine fundus from the contralateral port, to maximize the distance from the ureter to the uterine ves-

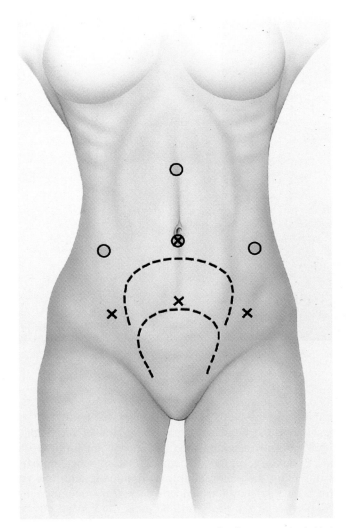

Figure 16-3.2 Trocar site placement is demonstrated. Note that the trocar sites move up in the abdomen as the uterine size increases.

Pearl 8. *Amputation of the cervix must begin at or below the level of the internal os and procede in a coring fashion down into the cervical canal.*

The surgeon should note that this division of the cervix is at or below the endocervical os. The remainder of the dissection is performed in a coring manner with removal of the upper end of the cervical canal. The uterine manipulator can facilitate this amputation. After removal of the uterus, the cervix is inspected and any areas of bleeding are co-agulated, using the bipolar cautery. The anterior and posterior folds of the perineum and the anterior pubo-cervical fascia and posterior cervix are plicated together using an interrupted mattress suture of 0-vicryl or using the EMS endoscopic stapler (Ethicon EndoSurgery, Inc.). Prior to peritoneal closure the endocervical canal should be ablated using the Nd:YAG laser, the bipolar cautery, or a mono-polar ball to decrease postoperative leukorrhea and reduce dysplasia risk. At this point, the abdomen is lavaged and inspected for signs of bleeding while decreasing intraab-dominal pressure to <8 mmHg. Any areas of bleeding are carefully attended to using the bipolar forceps or the Nd:YAG hemostasis tip. The uterus is then bifurcated or

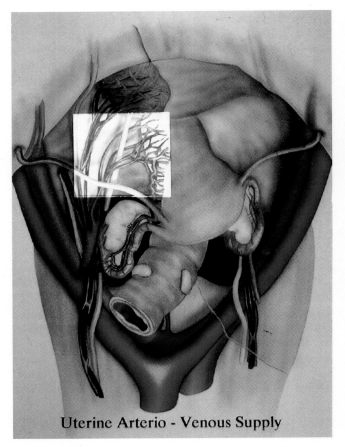

Uterine Arterio - Venous Supply

Figure 16-3.3 Ureter-uterine vessel relationship at the lower segment. Note that the effect of fundal countertraction is to increase the distance between the ureter and the vessels.

sels at their insertion into the uterus (Figure 16-3.3). After the uterine arteries have been dissected carefully and the ureter is identified well away from these structures, the uter-ine arteries are bipolar-desiccated and divided. Occasion-ally, suture ligatures or ligaclips may be placed if a pedicle can be developed in this area. However, high ligation of the uterine artery is usually unnecessary unless this area of anatomy has become obscured due to endometriosis, etc. Once these vascular structures have been occluded, the uterus will become cyanotic, denoting that the vascular sup-ply has been eliminated. At this time, the Nd:YAG laser scalpel is used to divide the uterine vessel and to cut down on the uterine manipulator which was placed preoperatively into the cervix. This procedure can also be performed with a monopolar spoon or needle using high power density cut-ting current or the harmonic scalpel.

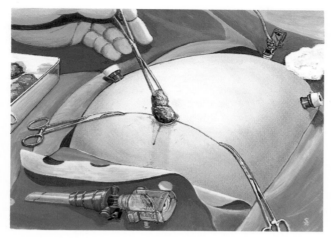

Figure 16-3.4 Specimen removal via the subumbilical port. The trocar has been removed to facilitate morcellation and removal at the abdominal wall.

morcellated, using sharp dissection with the ultrasonically activated scalpel or large scissors. Removal is accomplished through the subumbilical open laparoscopy port (Figure 16-3.4). This port is chosen because it can easily be extended to accommodate a larger uterine corpus. During this process, the scope is moved to the lower 10/11 trocar for direct visualization of removal of the uterus and/or other pathologic specimens. Appendectomy or other procedures may be performed as necessary at this time.

Pearl 9. *Posterior vault support should be provided in all cases of hysterectomy. We prefer to perform a High McCall's procedure to support the tissues well up in the pelvis, using permanent suture material.*

A modified McCall's posterior culdoplasty may be accomplished by plicating the uterosacral ligaments which remain intact and the posterior fascia using a O-Ethibond pursestring suture and an extracorpeal knotting technique (Figure 16-3.5). The patient is then allowed to recover with the Foley in place and is observed for approximately an 18-hour period postoperatively, prior to discharge.

Patients are allowed to return to normal activity at home within 2 to 3 days and are able to return to work within 7 to 10 days with normal activity. There is no evidence of significant vaginal discharge postoperatively, and intercourse may be resumed at 2 weeks.

RESULTS

In our clinic a total of 236 LSH procedures have been performed over a 4-year period from February of 1990 to February of 1994. Results of these patients are demonstrated in Table 16-3.1. A learning curve was demonstrated in Cases 1 to 50 which resulted in steadily decreasing operative times; however, this is the only variable which changed during this time period. Complications were no

more frequent in year one versus year four. Also, the learning curve may not have been as dramatic because laparoscopically assisted vaginal hysterectomy (LAVH or technically LH) had been performed in 25 cases prior to initiating LSH. It should be noted that at no time did procedures extend beyond four hours (average time now 85 minutes) and no injury occurred to bowel, bladder, ureter, or major vasculature. Febrile morbidity was less than 1%, no transfusions were required (average blood loss 55 cc) and hospital readmission occurred in only 3 patients. One patient underwent trachelectomy and node dissection two weeks postoperatively, due to the presence of a microscopic focus of endometrial carcinoma found on pathology exam following a hysterectomy for painful menses. There were no cases of conversion to open surgery despite a group of 30 patients with uteri weighing greater than 500 g (8 patients each had uteri greater than 1,000 g). Hospital stay averaged 16 hours in all patients and resumption of normal activity was within 2 to 3 days. Return to work was at 2 weeks in the entire series. Increasingly, late in the series, other procedures for pelvic support (Burch, rectocele, and enterocele repair) were performed, which, combined with LSH, gave this patient population a significant improvement in overall morbidity when combined with similar vaginal or abdominal approaches.

DISCUSSION

This treatise is intended to present a method of performing LSH as developed by one surgeon using readily

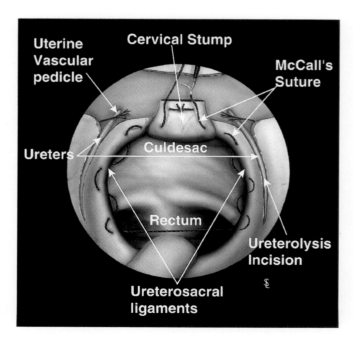

Figure 16-3.5 The High McCall's culdoplasty-suspension is represented.

Table 16-3.1 *Clinical outcomes of laparoscopic supra cervical hysterectomies*

Age = 43.4 yrs. (range: 27–86)
Parity = 2.1 (range: 0–9)
Weight = 68.7 Kg (range: 41–77)

	Preoperative	Postoperative	
Diagnosis	DUB 69%	Lieomyomata uteri 69%	
(Average uterine weight	Myomata 53%	Adenomyosis 68%	
178 gms.)	Pain 53%	Endometriosis 36%	
	Pelvic relaxation 45%	Pelvic inflammation 21%	
	Endometriosis 23%	Ovarian adenocarcinoma <1%	
	PID 11%	Normal pathology 31%	
	Ovarian cancer <1%		
Associated procedures			
Unilateral or bilateral salpingoopharectomy			117
McCalls/modified Moschowitz			216
Burch			54
Appendectomy			65
Adhesiolysis			205
Sacral colpopexy			2
High rectocele repair			12
Estimated blood loss	55 cc (25–125)		
Operating time	85 min (59–235)		
Hospital stay	17 hrs (3–38)		
Readmission	2 (Both patients had signs of bowel obstruction at 7–10 days postoperatively—spontaneous resolution with hydration)		
Conversion to open	0		
Recurrent bleeding	1 (Ceased with treatment of canal with Hg NO₃)		
Acute complications of surgery			
Infection	4 trocar site infections requiring drainage; 2 urinary tract infections		
Bleeding	0; no transfusions required		
Bowel injury	0		
Urinary tract injury	0		
Subcutaneous emphysema	1 mild		
Reoperations to remove cervix	3 (1 patient was found to have endometrial cancer on path at the time of surgery. 2 patients had subsequent reconstruction.)		

PID, pelvic inflammatory disease.

available materials, with attention to cost-effectiveness, and, most important, to the benefit of the patient. Experience has shown us that procedures done laparoscopically have decreased morbidity when compared to open, traditional, surgery. Experience can show us methods of further lowering that morbidity, using classic surgical axioms with application of new minimally invasive techniques.

Pearl 10. *The final pearl: When asked why I perform a task in a given manner, the answer is always the same—because I have done it wrong in a thousand other ways. Don't be afraid to innovate, but also, don't be afraid to let someone else make a mistake first and then benefit from it.*

Use the recommendations from this work to assist you in your laparoscopic hysterectomy cases. There certainly are many other ways to work through these procedures. Each surgeon will develop his or her own style, but we can all agree that minimally invasive procedures, when performed well, are to the greatest benefit of our patients.

ACKNOWLEDGEMENTS

I would like to acknowledge the artist Samuel A. Lyons Jr. for production of the illustrations used in this chapter. Also, Ethicon EndoSurgery and Johnson & Johnson Medical, Inc. provided grant assistance for the production of these illustrations.

I would like to thank Wendy K. Winer, RN, for her assistance in surgery, her innovative suggestions, and her help in preparation of this work.

SUGGESTED READING

Brumsted J, Kessler C, Gibson C, et al. A comparison of laparoscopy and laparotomy for the treatment of ectopic pregnancy. *Obstet Gynecol* 1986;71:889–92.

Cutler EC, Zollinger RM. *Atlas of Surgical Operations.* New York: Macmillan; 1949.

Gallup DG, Morley GW. Carcinoma in situ of the vagina: a study and review. *Obstet Gynecol* 1975;46:334–40.

Garry R. Laparoscopic hysterectomy: definitions and indications. *Gynaecol Endosc* 1994;3:1–3.

Jimerson GK, Merrill JA. Cancer and dysplasia of the posthysterectomy vaginal cuff. *Gynecol Oncol* 1976;4:328–32.

Kilkku P. Supravaginal amputation versus hysterectomy with reference to bladder symptoms and incontinence. *Acta Obstet Gynecol Scand* 1985;64:375–9.

Kilkku P, Gronoos M, Hirvonen T, et al. Supracervical uterine amputation vs. hysterectomy: effects on libido and orgasm. *Acta Obstet Gynecol Scand* 1983;62:141–6.

Kilkku P, Gronoos M, Taina E, et al. Culposcopic, cytological, and histological evaluation of the cervical stump 3 years after supravaginal uterine amputation. *Acta Obstet Gynecol Scand* 1985;64:235–40.

Kilkku P, Hirvonen T, Gronoos M. Supracervical uterine amputation vs. abdominal hysterectomy: the effects in urinary symptoms with special reference to pollakisuria, nocturia, and dysuria. *Maturitas* 1981;3:197.

Kilkku P, Lehtinen V, Hirvonen T, et al. Abdominal hysterectomy vs. supravaginal amputation: psychic factors. *Ann Chir Gynecol* 1987;202:62–6.

Levy BS, Hulka JF, Peterson HB, Phillips JM. Operative laparoscopy: AAGL 1993 membership survey. *J Am Assoc Gynecol Laparosc* 1994;1:301–5.

Liu CY. Laparoscopic hysterectomy: report of 215 cases. *Gynecol Endosc* 1992;1:73–7.

Lyons TL. Laparoscopic supracervical hysterectomy: proceedings of the 20th annual meeting AAGL, Las Vegas, November 1991.

Lyons TL. Laparoscopic supracervical hysterectomy: a comparison of morbidity and mortality results with laparoscopically assisted vaginal hysterectomy. *J Reprod Med* 1993;38:763–7.

Lyons TL. Subtotal Hysterectomy. In: Daniell J, Diamond M, Jones H (eds.). *Hysterectomy.* Boston: Blackwell Scientific, 1994:88–98.

Maher PJ, Wood EC, Hill DJ, et al: Laparoscopically assisted hysterectomy. *Med J Aust* 1992;156:316–8.

Martin DC. *Laparoscopic Appearance of Endometriosis.* Memphis: Resurge Press; 1990.

Ou CS, Beadle E, Presthus J, Smith M. A multicenter review of 839 laparoscopically assisted vaginal hysterectomies. *J Am Assoc Gynecol Laparosc* 1994;1:417–22.

Semm K. Hysterectomy via laparotomy or pelviscopy: a new CASH method without culpotomy. *Geburtshilfe Frauenheilkd* 1991;51:996–1003.

Stuart GCE, Allen HH, Anderson RJ. Squamous cell carcinoma of the vagina after hysterectomy. *Am J Obstet Gynecol* 1981;139:311–5.

Thompson JT. In: *Telinde's Operative Gynecology.* Thompson JT, Rock J. (eds.). Philadelphia: Lippincott, 1992:758–9.

Operative Laparoscopy, Second Edition
The Masters' Techniques in Gynecologic Surgery
Lippincott–Raven Publishers, Philadelphia © 1998.

17

Urogynecologic Procedures

Thierry G. Vancaillie

Urogynecology is defined as a specialty dealing with the pelvic floor physiology and pathology of women. It is a field encompassing a vast array of problems. The most commonly presenting pathologies are those of urinary incontinence and pelvic floor relaxation.

Historically, there has been a continuing debate as to whether these problems should be addressed vaginally versus abdominally, provided there is an indication for surgical correction.

This debate is not likely to disappear soon. In general, a surgical procedure should be performed to the best of the surgeon's ability and to the greatest of the patient's comfort. Although hard data are not legion, it is generally considered that vaginal surgery is less morbid for the patient, compared to abdominal surgery. On the other hand, most surgeons are more comfortable dealing with abdominal procedures than vaginal procedures in any area of gynecology, mainly because of greater freedom of access to the various regions of the pelvic anatomy, with the exception of the lower vaginal tract.

A new parameter was introduced with the finding by Benson that vaginal surgery for complex pelvic floor relaxation caused significantly more neurovascular damage than did abdominal procedures. How well the patient recovers from this damage in the long term still needs to be evaluated. However, this finding should prompt us to continue exploration of new venues in treating surgically the defects of the pelvic floor.

Laparoscopy offers a low-morbidity alternative to laparotomy for access to the pelvic floor. It should be stressed that low morbidity does not mean low complication rate; it is more than likely that the complication rate overall is higher for laparoscopy than for laparotomy, because of the greater demand on the surgeon's skill. For procedures with a low incidence, such as sacral colpopexy, one should question the validity of using the laparoscopic approach, in view of the real specter of serious hemorrhagic complications. The majority of procedures are a great indication for use of the laparoscopic approach, especially because laparoscopy offers the advantage of improved evaluation of the topographical anatomy. Greater knowledge of anatomical detail should, theoretically, lead to better surgical repair. The problem is in the surgeon's ability to perform suturing. I continue to believe that no technical gimmick will replace the use of sutures in the foreseeable future, and that surgeons should stop procrastinating and start learning how to suture laparoscopically. Manipulating sutures laparoscopically at any opportunity, such as during LAVH, provides needed training.

REVIEW OF THE FEMALE PELVIC ANATOMY

The pelvic anatomy of a patient should be reviewed while recalling organ position when the person is upright. Certain specific aspects of the anatomy are reviewed with emphasis on their use in surgical correction of anatomic defects.

The Bony Pelvis

In the upright position, the patient's pubic symphysis is the lowest point of the pelvis; the ischial spine, a landmark which can be palpated in almost every female patient because of vaginal access, is in a plane above the symphysis pubis.

The Fascial Pelvis

Several ligaments span the different bony protuberances within the pelvis, in an effort to reduce the open space. The two important structures, in view of their potential use for correction of defects, are the arcus tendineus fasciae pelvis and the sacrospinous ligament.

There are actually two "white lines" along the obturator fascia, one where the pubocervical fascia attaches and one where the levator muscle attaches. In most patients, it is close to impossible to differentiate both entities. This differentiation is of academic importance only.

The second important ligamentary structure is the sacrospinous ligament bridging the distance between the ischial spine and the sacrum. In the patient in the upright position, this ligament has a near horizontal course. The ligament runs in a plane which is parallel to the upper third of the vagina. Attachment of the vaginal vault to the ligament, therefore, positions the vaginal vault in a near physiologic position.

The Muscular Pelvis

The most important muscle of the pelvic floor is, without contest, the levator ani. Together with the sphincter muscles, the levator assures continence of urine and feces. The levator muscle describes the shape of a deep plate with a wedge, called the levator hiatus. The levator is attached to the bony and fascial pelvis all around, and in the contracted state elevates the contents of the pelvis to the level of the ischial spine, which is above the level of the symphysis pubis in the upright position. Contraction of the levator will also cause a narrowing of the levator hiatus. Therefore, contraction of the levator is an active tool in the prevention of prolapse of the pelvic viscera.

The Vascular Pelvis

The hypogastric artery separates the posterior pelvis from the anterior pelvis, and points toward the ischial spine. When viewing the pelvis in the upright position, one notes that the hypogastric artery runs perpendicular to the pelvic floor.

The second vessel of importance, because it must be avoided, is the obturator artery and vein. These vessels run through the obturator canal and will retract within this bony channel, with almost no chance of getting to them if sectioned. One should again emphasize the relation between the ischial spine, which can be palpated, and this anatomic structure, which is very often quite evident at laparoscopy. The two structures are situated on a horizontal line, when the pelvis is in the upright position. This is a great help. When one of the two structures is identified, it should be no challenge to find the other.

Knowledge of the positions of several other vessels is important to the surgeon, including the medial hemorrhoidal artery, which may be encountered when dissecting an enterocele. Bleeding from this artery is quite impressive; there is good collateral vascularization. The rectal pillars, which are dissected to a certain extent when performing a rectocele repair, are densely vascularized and injury of these structures can lead to postoperative hematoma formation within the rectovaginal space. The vascularization of the rectal pillars is dependent on the medial hemorrhoidal artery, itself a branch of the pudendal artery, or directly from the hypogastric artery. The main branch of the pudendal artery runs underneath the levator muscle together with the pudendal nerve along the side wall in the so-called Alcock's canal. It splits into branches, penetrating the levator muscles and surrounding loose connective tissues and skin from below. To avoid injury to the pudendal vessels, one should avoid placing sutures into the obturator fascia, below the level of the arcus tendineus.

The Neural Pelvis

The innervation of the pelvic organs follows vascularization in the same manner as in most other anatomic regions. The main nerve for the pelvic floor is the pudendal nerve, which, fortunately, runs mainly underneath the levator and therefore out of harm's way for the vaginal surgeon. Obviously, peripheral branches of the pudendal nerve are injured during vaginal surgery, more so than during abdominal surgery.

Innervation of bladder, uterus, and rectum is channeled mainly through the pelvic nerves of the hypogastric and pelvic plexus. The branches destined for the levator muscles run above the levator plate and can be injured during surgery involving the levator muscle itself. Bladder, uterus, and rectum innervation follows the sacrouterine ligaments, the hypogastric artery, and its tributaries. Injury to these neural paths is common during hysterectomy, most often in the so-called "extrafascial" procedure.

The Visceral Pelvis

The pelvic floor and more particularly, the levator hiatus, allow three structures to pass through: the urethra, the vagina, and the rectum. In the upright position, the initial course of all three structures is perpendicular to the pelvic floor. Immediately after passage of the levator hiatus, all three structures will start leaning to the hollow of the sacrum. The degree of bending increases from the front to the back. Contraction of the levator muscle exacerbates this bend and results in the typical telescoping effect of increased intraabdominal pressure upon the visceral pelvis.

The visceral pelvis is supported by a modified "mesenteric" structure which we call endopelvic fascia. The overall structure of this "mesentery" is, however, similar to any other mesentery in the abdominal cavity: it originates from the bony structures of the back and it contains the neurovascular channels necessary to the viscera it supports. The endopelvic fascia originates along the sacroiliac joints and the presacral fascia. Fibers extend all the way to the ischial spine and along the levator and obturator fascias. The hypogastric artery runs along these support structures in the tradition of the mesenteric structures. The ureter perforates the endopelvic fascia at the level known as the ureteral canal within the cardinal ligaments, but is otherwise not involved with the endopelvic fascia. The cardinal and sacro-uterine ligaments are densities of the same endopelvic fascial structure that is sometimes referred to as the Mackenrodt ligament. One particularity of the endopelvic fascia is that it totally enwraps the vagina, more so than the bladder or rectum. It appears that the vagina plays the role of the stronger of the three structures which pierce through the levator plate. Between the vagina and the bladder and rectum there are spaces, called the vesicovaginal and the rectovaginal spaces. The role of these spaces is unknown. One may, however, postulate that these spaces facilitate the expansion of both the bladder and the rectum, which have both a reservoir function.

The role of the endopelvic fascia in maintaining integrity of the pelvic floor should be considered. Little is known about the mechanisms of pelvic floor relaxation; the pathogenesis I most adhere to is the one based on the principle of active and passive support of the pelvic floor. The passive aspect of support is provided for by the peculiar anatomic construction of the human pelvic bony and ligamentary structures, whereas the active aspect is provided by the contractions of the levator muscles. It seems sensible, therefore, during surgery, to define the endopelvic fascia and to repair defects, if present. The fascial structures can also be strengthened by the use of tissue enhancers such as mesh— absorbable or not—and autologous grafts of fascial tissues such as vaginal total thickness grafts, fascia lata grafts, and so on.

PROCEDURES

The different procedures which involve the pelvic floor can be divided into two categories: anterior and posterior. Anterior procedures involve support of the anterior vaginal wall and the overlying urethra and bladder neck. Most of these procedures are intended to cure or to improve urinary incontinence. Among these procedures are the Marshall-Marchetti-Kranz urethropexy, the Burch-Tanagho urethropexy and the paravaginal repair. Plication of the pubourethral ligament combined with paravaginal repair is a variation of the latter procedure. More recently there have been attempts at reproducing abdominal sling procedures.

The posterior procedures include the rectocele repair, the enterocele repair such as the Moschcowitz or McCall procedure, and the sacral colpopexy. The most common of all posterior procedures is the enterocele repair. The difference between a high rectocele and an enterocele is usually one of semantics only. The sacral colpopexy is rather uncommon and does present with potentially serious complications. The procedures with which I am familiar are discussed below.

Urethropexy by Plication of the Pubourethral Ligament and Paravaginal Repair

The initial incision is made along the medial border of the patient's left umbilical ligament. The incision starts at the level of the upper border of the pubic bone and is continued until the midline trocar is reached and passed; thus the midline trocar becomes extraperitoneal. The loose areolar tissue and fascial planes are bluntly passed, until the pubic bone is reached.

Once the posterior aspect of the pubic bone is identified, the assistant can retract the bladder toward the right side, away from the field, lowering the risk of injury to the bladder while providing access to the Space of Retzius. The surgeon enters the retropubic space and dissects the pubic arch, either with scissors or with dissecting spatula. The fat within this space is gently removed to expose the anatomy of the region. The detail in which one can examine the bladder neck, urethra, and surrounding anatomy is astounding.

Vessels, mainly capillaries and veins, are distinguished easily in part because of the magnification inherent in all fixed-focus optical systems. Meticulous hemostasis is mandatory, because fluids tend to pool in the Space of Retzius and because blood tinges the tissues, making visual identification more difficult. Blunt dissection is continued, using scissors and irrigation probe, until the anatomy is clearly defined. In particular, it is necessary for the surgeon to be able to discern the pubourethral ligaments, the endopelvic fascia, the obturator fascia and Cooper's ligament. The pubovesical ligament, which is a single midline structure, has no role in the support of the bladder and/or urethra.

With the anatomy clearly identified, the operator now inserts a suture through the suprapubic trocar. I use Ethibond 2/0 (Ethicon, Sommerville, NJ) because it is long and nonabsorbable. Suturing, technically, is the difficult part of the procedure.

The right side suture is placed first. Placing the needle is done while the surgeon has his left hand in the patient's vagina, allowing him to displace the urethra to the left, so as to increase the available space. The groove between urethra and vagina is well delineated, even more when the surgeon pushes the vaginal wall up. During actual placement of the needle, however, there is more mobility for the needle and needle-holder, if the surgeon displaces the vagina to the left, rather than toward the pubic bone. The needle is placed through the middle of the pubourethral ligament, at about 1 to 1.5 cm from the lateral edge of the urethra. It is passed through the ligament from back to front. Care is taken to avoid the venous plexus, which runs in front of the urethra, (the dorsal vein of the clitoris). The needle is passed through the ligament only once. Whether a figure-eight approach would be better is not known. Next the needle is passed through the ligament of Cooper at the level of the pubic tubercle on the ipsilateral side. The needle is driven through the ligament from inside to outside and from posterior to anterior. This creates a simple loop between the two ligamentary structures. The free ends and the needle are pulled through the midline trocar. An extracorporeal knot is made and slipped down. The knot slides down and can be arrested at any level by pulling the short and long ends at 180°. That means that this slip knot can be positioned by the surgeon at almost any level he or she chooses. That is important in this case, because overcorrection is a complication most surgeons want to avoid. I do not implement a particular quantifiable method of evaluation of the bladder neck elevation, other than my best judgment.

The next suture connects the left pubourethral ligament with the left ligament of Cooper. Passage through the pubourethral ligament on the left is difficult because it requires mastering the backhand technique familiar to most microsurgeons. Alternatively, the surgeon may opt to use the needle-holder through the right lower port instead of the left. This will position the needle tip at straight angle with the ligament, ready for a simple forehand stitch.

Once the first pair of sutures is placed, the surgeon evaluates the need for additional support for the bladder base. I believe at least one additional suture should be placed to approximate the endopelvic fascia and the obturator fascia on both sides; I increase the number to three in cases with large paravaginal defects. Whether it is easier to place the most distal first (i.e. toward the ischial spine), is unclear. It is technically possible to place all sutures along one side,

without tying the knots until all sutures are placed to the satisfaction of the surgeon.

The insertion of vicryl mesh follows. This mesh is absorbable and will be replaced by natural scar tissue within 6 to 12 weeks after insertion. Two strips of 7-by-4 cm mesh are inserted and positioned along the suture lines, covering both the vaginal fascia and the obturator fascia, not the bladder (Figure 17-1).

After control of hemostasis, the peritoneal incision is closed with one or two sutures.

The procedure as described above has been performed by the author since early 1993. This was the second modification of the original procedure, performed since early 1990 and published in 1991. Surgical complications occurred in three cases, all of them bladder injuries. A laparotomy was performed to repair the injury in the first two. Subsequently, the bladder injury was treated by indwelling catheter only. One patient underwent a laparoscopy for a different problem approximately 18 months after the laparoscopy for correction of her urinary incontinence; herniation of small bowel within the Space of Retzius was noted. This was asymptomatic in this patient. Since this case, we close the incision of the parietal peritoneum. Two of the

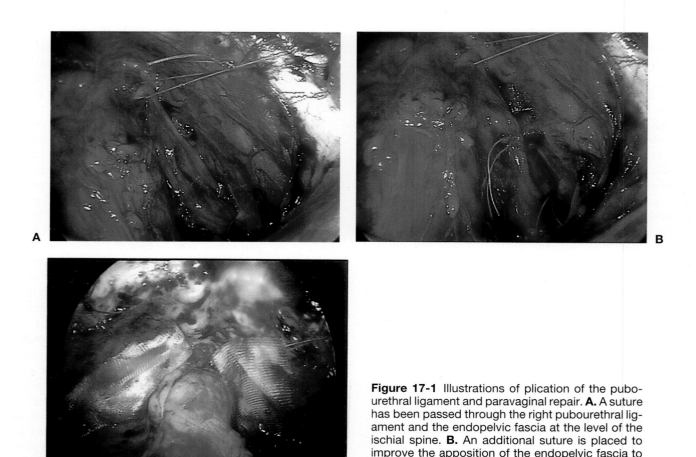

Figure 17-1 Illustrations of plication of the pubourethral ligament and paravaginal repair. **A.** A suture has been passed through the right pubourethral ligament and the endopelvic fascia at the level of the ischial spine. **B.** An additional suture is placed to improve the apposition of the endopelvic fascia to the obturator fascia. **C.** Vicryl mesh covers the suture line. View at the end of the procedure.

first four cases could not be finished under laparoscopy; laparotomy was required to complete the procedures.

In a cohort of 42 patients, who were operated upon between June 1991 and December 1992, 24% experienced continuing or de novo urgency symptomatology. In this same series, 40 patients were satisfied with the result of the surgical procedure. Although the surgical procedure was slightly different from the one presented (briefly, the urethropexy consisted of a single suture connecting the pubourethral ligament with Cooper's ligament), it may be safely assumed that the results after the procedure described above will be similar.

ENTEROCELE REPAIR

Once the laparoscope is introduced and the anatomical landmarks asserted, the first surgical step consists of resection of the hernia sac. The peritoneum of the hernia is placed under tension by traction with forceps. Scissors are used to incise the peritoneum along the sacrouterine ligaments and the posterior aspect of the vagina. Thus a flap of peritoneum is created, which is attached posteriorly to the rectum. The rectum is, partly sharply, and partly bluntly, detached from the peritoneum and the flap resected. The defect in the rectovaginal septum is now visible. Closure of the defect will result in occlusion of the enterocele and at the same time suspend the vagina at a higher level. This lengthens the vagina, which has a tendency to be shortened after posterior repair. The first suture is applied posteriorly, 2 to 3 cm in front of the dorsal insertion of the sacrouterine ligaments. The needle is first driven through the right ligament and then along the anterior wall of the rectum toward the left ligament. Care is taken not to strangle the rectum. Once the suture is tied, the position of the ureters is checked. Invariably, there is some degree of medial displacement. Should this move be judged excessive, a relief incision is made into the peritoneum below the ureter. The incision need not be deep, because the ureter lies immediately below the peritoneum at that level, and above the endopelvic fascia. These relief incisions will therefore not weaken the newly created pelvic floor. The next stitches incorporate the posterior vaginal wall, thereby reattaching the Denonvilliers' fascia with the sacrouterine ligaments. Finally, the peritoneal defect is closed with a few additional sutures.

This enterocele repair causes elongation of the vaginal conduit, but also reduces the pressure transfer from the abdomen to the urethra and may worsen a pre-existing urinary incontinence. One should also consider that if significant tension is necessary to approximate the sacrouterine ligaments, it may be better to incorporate one form of graft to bridge the gap between the ligaments.

During 1992, 18 patients underwent the above procedure. One case could not be completed for technical reasons, another patient continued to complain of a pressure sensation in the vagina despite a normal physical examination, and is considered a failure. The other 16 patients continue to do well.

ENTEROCELE REPAIR AND VAULT SUSPENSION USING VAGINAL SKIN GRAFT

The purpose of the procedure is to define the borders of the herniation which is the origin of the prolapse. The defect in the support structures is closed with the help of a vaginal skin graft; then the vagina is repositioned in a physiologic plane.

In order to strengthen the repair of the posterior compartment, it appears logical to reinforce the Denonvilliers' fascia with a graft, either autologous (vaginal skin) or artificial (vicryl mesh). The use of vaginal skin has been promoted by Zacharin. It makes perfect sense, because excess vaginal skin is resected in most cases and is therefore available. It does not cause a foreign body reaction, and the fear that epidermal inclusion cysts may become a problem has not yet materialized.

The procedure is started vaginally. If an anterior defect exists, the repair is performed prior to the posterior wall dissection. A transverse incision is made at the posterior fourchette to isolate the perineum from the vaginal mucosa. A strip of vaginal mucosa is prepared from the posterior wall, approximately 3 cm wide. The dissection is continued up to the vaginal vault, where the graft is separated and kept for later use in saline. The lateral walls of the vagina are then separated from the underlying connective tissues to identify the endopelvic fascia, or at least what is left of it. The rectal pillars are dissected free during this process. To reduce bleeding, the dissection is carried along as close to the vaginal wall as possible. The dissection is continued until the entire enterocele defect is dissected free; care is taken not to pierce the peritoneum.

The remnants of the Denonvilliers' fascia are identified and if still solid, used to close the rectocele and enterocele defects. If little strong tissue is identified, the surgeon will place sutures to approximate the levator muscles in front of the rectum. It is not necessary to actually pull the muscles together; a gap can be left. This gap is then bridged by placing the graft. The graft is placed, mucosal face down, on top of the fascia or muscle and attached to the perineal bodies proximally and to the levator plate laterally.

Next the vaginal wall is closed. Sometimes a small drain is inserted into the rectovaginal space and placed on low suction.

The laparoscopy is started in the usual fashion. A total of four trocars is used: 2 10-mm trocars in the midline and 2 5-mm trocars laterally. The pelvis is visualized and inspected. The enterocele sac which has been dissected already is cut out. The anatomic landmarks are identified: rectum, pararectal gutters, vagina, graft, bladder, and ureters. The remnants of the ligaments are retracted along the bottom of the broad ligaments. Next sutures are

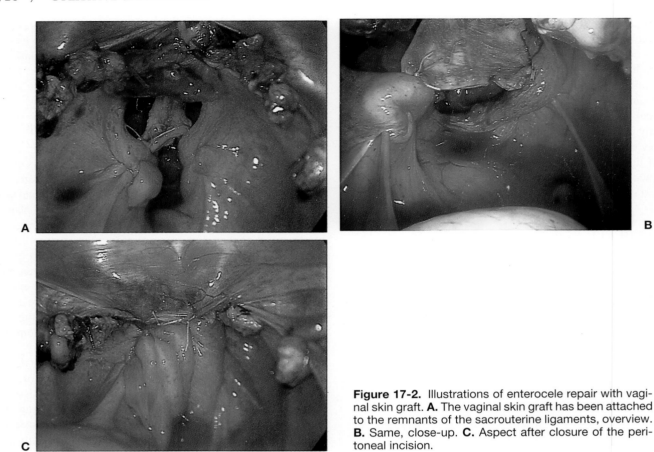

Figure 17-2. Illustrations of enterocele repair with vaginal skin graft. **A.** The vaginal skin graft has been attached to the remnants of the sacrouterine ligaments, overview. **B.** Same, close-up. **C.** Aspect after closure of the peritoneal incision.

placed which will connect the graft to the remnants of the sacrouterine ligaments on both sides. Once the graft is securely attached, the vagina is attached to the graft with no tension whatsoever. The peritoneum is then closed (Figure 17-2).

From January till December 1994, 12 patients underwent repair of an enterocele with or without vault prolapse, using a vaginal skin graft technique in a combined vaginal and abdominal approach. Two of them developed small inclusion cysts, which have remained asymptomatic. The repair of the posterior compartment appears to be holding. Four patients present with some degree of persisting anterior compartment defect, pointing to the need for better identification of the defects and more specific repair.

The major complications that arise in repair of the enterocele and vault prolapse involve the ureters. In some isolated cases, it may be necessary to define the course of the ureter surgically, especially on the left side. Although the hypogastric vessels are more cephalad to the space involved, vascular complications involving these vessels have occurred. Further, complications can occur in dissection of the hernia sac because it is situated close to the anterior border of the rectum; laceration of the rectum can occur. If this laceration is below the peritoneal reflection, primary closure, even in the absence of bowel preparation, is stan-

dard. Lacerations above the peritoneal reflection are, fortunately, less common, because their primary repair is prone to breakdown in the absence of a bowel preparation. For this reason, mechanical bowel preparation is highly recommended before the procedure begins. This practice, in addition to facilitating primary repair of rectal lacerations, also will increase the space available within the pelvis, because the bowel is empty. In the small series of 12 patients presented, there were, fortunately, none of these complications.

SACROCOLPOPEXY

It is unfortunate, in a sense, that true vaginal vault prolapse is such a rare condition, because this precludes us, as surgeons, from reaching proficiency in dealing with the condition. In my opinion, sacrocolpopexy is not an easy procedure and carries potentially fatal complications secondary to severe hemorrhage.

The procedure itself is an extension of the enterocele repair. The initial dissection is the same, but is carried upward along the right pararectal gutter to the promontorium. The graft used for this procedure should be longer, as it has to cover the distance between the perineal bodies and the promontorium. It is reasonable to use the vaginal skin for replacement of Denonvilliers' fascia and a mersilene mesh or vicryl mesh for replacement of the sacrouterine ligament. Variations are legion with reinforcement of the endopelvic fascia in various additional places, such as the upper anterior vaginal wall. The general principles of hernia surgery, i.e., avoidance of tension and generous use of tissue enhancement, continue to apply.

SUGGESTED READING

Benson JT (ed.). *Female Pelvic Floor Disorders: Investigation and Management.* Norton Medical Books.

Cusumano PG, Deprest JA (eds.). *Advanced Gynecologic Laparoscopy: A Practical Guide.* New York: Parthenon.

Nichols DH (ed.). *Gynecologic and Obstetric Surgery.* St. Louis: Mosby–Year Book, 1992.

Walters MD, Karram MM (eds). *Clinical Urogynecology.* St. Louis: Mosby–Year Book.

Operative Laparoscopy, Second Edition
The Masters' Techniques in Gynecologic Surgery
Lippincott–Raven Publishers, Philadelphia © 1998.

18

Laparoscopic Lymph Node Dissection

Joel M. Childers

The operative technique described in this chapter is radically different from that of most gynecologic operative laparoscopic procedures. It is a retroperitoneal procedure, and requires the surgeon to have solid knowledge of this anatomy, and a high level of comfort with retroperitoneal operative techniques. It also requires the surgeon to change his way of operating.

This paradigm shift is required for both laparoscopists and laparotomists. The laparotomist will no longer be able to use retractors in the retroperitoneal space, and will no longer need multiple clips. The laparoscopist will not need standard laparoscopic instruments or techniques. Bipolar electricity need not be on the operating table; aquadissection is never utilized; lasers are of no benefit; irrigation may be performed only at the end of the procedure, if at all; preoperative bowel preparation of the patient is mandatory.

The technique described in this chapter relies heavily on proven surgical principles: traction and countertraction, use of proper surgical planes, sharp and blunt dissection, and a surgeon operating with both hands. It also requires the surgeon to become a virtuoso with the oldest, least expensive, most common, and, in my opinion, the best energy source available to surgeons: monopolar electricity. Horror stories about monopolar electricity outdate us all. Electrical "gurus" shun its use, based on theory. Medicolegal experts are poised, ready to "fry" those who try. However, with this procedure, monopolar electricity is safe and efficient if certain principles are understood and important anatomical structures are kept out of harm's way.

If the operative laparoscopist performs the lymph node dissection outlined in this chapter, only two instruments will be used (scissors and graspers), only one instrument will be removed from its port during the entire procedure (a grasper to extract nodes as they are dissected), the surgeon will operate with both hands, and the assistant will provide exposure and visualization. A 30-minute operation quickly becomes a 2-hour operation if this paradigm shift is not made.

Lymph nodes from the abdominal aorta to the pelvic floor can be the primary sites of metastases in cervical, vaginal, endometrial, ovarian, and fallopian tube carcinomas. Most gynecologic malignancies are either staged surgically or managed surgically, and lymphadenectomy is the foundation of surgical staging for gynecologic malignancies.

Most gynecologic oncologists perform a selective lymphadenectomy or a lymph node sampling for gynecologic malignancies, with the exception of early carcinoma of the cervix, in which a complete or therapeutic lymphadenectomy is performed. Most of the regional lymph nodes are removed during a lymph node sampling procedure. However, emphasis is not placed on skeletonizing the vessels, as is done in a therapeutic, or complete, lymphadenectomy. For practical purposes, the procedure described in this chapter will be that of a selective lymphadenectomy.

Once the gynecologist has mastered the technique of laparoscopic lymphadenectomy, a whole new world opens up. The vast majority of early gynecologic malignancies and some advanced carcinomas can now be surgically managed by laparoscopy. As vaginal and laparoscopic operative skills improve, up to 75% of laparotomies may be avoided. This shift is already taking place in many practices, and it is safe to say that the gynecologic oncologist of the early twenty-first century will be an operative laparoscopist.

THE EVOLUTION

The technique described in this chapter is a transperitoneal approach to both pelvic and paraaortic lymph nodes that Dr. Earl Surwit and I developed beginning in 1990. However, it was the extraperitoneal approach of Daniel Dargent that ushered modern operative laparoscopy into the world of gynecologic oncology. The first transperitoneal lymphadenectomies were reported in 1991 by Querleu, et al. Reports on low laparoscopic paraaortic lymphadenectomy in patients with cervical, endometrial, and ovarian cancer, soon followed. The final phase of development of laparoscopic lymphadenectomy came with the ability to perform high paraaortic or infrarenal lymphadenectomies, which is necessary for the staging of patients with ovarian and fallopian tube cancer.

Preoperative Considerations

Obviously, routine preoperative preparation is necessary, and issues such as informed consent and proper patient selection will not be discussed here. However, one subject worthy of mention, since most gynecologists do not routinely perform this, is that of bowel preparation. Evacuating the large and small bowel facilitates the laparoscopic lymphadenectomy and, potentially, reduces the likelihood and morbidity of enterotomy. This is easily accomplished by having the patient on a liquid diet for two days prior to the procedure and administering one bottle (240 cc) of magnesium citrate one and two days prior to the procedure. An enema on the morning of admission will aid in the evacuation of the lower colon.

Anesthesia and Operating Room Considerations

General anesthesia is used. An endotracheal tube is placed and end-tidal carbon dioxide is monitored. A nasogastric or oral gastric tube is inserted to empty the stomach contents prior to placement of the primary trocar or Veress needle. A pulse oximeter is used and a Foley catheter is placed. The patients' arms are tucked to the sides, with consideration for padding of the ulnar nerve. Sequential compression stockings are currently used.

Instrumentation

In general, the procedure can be accomplished with a few simple laparoscopic instruments. It is necessary to have: (a) *sharp scissors* with monopolar electrocautery capabilities (these should be with Metzenbaum-like tips); (b) grasping forceps with tips large enough to grab large nodal bundles and extract them through a 12-mm laparoscopic sleeve; (c) an irrigation-suction apparatus. A 10-mm laparoscopic telescope with a 0° lens is preferable for most cases. On occasion, the laparoscopic clip-applier may be needed. This is most commonly used for perforating veins over the vena cava.

OPERATIVE TECHNIQUE

Port Placement

Four laparoscopic ports are needed to perform this procedure (Figure 18-1). The primary port is placed in the umbilicus and should be at least 10 mm in size for use with a 10-mm telescope and camera. I believe it is important to place the umbilical port in the base of the umbilicus at a 90° angle to the abdominal wall, as opposed to a subumbilical insertion at a 45° angle. The latter method of subumbilical port placement can lead to a large amount of abdominal tissue between the site of insertion on the skin and the site of entrance into the intraperitoneal cavity. This large fulcrum of skin makes it difficult to direct the laparoscopic camera to the upper abdomen or to the paraaortic area. With placement through the base of the umbilicus, the umbilical port can easily be directed to the pelvis or the upper abdomen. Furthermore, with a skin incision made in the base of the umbilicus by a No. 11 blade scalpel and with upward traction on the anterior abdominal wall by towel clips, the peritoneal cavity is, in most instances, entered. When this is done, the umbilical sleeve can be placed into the intraperitoneal cavity without a trocar. This is safer than direct trocar insertion and quicker than open laparoscopy. The three ancillary ports are placed under direct laparoscopic visualization. Two 5-mm trocars and sleeves are placed lateral to the inferior epigastric vessels and the rectus muscle bilaterally. The third ancillary port is placed in the midline above the symphysis and should be 12 mm in size to allow removal of the nodal tissue, which at times can contain sizeable specimens.

Inspection of the Intraperitoneal Cavity

After the laparoscopic ports are in place and before the patient is placed in Trendelenburg position, it is important to explore the entire intraperitoneal cavity. This should be done in a systematic fashion and should specifically include areas to which gynecologic malignancies metastasize. If pelvic washings are to be taken, they should be obtained before any operative procedures are undertaken.

Laparoscopic Pelvic Lymphadenectomy

Laparoscopic lymphadenectomy, like lymphadenectomy performed at laparotomy, can be accomplished in a number of ways. In general, however, it is easier if the surgeon stands on the side opposite that of the nodes to be dissected. The telescope is placed through the umbilical port and is held by the assistant. The assistant also uses a grasper, placed through the lateral port on the side where he or she is standing. The surgeon, on the opposite side, uses a grasper through the lower midline port and scissors with monopolar cautery capability through the lateral port.

The peritoneum is picked up and incised over the psoas muscle near the external iliac artery, between the round and infundibulopelvic ligaments. These ligaments can be left intact, but greater exposure is offered if they are transected. The broad ligament is opened and the obliterated umbilical artery is identified. This built-in retractor is retracted medially, opening the paravesical and obturator spaces. The obliterated umbilical artery can easily be identified in the pelvis of thin patients adjacent to the external iliac vein. In

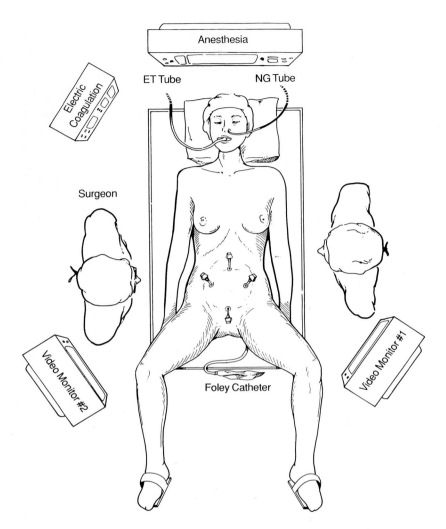

Figure 18-1 Four laparoscopic ports are needed to perform the lymphadenectomy described in this chapter. The umbilical port needs to be large enough to accommodate a 10-mm telescope. It is recommended that the suprapubic port be 12 mm in size to accommodate easy removal of large lymph-node bundles. The lateral ports are 5 mm in size and are placed lateral to the rectus muscle and inferior epigastric vessels. The patient's arms are tucked at her sides, with careful emphasis on protecting the ulnar nerve. A Foley catheter has been placed in the bladder and the stomach has been decompressed.

patients with more adipose tissue, the umbilical artery can be identified in the pelvis by pushing on it at the anterior abdominal wall and watching for its movement in the pelvis. The avascular plane between the obliterated umbilical artery and external iliac vein is easily opened, exposing the obturator space very nicely.

It is advisable to perform the obturator lymphadenectomy first, because blood, lymph fluid, or irrigation fluid can accumulate in this dependent area and may obscure visualization somewhat if these nodes are not removed first. The obturator nerve is identified and the nodal tissue on the anterior surface of the nerve is dissected off, bluntly. The nodal tissue along the medial aspect of the external iliac vein is then dissected off, along the length of the vein. In performing this dissection, care should be taken not to damage any aberrant or accessory veins emptying into the external iliac vein. The proper plane between the nodal tissue and the vein can be identified easily by seizing nodal tissue with the grasper and retracting it medially. The scissors tips

can be placed into the space and opened, and the remaining tissue can easily be bluntly separated.

It is my preference then to follow the nodal bundle distally to the pelvic wall and transect the nodal package at the pelvic wall with monopolar electrocautery. I use a fulgurating technique in which the scissors tips are held adjacent to the nodal tissue to be transected and the spark is allowed to jump to the nodal tissue. Traction on the nodal bundle is mandatory. Once this is completed, the only remaining attachment of the obturator nodal package is at the junction of the hypogastric and external iliac arteries. This is usually the most difficult part of removing the obturator nodes. Adequate visualization can be difficult to obtain because the nodal bundle starts to course laterally. Furthermore, the ureter crosses the iliac vessels in this area, making the ureter more likely to be injured during this portion of the dissection. The safest way to extract the cephalad extent of this bundle is by blunt traction, pulling the node away from the vein and underlying obturator nerve. The nodal bundle is removed intact through the lower 10 to 12-mm port using the large forceps.

Removal of the external lymph nodes is performed in a fashion similar to that of laparotomy. The assistant retracts the distal transected round ligament, offering exposure to the distal external iliac vessels, and the surgeon substitutes monopolar electricity for surgical clips. This dissection is accomplished by creating a plane in the adventitia of the external iliac artery and dissecting it up to the circumflex iliac artery. Effort must be made to avoid damaging the genitofemoral nerve laterally. The dissection can be extended proximally to the point where the ovarian vessels and/or the ureter cross the iliac vessels. Here, the assistant must retract the ureter in a cephalad and medial direction. The nodal dissection can be continued then, up the distal common iliac artery (Figures 18-2 and 18-3).

When the surgeon removes the left pelvic lymph nodes, he or she must take down the rectosigmoid from the left pelvic sidewall. This can be accomplished by incising the peritoneum in this area along the white line of Toldt, which will give access to the retroperitoneal space. If mobilization of the rectosigmoid is not required, the same incision, as previously described, is made between the round ligament and the ovarian vessels. The surgeon stands on the right side of the patient and operates through the midline port with graspers and the lateral port with scissors.

At the end of the procedure, the operative site can be irrigated and inspected to ensure that hemostasis is adequate. The peritoneum is left open and no drains are used.

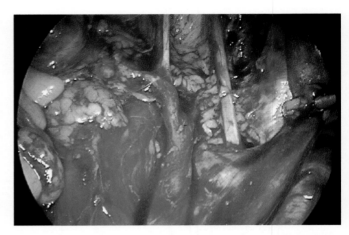

Figure 18-3 This closeup photograph was taken after a right-side pelvic lymphadenectomy. The external iliac artery and vein are being retracted laterally by the tip of a grasper, seen on the right side of this photograph. The internal iliac artery is seen running vertically in the center of the photograph. Note that it gives rise to the uterine artery, which branches medially, and continues to the top of the photograph as the obliterated umbilical artery. This is an unusual view of the internal iliac vein emptying into the external iliac vein, and the obturator nerve can be seen exiting from behind this vein, running vertically to the top of the photograph.

Laparoscopic Paraaortic Lymphadenectomy

Sampling of the paraaortic lymph nodes cannot be accomplished without adequate exposure, which requires placement of the omentum, transverse colon, and small bowel into the upper abdomen. The laparoscope can be placed temporarily through the suprapubic port to obtain a more panoramic view. The omentum can be flipped on its pedicle and placed atop the liver. The stomach should be adequately decompressed. Next, the small bowel should be flipped on its mesenteric pedicle in a cephalad direction and splayed out across the upper abdomen. Trendelenburg position, a good bowel preparation, and, occasionally, lateral tilt of the operating table, assist in keeping the bowel in the upper abdomen. It is during this process that the small bowel can be inspected for metastatic disease. This "packing" of the bowel is extremely important, and time should be taken to accomplish this correctly, lest time be lost later. Occasionally, the use of additional 5-mm left or right upper quadrant ports to keep the bowel in the upper abdomen may be required to accomplish a paraaortic lymphadenectomy, especially in heavier patients. Depending on the patient's anatomy, the transverse duodenum can often be visualized as it crosses the vena cava and aorta. Lifting the mesentery of the small bowel as it crosses the aorta will aid in visualizing the third portion of the duodenum. Sometimes the peritoneum over the aorta and proximal right common iliac artery will need to be incised and mobilized before the transverse duodenum can be visualized. The aorta, right

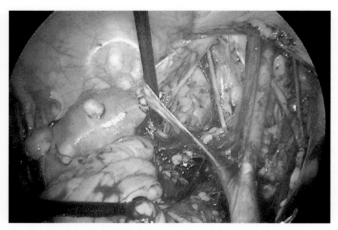

Figure 18-2 This photograph was taken after a right pelvic lymphadenectomy had been performed. The laparoscopic instrument in the top center of the photograph has been placed through the suprapubic port and is retracting the obliterated umbilical artery medially. Note that the obliterated umbilical artery is an extension of the hypogastric artery, a branch of the common iliac artery, seen on the bottom right portion of the photograph. Retraction of this vessel opens the obturator space. The obturator nerve can be seen running vertically in this photograph between the obliterated umbilical artery on the left and the external iliac artery and vein on the right.

common iliac artery, and the ureter as it crosses the right iliac vessels, are landmarks that should be identified before the dissection begins.

Right-side Paraaortic Lymphadenectomy

There are a number of ways to sample the paraaortic lymph nodes laparoscopically. The surgeon can stand on the side of the patient, or between the patient's legs. The telescope can be placed through the umbilical or suprapubic port. The technique described here mimics that of the procedure performed at laparotomy, and is therefore easy to learn.

The surgeon, on the left side of the patient, performs the procedure with graspers in the lower midline port and scissors in the left lateral port, identical to the positions in the pelvic dissection. The assistant holds the camera in the umbilical port and uses graspers in the right lateral port. It is helpful to rotate the camera so that the aorta and vena cava are horizontal on the color monitor, with the patient's head to the right of the monitor. It is also helpful to move the monitors from the foot of the operating table to the side of the patient, either near the umbilicus or near the patient's head. In this situation, two monitors may be necessary.

An incision is made in the peritoneum, over the aorta. This incision is extended down the right common iliac artery to where the ureter crosses the iliac vessels, and up the aorta to the mesentery of the small bowel or the transverse duodenum. The peritoneum is lifted with graspers, and blunt dissection is performed laterally toward the right psoas muscle. The right ureter is identified and lifted away from the underlying psoas muscle. The grasper in the midline port is used then to elevate the ureter anteriorly and laterally. The right psoas and tendon of the psoas should be easily seen.

The assistant then places his or her grasper (in the right lateral port) beneath the ureter to retract it anteriorly and laterally out of the operative field. This also creates a small ''tent,'' which helps prevent small bowel from falling into the operative field.

The surgeon then dissects the nodal and fatty tissue off the aorta, by first sharply developing the adventitial plane of the aorta. This arterial dissection is continued in a cephalad and caudad direction, up the aorta and down the common iliac artery, using the scissors and electrocautery as needed. Lateral dissection is then performed toward the psoas muscle, so that the nodal bundle is separated from the underlying vena cava. Care should be taken to avoid lacerating perforating vessels when unroofing the vena cava. It is uncommon to encounter a perforator from the vena cava that cannot be controlled with monopolar electricity. Only through experience will the surgeon gain an appreciation for which perforating vessels should be clipped. If there is any doubt, the clip applicator should be used; but as stated, with experience this is an uncommon

event. Dissection is continued up and down the vena cava. Small vessels and lymphatic channels are coagulated easily with monopolar electricity.

One end of the nodal bundle is then transected. This can be easily and quickly performed by using short bursts of monopolar electrocautery in a fulgurating fashion. Once the nodal package is transected at one end, it is easy to peel the bundle off the vena cava toward the opposite end. Transection of the remaining end is again accomplished by monopolar electrocautery. When transecting the cephalad end of this bundle, the surgeon avoids injury to the transverse duodenum, and when transecting the caudad end of the bundle, to the right ureter. The nodal tissue is extracted by using the large forceps through the lower midline port. The operative field is irrigated and hemostasis is secured (Figure 18-4).

If the nodal tissue over the right common iliac artery is to be removed as well, this can be accomplished through the same peritoneal incision. The assistant uses his or her grasper to retract the ureter atraumatically in a caudad direction. This will provide exposure to the nodal tissue over this artery and beyond its bifurcation. The nodal dissection is then continued down the common iliac to the proximal internal and external iliac vessels.

Left-Side Paraaortic Lymphadenectomy

The surgeon, on the right side of the patient or between the patient's legs, performs this procedure using a grasper placed through the lower midline and scissors through the right lateral port. The assistant holds the telescope and camera through the umbilical port. The camera is rotated so that the surgeon is comfortably oriented.

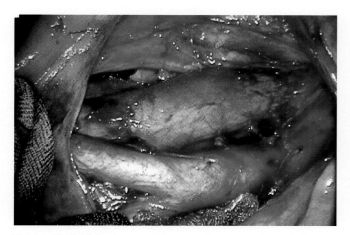

Figure 18-4 This photograph was taken after completion of a low right paraaortic lymphadenectomy. The aorta and right common iliac artery run horizontally across the screen. The lymph-node bundle overlying the vena cava has been completely removed. Note the blue tape of a mini-laparotomy pad on the left side of the photograph. It has been placed intraperitoneally to assure hemostasis.

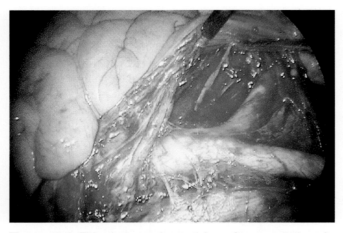

Figure 18-5 This photograph was taken after completion of a low left paraaortic lymphadenectomy. The aorta is running horizontally in the picture and gives rise to the right and left common iliac artery, seen on the right side of the photograph. The dark laparoscopy instrument at the top of the photograph is placed through the left lateral port and is retracting the inferior mesenteric artery, the mesentery of the rectosigmoid, and the left ureter and ovarian veins. Note that the nodal tissue over the proximal one-half of the left common iliac artery has been removed.

If the peritoneal incision has not already been made, an incision is made similar to that used for the right-side para-aortic lymphadenectomy. This incision over the aorta is extended in the cephalad direction as far as possible. The mesentery of the small bowel or the third portion of the duodenum will limit the cephalad extent. The incision is extended in a caudad direction over the proximal left common iliac artery.

The surgeon first dissects in the adventitial plane of the aorta in a cephalad and caudad direction. It is important to extend this adventitial dissection as far as possible in both directions, to allow ample room to safely perform the lymphadenectomy. On the left side, the cephalad extent will be limited by the inferior mesenteric artery. Care should be taken to avoid injuring this artery, as its origin on the abdominal aorta is often difficult to identify. The more the aorta and left common iliac are "cleaned off," the more space and visibility the surgeon will have.

Only *after* the adventitia over the aorta has been adequately dissected free should lateral dissection toward the left psoas muscle be carried out. I believe this greatly assists in the identification of the proper surgical plane for lateral dissection. Using this plane, the surgeon can dissect safely beneath the left ureter and mesentery of the rectosigmoid. This differs from the right-sided paraaortic lymphadenectomy, where lateral dissection is carried out after making the peritoneal incision but before dissecting the aortic adventitia. Identification of the proper plane is critical. If the surgeon dissects laterally anterior to the proper plane, which is easy to do, the left lumbar ureter or inferior mesenteric

artery may be left posterior and subsequently injured during extraction of the nodes.

Lateral dissection is performed until the psoas muscle and its tendon are identified. The assistant now places the grasper (left lateral port) into the dissected space beneath the mesentery of the rectosigmoid and the left ureter. This retraction is paramount for adequate exposure, which is mandatory, because the left-sided paraaortic lymph nodes in this area are lateral to the aorta.

Once adequate exposure has been created, the surgeon grasps the nodal bundle adjacent to either the aorta or the proximal common iliac artery, and lifts anteriorly while simultaneously pushing down slightly on the aorta with the scissors. This frees the loose attachments between these two structures and assists in dissecting beneath the nodal chain. This blunt dissection creates a window beneath the nodal chain at its caudad end. Transection of the nodal chain is easily accomplished with scissors and electrocautery. The dissection is then extended in a cephalad direction, using blunt and sharp dissection, and electrocautery with the scissors, as needed. The nodal chain is then transected at the cephalad end near the inferior mesenteric artery. The specimen is removed through the lower midline 12-mm port and the operative field is irrigated and inspected for hemostasis (Figures 18-5 and 18-6).

Infrarenal Paraaortic Lymphadenectomy

To sample the paraaortic lymph nodes above the inferior mesenteric artery, the avascular plane between the transverse duodenum and the vena cava and the aorta is opened by blunt and sharp dissection. The surgeon continues this dissection in a cephalad and *lateral* direction. The assistant provides exposure by maintaining upward retraction on the

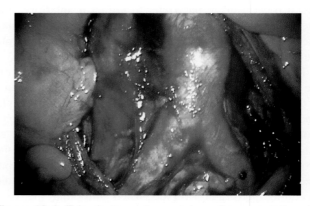

Figure 18-6 This photograph was taken after completion of a low left and right paraaortic lymphadenectomy. The nodal tissue below the inferior mesenteric artery overlying the vena cava and lateral to the left side of the aorta has been completely removed. Note that the nodal tissue over the proximal common iliac arteries is also removed during this step of the operation.

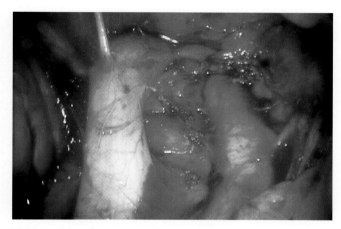

Figure 18-7 This photograph was taken from the umbilicus during an infrarenal lymphadenectomy. The vena cava is seen running vertically on the left side of the photograph, and the right ovarian vein can be seen emptying into the vena cava at the top portion of the photograph. The aorta runs vertically and on the right side of the photograph. The renal vein can be seen crossing the aorta at the top of the photograph, emptying into the vena cava, and the origin of the inferior mesenteric artery can be seen on the left side of the photograph. Note that in elevating the transverse duodenum, the vena cava can be lifted slightly from its underlying vertebral bodies and the aorta and the vena cava can be separated somewhat, simplifying removal of the lymph-node tissue between these great vessels. Note that the nodal tissue between the inferior mesenteric artery and the left renal vein has not yet been extracted.

transverse duodenum. These higher nodes can be removed with the surgeon standing on either the left or right side of the patient or between the patient's legs.

After adequate cephalad exposure is obtained, the nodal dissection is begun. On the right, this is simply a matter of continuing the previously performed lymphadenectomy up to the origin of the ovarian vein, which may enter the vena cava distal to, or very near, the left renal vein. On the left, the surgeon is faced with the lateral location of the nodal chain, and working around the inferior mesenteric artery. It is extremely important to identify the left renal and ovarian veins as soon as possible. They are often disguised in the endoabdominal fascia and could be easily damaged. Once these vessels are located, dissection in the adventitia of the aorta should be carried out. With generous use of monopolar electricity, annoying small bleeders will be minimized. The ovarian artery may need to be sacrificed; this can be done with clips or bipolar or monopolar electricity. The nodal bundle is transected near the left renal vein. This entire dissection can be performed with scissors and monopolar electricity (Figure 18-7).

The peritoneum is not closed and no retroperitoneal drains are placed. The mesentery of the small bowel is repositioned over the paraaortic incision site at the end of the dissection. Patients undergoing laparoscopic lymphadenectomy only are given a regular diet on the day of the procedure.

PITFALLS

If performed properly, laparoscopic lymphadenectomy is a two-person, four-port operation. Once the operation begins, the only instrument to be removed from a port is the grasper, through the suprapubic port site, and this is done only to remove lymph nodes as they are dissected.

Like most operations, laparoscopic lymphadenectomy can be accomplished in a number of ways. One of the biggest pitfalls, however, is utilizing traditional laparoscopic surgical techniques for this procedure. This usually results in irrigating and aspirating too frequently and over-utilization of clip applicators and bipolar electrocautery forceps. For this operation, these steps are time-consuming and generally unnecessary. This constant changing of laparoscopic instruments only slows the process.

Another common pitfall is the inappropriate use of monopolar electricity. The greatest mistake is using another instrument to accomplish what monopolar electricity can accomplish. This only results in loss of valuable time and possible increase of the cost of the operation (e.g., disposable clip applicators). In my experience, bipolar energy and clip applicators are virtually never needed for pelvic lymphadenectomies and only rarely for low paraaortic lymphadenectomies. Another mistake with monopolar electricity is its misuse. When it is used appropriately, only short bursts of electrical energy are required. In most instances, the fulgurating technique is all that is needed. Occasionally, large vessels will need to be coapted. In these instances, the vessel is grasped and the scissors apply "cutting" current to the grasper.

As the surgeon becomes adept at this process, the lymph-node bundles removed will be virtually intact. Some of these bundles, like the obturator nodal bundle, can be quite large, and for that reason, use of a 12-mm suprapubic port is strongly recommended. Large lateral ports are not necessary and only increase the incidence of postoperative pain and the likelihood of postoperative bowel herniation.

If the surgeon is not careful with hemostasis, the retroperitoneal tissue is readily bloodstained, which absorbs light, and, even with excellent cameras, visualization is decreased. Preoperative bowel preparation is mandatory.

In the pelvis, the most common complications will be injury to the genitofemoral nerve and injury to an aberrant or accessory obturator vein. Experience and attention to detail will minimize the frequency of these complications. Injury to the left pelvic ureter near the bifurcation of the common iliac vessels can be prevented by a good assistant who without trauma retracts the ureter medially while the surgeon is operating in this area.

Proper identification of the appropriate surgical planes is mandatory. In the pelvis, the key is in learning to identify quickly the obliterated umbilical artery. This key landmark is the door to the avascular plane that opens the obturator space. In the right paraaortic area, the crucial plane is between the ureter and the ovarian vessels anteriorly, and the vena cava nodal pad and psoas muscle posteriorly. The right ureter must be separated from the psoas muscle to avoid injury. In the left paraaortic area the crucial plane is beneath the inferior mesenteric artery, the ureter, and the ovarian vessels. This plane is more posterior than one may think. If the adventitial plane over the aorta and left common iliac artery are not cleaned off first, it is easy for the surgeon to dissect laterally toward the psoas muscle in the wrong plane. It is here where the left lumbar ureter and inferior mesenteric artery can easily be damaged during lymph node dissection. When removing the infrarenal lymph nodes it is mandatory that enough blunt and sharp dissection be performed to allow identification of the left renal vein as it crosses the aorta and the left ovarian vein as it empties into the left renal vein, prior to performance of the lymphadenectomy. If the lymph nodes are attacked before proper identification of these landmarks is made, disastrous results may ensue.

Finally, it should come as no surprise that there is a learning curve associated with this surgical procedure. It is unlikely that this procedure will be mastered by the surgeon with no experience in open pelvic and paraaortic lymphadenectomy, or by the experienced oncologic surgeon who performs this laparoscopic procedure only occasionally. Only the experienced, committed, laparoscopist will master the laparoscopic pelvic and paraaortic lymphadenectomy.

SUGGESTED READING

Childers JM, Hatch KD, Surwit EA. Laparoscopic paraaortic lymphadenectomy in gynecologic malignancies. *Obstet Gynecol* 1993; 82:741–47.

Childers J, Hatch K, Surwit E. The role of laparoscopic lymphadenectomy in the management of cervical cancer. *Gyn Oncol* 1992;47:38–43.

Childers J, Lang J, Surwit E, Hatch K. Laparoscopic surgical staging of ovarian cancer. *Gynecol Oncol* 1995;59:25–33.

Querleu D. Laparoscopic paraaortic node sampling in gynecologic oncology: a preliminary experience. *Gynecol Oncol* 1993;49:24–9.

Querleu D, LeBlanc E. Laparoscopic infrarenal paraaortic node dissection in the restaging of carcinomas of the ovary and fallopian tube. *Cancer* 1994;73:1467–71.

Querleu D, LeBlanc E, Castelain B. Laparoscopic pelvic lymphadenectomy in the staging of early carcinoma of the cervix. *Am J Obstet Gynecol* 1991;164:579–81.

Spirtos N, Schlaerth J, Spirtos T, Schlaerth A, Indman P, Kimball R. Laparoscopic bilateral pelvic and paraaortic lymph node sampling: an evolving technique. *Am J Obstet Gynecol* 1995;173:105–11.

Operative Laparoscopy, Second Edition
The Masters' Techniques in Gynecologic Surgery
Lippincott–Raven Publishers, Philadelphia © 1998.

19

Laparoscopic Retropubic Urethrocolpopexy

Marshall L. Smith, Jr.

While the anterior colporrhaphy has been utilized for many years for the problem of anatomical urinary stress incontinence, most authorities at this point agree the more effective and longer lasting surgical treatment for incontinence is the retropubic approach. There have been numerous techniques described by this approach, but the procedure as described by Burch seems to be most widely accepted as the "gold standard." This involves placement of sutures in the pubocervical fascia lateral to the urethral vesical angle and suspending them into Cooper's ligament. Traditionally, this has been performed through an abdominal incision with open dissection into the Space of Retzius. But, again, the patient is subjected to the morbidity and prolonged recovery of the abdominal incision. The retropubic urethropexy was first performed laparoscopically by Dr. Vancaillie and Dr. Liu, and most techniques today use modifications of their approaches.

While the workup leading to the decision to perform a retropubic urethropexy is beyond the scope of this chapter I would emphasize the fact that this decision should be independent of the type of approach utilized. As with most laparoscopic procedures the procedure should be performed no more frequently just because it can be accomplished laparoscopically.

INDICATIONS

I utilize preoperative urodynamics liberally in evaluating these patients, and in addition always evaluate the mobility of the urethra with transperineal ultrasound. Once I feel comfortable that hypermobility of the urethra is a major component of the patient's problem and all other treatments have been either tried or offered, I discuss with the patient the surgical approach for her incontinence. As long as there are no contraindications, I tell her that the procedure can be performed laparoscopically; that it is a well-established procedure, and that the technique of suture placement is identical to the open one, except that we use smaller incisions.

In actuality, I feel I can place the sutures more precisely now through a laparoscopic rather than through an open incision; because technical advances have improved visibility greatly in laparoscopy. I explain that the sutures are placed in the identical location whether it is done through an open procedure or a laparoscopic one. I then go over the usual counseling before a procedure; the alternatives to surgery, the patient's expectations, the risks and complications, and the failure rate.

Previous abdominal incisions are not a contraindication to a laparoscopic urethropexy even when planning a preperitoneal approach. The dissection into the Space of Retzius may be a little more difficult and more tedious, but it can be accomplished in most patients. A previous needle suspension procedure or even a Marshall-Marchetti-Krantz (MMK) is also not a contraindication, although it is more difficult and requires more laparoscopic dissection. I would not recommend this approach for your initial case. If I can review the operative notes and ensure that it was indeed an MMK, then the more lateral areas of the Space of Retzius are usually not so dense with adhesions and can be dissected out. If a patient has had extensive surgery with problems in the retropubic space (e.g. previous Burch procedure with an infection or hematoma), I resort to an open procedure; there are just some times when discretion is the better part of valor. And, regardless of her previous surgical history, I always counsel the patient when discussing the surgery that we may have to resort to an abdominal incision if we cannot accomplish the procedure laparoscopically. Most patients seem to accept this contingency because it would be the surgical alternative.

INTRAOPERATIVE

After the patient is taken to the operating room and general anesthesia has been initiated, I personally place the patient's legs in the stirrups. I use an Allens-type stirrup and pad the patient's legs with foam rubber; the patient is placed in a modified dorsal lithotomy position. A Foley catheter is placed and I utilize a 5-cc bulb with 10 ccs of fluid placed in the bulb. I do not like a 30-cc bulb because it restricts my dissection and access to the paravaginal areas. The catheter is attached to a partially empty IV bag of fluid via a step-down adapter and cysto tubing. Part of the fluid from the IV bag is emptied to allow urine to drain during the procedure; the bag is placed on the floor and the tubing opened. This functions as a catheter bag during the surgery, but by simply lifting the bag to an IV stand the bladder can be filled quickly. When I was using the transperitoneal approach, I would put dye in the bag and use the partially filled bladder as a landmark for dissection. The setup should be double-checked to make sure that the tubing is open, because the tendency is to keep the tubing closed when connecting it. If you forget to open the drainage system to allow the bladder to drain, the distended bladder can make it extremely difficult to dissect the pubocervical fascia. I always double-check to ensure the catheter has been open when I have difficulty dissecting down into the Space of Retzius (it only has to happen to you once). Once the bladder is drained and the Foley catheter opened to ensure continuous drainage, I begin the surgery.

I have changed my techniques since I began performing the procedure several years ago. Initially, nearly everyone using the laparoscopic approach entered the abdominal cavity and then exited via a transverse peritoneal incision over the cephalic margin of the bladder. The dissection was carried over the bladder through the preperitoneal area into the Space of Retzius. This technique does provide a larger opened area in which to work and is actually easier to suture and sew in because of the angle of the trocars and instruments. However, in my practice I have found this approach to be both more bloody and more time-consuming; there are numerous vessels that have to be controlled during this preperitoneal dissection. It also requires closure of the peritoneum afterward, which is another time-consuming step. Nevertheless, if you are already inside the abdominal cavity or just beginning to learn the technique, this approach can be readily utilized. A semi-lunar transverse incision between the umbilical ligaments is performed in the parietal peritoneum approximately two cm above the cephalic margin of the bladder (Figure 19-1). I usually enter in the midline, where there is a vessel associated with the urachus which must be addressed and controlled. When the preperitoneal fatty area is entered, you must dissect into this layer slightly to find the correct plane. I describe it as a thin, weblike layer of tissue. When this plane is entered, it opens up readily, down to the pubic bone. The whiteness of the pubic bone is easily visible as you approach it, and once I have located the bone and oriented myself I take the dissection laterally. There are always some small but troublesome vessels in this lateral dissection, but there should be no major vessels as long as you stay medial to the umbilical ligaments. Once the pubic bone and rami are visualized, the areas for suture placement are dissected out and the pro-

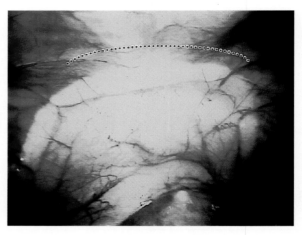

Figure 19-1 Line of incision in the parietal peritoneum when dissecting into the Space of Retzius from inside the abdominal cavity. The incision should be made approximately 2 cm above the cephalic margin of the bladder and kept between the umbilical ligaments.

cedure performed as described below. At the end of the procedure, the peritoneum has to be reattached. There are some surgeons who do not close the peritoneum, but my concern is a loop of bowel becoming attached or strangulated down into this defect. I utilized a hernia stapler to close the peritoneum when I used this technique, but with this method, you have the problem of cost and larger trocars. Suturing the peritoneum is certainly another option, if you can do it in a timely fashion.

The next technique I utilized was the preperitoneal approach with a balloon dissector; in this way I avoided having to enter the abdominal cavity. Staying preperitoneal is a distinct advantage, but I found the balloon to be cumbersome at times. Insertion required an open dissection down to the rectus muscle, and precise placement in the preperitoneal space was not always possible. Expense was another consideration. I stopped using the balloon and began to use an optical trocar for dissection into the preperitoneal area. I presently use the Visiport and I have found this to be much easier, quicker, and a less expensive method of gaining access to and opening the Space of Retzius by a preperitoneal approach.

Once the abdomen is prepped and draped, I utilize a subumbilical skin incision. I do not perform the incision at the depth of the umbilicus, as I want to avoid the areas of fusion of the fascial layers immediately underneath the umbilicus. After the incision in the caudal portion of the umbilicus, I place the laparoscope and the Visiport through this incision. I am very careful not to enter the fascia, but to stay in the subcutaneous fat. Utilizing primarily blunt dissection with the trocar, I carry this dissection down in the subcutaneous fat to a location three to four cm caudal to the umbilicus and two to three cm lateral to the midline. Note that I can see exactly where I am at all times through the end of the

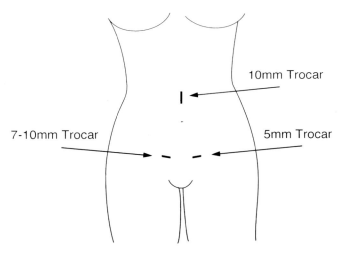

Figure 19-2 Trocar placement for a laparoscopic retropubic colpopexy with an extraperitoneal approach to the Space of Retzius. Note that the sites are much lower and closer to the midline than the usual operative sites. The trocars should be placed just at the lateral margin of the rectus muscles and angled medially and caudally.

optical trocar. At this point, I dissect vertically until I see the anterior fascial layer of the rectus sheath. I then cut through the anterior fascial layer with the blade on the Visiport, and at this time I am looking at the anterior surface of the rectus muscle. I have taken care to move lateral to the midline so as to avoid the area of fusion of the fascial layers in the midline and to ensure that I enter the rectus sheath. Once I visualize the rectus muscle I know I am inside the muscle sheath. Just by pushing the blunt trocar, I carry the dissection around the medial edge of the rectus muscle until I am on the underside of the muscle. The posterior fascial sheath is easily visible at this level and helps to prevent going any deeper at this point. I angle the trocar up until it is on the underside of the muscle and then slide it down toward the pubic bone, staying immediately adjacent to the underside of the muscle. This plane separates very easily as long as the trocar is kept exactly at the junction of the muscle and the underlying fatty tissue layer. If it is allowed to veer away from the muscle and down into the preperitoneal fat, the landmarks become much more difficult to locate. In addition, it is much easier to dissect down to the pubic bone laterally underneath the muscle, rather than in the midline. I gently set my other hand on the abdominal wall to monitor the location of the tip of the trocar, and then push it caudally until it hits the pubic bone. A tendency we all have is to lift the abdominal wall with our other hand, and I have found that this distorts the layers and actually makes the dissection more difficult. Usually this dissection goes very easily, but sometimes where there are previous surgery adhesions difficulty may be encountered. As long as you are immediately beneath the muscle, then the blade in the Visiport can be rotated horizontally and

fired to cut through the scar tissue. I look for the pubic bone to come into view; once the landmarks are learned they are usually recognized readily. The other hand resting on the abdominal wall also helps to determine where the tip of the trocar is. When the underside of the pubic bone is reached, I use the trocar to bluntly dissect laterally and to push the bladder down away from the underside of the pubic bone.

I begin insufflation at this point, but only to a maximum pressure of 12 mmHg so as to prevent its subsequent spread into the subcutaneous tissue. The space is being opened by the blunt dissection of the laparoscope and trocar, because the insufflation will not primarily dissect the tissue; however, the pressure will hold the space open once it is dissected. As soon as an opening is accomplished, I take the Visiport out, reinsert my laparoscope and visualize the area. Usually the best landmark is the underside of the symphysis pubis; this is often readily seen. The bleeding is usually minimal, so the laparoscope itself is utilized to dissect and enlarge the space, carrying the dissection laterally along each pubic ramus and dissecting down to the bladder beneath it. I dissect with the laparoscope only enough to be able to place my trocars and then complete the dissection with instruments. I utilize a short 5-mm trocar on the left and a 7 to 10-mm disposable trocar on the right (Figure 19-2). The larger trocar is utilized on the right because the suture and needle are inserted into the space through this trocar. The placement on the abdominal wall is also somewhat different; the trocars are inserted much lower than with intraabdominal laparoscopic procedures. Prior to placing the trocars, I insert a spinal needle along the same track as the trocar to orient myself and ensure proper direction of the trocar. The space which has been opened and where the suturing is performed is much smaller and more

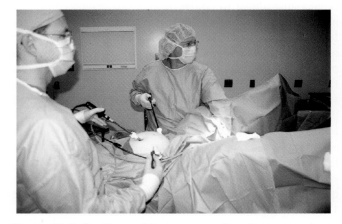

Figure 19-3 Positions of the surgeons for a laparoscopic retropubic urethropexy. Note I am standing on the left side of the table, operating an instrument or needle holder through the trocar in the left lower quadrant with my right hand, and elevating the pubocervical fascia with my left hand. My assistant is standing on the right, operating a needle holder through the right lower trocar with his right hand, and holding the camera with his left hand.

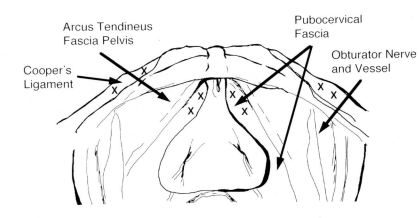

Figure 19-4 A laparoscopic view of the Space of Retzius. The entire area can be viewed simultaneously by both the surgeon and assistant. The pubocervical fascia and the location of the bladder, urethra and urethrovesicle junction, as well as Cooper's ligament, can be better evaluated for exact placement of the sutures (see X's). The obturator foramen and its contents can be located to avoid complications.

crowded than the abdominal cavity, and trocar placement is crucial to maneuvering the instruments. In addition, it is sometimes harder to hit the space with the trocar, and the initial insertion and visualization of the spinal needle makes the orientation and subsequent trocar insertion much easier. As a general rule, the trocar incisions are usually placed just above the lateral and superior aspects of the triangle of pubic hair and directed both medially and caudally from the skin incision.

Once my two trocars are in place, I continue the dissection and open the Space of Retzius further. I place my left hand into the vagina, and operate an instrument with my right hand through the lower left trocar. My assistant then takes the laparoscope in the left hand and works the instrument in the right lower trocar with the right hand (Figure 19-3). I utilize a bipolar instrument to coagulate any bleeding along the region, but as a general rule the bleeding is minimal. However, I often perform the dissection with the bipolar instrument to coagulate quickly any bleeding that may develop. The cleaner the space can be kept, the better I can visualize landmarks for placing sutures. I push up with my fingers in the vagina and move the bladder and urethra out of the way to facilitate the dissection of the pubocervical fascia. When either dissection is being performed or the sutures are being placed, it is easy to concentrate so hard that you forget it is your own left hand, and you tend to relax, thus not elevating the fascia adequately. Significant elevation of the pubocervical fascia with the fingers of the left hand makes both the dissection and the suturing much easier. I dissect out and visualize the arcus tendineus, pubocervical fascia and Cooper's ligament bilaterally (Figure 19-4). I determine where the obturator foramens are located, so as to avoid them, but I usually do not dissect them out completely. You do have to be careful on Cooper's ligament above the foramen. There is occasionally an aberrant obturator vein coming from the foramen which courses up and over Cooper's ligament, and it can be quite large. If this is torn while cleaning Cooper's ligament, it can be a real nuisance to control. Once the pubocervical

fascia and Cooper's ligament are visualized and cleaned of adipose tissue bilaterally, I am ready to begin suturing.

SUTURE PLACEMENT

With a needle holder, my assistant inserts a suture of O-Gortex through the right lower trocar. Once the needle is inside, I take it with a needle holder from the left lower trocar. My assistant then closes his or her needle holder and with it retracts the bladder medially from the pubocervical fascia, exactly as is done with a stick sponge in an open procedure. Elevating the fascia with the fingers of my left hand, I take a bite through the pubocervical fascia, and my assistant then grasps the tip of the needle as it protrudes through the fascia. I release the needle while my assistant holds the needle steady, sweep the tissue from the needle and regrasp it. With my assistant holding the needle in the same orientation without moving it, the regrasp is very simple (Figure 19-5). I place two passes of the suture through the fascia and then one through Cooper's ligament. My assistant then takes the needle back out through his or her port and places at least eight throws, using the extracorporeal tying method. I elevate the urethra to the level I want with my intravaginal hand and my assistant then throws the knots down to suspend it there. By elevating the pubocervical fascia with my fingers, the suture is not used to lift the tissue; my assistant simply advances the knots so the suture is taut. Also, the pubocervical fascia is not pulled all the way to Cooper's ligament, as this is known to cause significant problems by overcorrection of the defect. My goal is to have approximately 1 to 2 cm, or one finger breadth, between the bladder and urethra and the symphysis pubis.

I usually place two sutures per side with a total of four sutures for the procedure. In some cases if the urethra appears to be very short or I am unable to dissect out a large portion of the pubocervical fascia, I place only one suture per side. I place, tie, and cut each suture before placement of the next one and have not found this to limit my ability

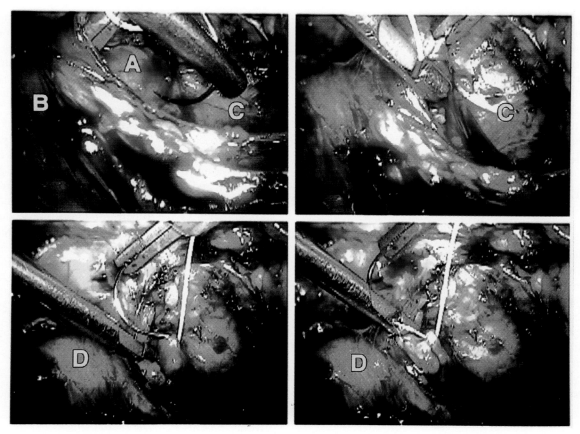

Figure 19-5 Technique of laparoscopic suturing in the Space of Retzius. **Upper left:** In the right paravaginal region, my assistant's needle holder (from the right trocar site) is moving the bladder and urethra to the left, exposing the right pubocervical fascia. I am elevating the fascia with the fingers of my left hand in the vagina, and holding the needle in my right hand through the left trocar site. **Upper right:** I have passed the needle through the pubocervical fascia, and my assistant has grasped the tip and is holding it steady. **Lower left:** I have released the needle and swept the tissue off the needle while my assistant continues to hold the needle steady. **Lower right:** I easily regrasp the needle as it is still oriented the same way as it was when I released it. (A) Pubocervical fascia; (B) bladder and urethra, pushed medially by my assistant; (C) obturator internus muscle; (D) Foley bulb.

to place subsequent sutures. It is sometimes more difficult to place the suture through the pubocervical fascia on the left when standing on the patient's left. I sometimes backhand this suture through the fascia, because the angles are somewhat difficult. On occasion, I have even had my assistant place the suture because he or she has a more favorable orientation for placement, especially through the pubocervical fascia. Once the four sutures are all in place and cut, I check again for satisfactory elevation of the urethra and adequate hemostasis in the space.

I then fill the bladder in preparation for placement of the suprapubic catheter by simply elevating the IV bag, attached to the Foley catheter, to an IV stand. Once approximately 300 cc have been infused into the bladder, I place a Bonnano catheter under direct visualization through the anterior abdominal wall into the dome of the bladder. The space is then desufflated after the instruments are removed. The trocars are removed and only the skin is closed; the

fascia is not closed because I have not entered the abdominal cavity. After this, I address the vaginal area. I perform a cystourethroscopy to ensure proper elevation of the urethral vesicle junction and to assure that there are no sutures in the bladder or bladder wall. At that time, I usually perform a posterior repair, as pelvic support defects are rarely isolated and there is usually concurrent posterior loss of support. During the posterior repair, I make a concentrated effort to see if there is any tendency toward a weakening in the area of the posterior cul-de-sac. If any is detected, I either reinforce this area or complete an enterocele repair. This is performed to reduce the incidence of subsequent posterior vaginal defects; they are known to occur with retropubic suspensions.

I feel mention should be made of a different technique being performed presently at some centers. Ou et al has described a technique which involves placing a piece of mesh into the space and using staples to attach the mesh to both the pubocervical fascia and Cooper's ligament, thus suspending the urethra and bladder. This technique offers an advantage: it is an alternative method for surgeons who have difficulty with suturing laparoscopically, and it also appears to be quicker than suturing. Initial data is just now being published and it appears to have an acceptable effectiveness rate, but it is not as time-tested as the more conventional techniques of suspension with sutures. However, as more long-term results and effectiveness rates are accumulated, it may become a viable alternative to suturing.

POSTOPERATIVE CARE

Most patients are then discharged within 24 hours following the procedure. I send them home with the suprapubic catheter in place after discussing with them how to bladder-train themselves at home. With the lateral type suspension that is performed (lateral to the bladder and urethra) probably a large percentage of these women could have the catheter removed prior to discharge and do well. However, a small percentage of patients will develop urinary retention; leaving the suprapubic catheter in place prevents them from having to return to either the office or the emergency room for reinsertion of a Foley. Consequently, I leave the suprapubic catheter indwelling and my nurse calls them on a daily basis to discuss bladder-training and their voided volumes. Once their residuals are less than 100 cc and less than one-third of the total voided volume I have the catheter removed. Because it comes out so easily, the patient can usually be talked through the removal at home, and most patients are willing to do that because there are only four small skin sutures holding the catheter in place. It usually comes out within 24 to 48 hours after leaving the hospital and having a nurse who calls them on a daily basis

and talks them through the removal of the catheter saves them another visit to the office. They can return to normal activity at their own rate. However, I do request that they do not perform any activity that requires strenuous exertion, including a Valsalva maneuver, for a period of six weeks. Most patients are able to return to work and normal activity within a week or so and usually do quite well.

One of the benefits of performing the colpopexy suspension laparoscopically is the improved visibility. Laparoscopic dissection and visualization of the Space of Retzius provides a much better view of the landmarks, placement of sutures, and evaluation of bleeding sites, than the traditional open procedure does. I have actually become quite spoiled; when I have to perform an open procedure now, I am frustrated with the lack of exposure compared to what I am used to with the laparoscopic dissection.

In addition, the data being accumulated is showing that the laparoscopic technique is just as efficacious as that of the time-honored open procedure. When this is combined with the dramatically improved recovery and quicker return to normal activity, it is obvious that our patients derive the benefits.

SUGGESTED READING

Erickson BC, Hagen B, Eik-Nes SH, et al. Long-term effectiveness of the Burch colposuspension in female urinary stress incontinence. *Acta Obstet Gynecol* 1990;69:45–50.

Liu CY, Paek W. Laparoscopic retropubic colposuspension (Burch procedure). *J Am Assoc Gynecol Laparoscop* 1993;1:31–6.

Ou CS, Presthus J, Beadle E. Laparoscopic bladder neck suspension using hernia mesh and surgical staples. *J Laparoendosc Surg* 1993;3:563–6.

Smith ML Jr, Perry C. Simplified visual preperitoneal access to the space of Retzius for laparoscopic urethrocolpopexy. *J Am Assoc Gynecol Laparoscop* 1996;1:295–9.

Tanagho EA. Colpocystourethropexy: the way we do it. *J Urology* 1976;116:751–3.

Vancaillie TG, Schuessler W. Laparoscopic bladder neck suspension. *J Laparoendoscop Surg* 1991;3:169–73.

Operative Laparoscopy, Second Edition
The Masters' Techniques in Gynecologic Surgery
Lippincott–Raven Publishers, Philadelphia © 1998.

20

Complications of Operative Laparoscopy

Richard M. Soderstrom, Carl J. Levinson, and Barbara S. Levy

COMPLICATIONS OWING TO EQUIPMENT

Uterine Manipulator

It is safe to say that complications from the uterine manipulator are not serious. Bleeding from cervical tenaculum marks can be controlled with absorbable sutures, electrical or photocoagulation, or compression. On rare occasion, one can use local infiltration of dilute Pitressin.

As with dilatation of the cervix, perforation of the lower or upper uterine segments can occur during insertion or manipulation of the intrauterine manipulator (Figure 20-1). Once this is noted, the manipulator should be removed and the puncture wound observed. In most instances, the bleeding site will become dry spontaneously. If not, a Pitressin injection or electrophotocoagulation can be used. It would be an unusual circumstance where laparotomy would be necessary.

There are a number of uterine manipulators on the market, some for manipulation only, some that allow chromotubation. Personal preference selects the instrument, as there is no evidence of one being safer than another.

Insufflation

Subcutaneous or retroperitoneal insufflation has occurred to every laparoscopist. This in itself is not a complication, but the placement of the needle into the proper location (peritoneal cavity) may be difficult if the properitoneal space has been distorted by a large bolus of instilled gas. Watching the flow rate and pressure during insufflation will alert the experienced laparoscopist that improper insufflation is probable. If so, stop insufflation and remove the needle.

Replacing the needle in the left upper quadrant of the abdomen is an easy way to overcome the problem of reinsertion of the needle in the same area where improper insufflation has occurred. This approach, commonly used in Europe, places the needle about 3 cm below the left costal margin and 4 to 5 cm to the left of the midline near the left

anterior axillary line, depending upon the patient's size. With one hand stretching the patient's skin caudally, making the skin taught, the needle is pushed gently in at a 15° angle cephalad, but staying parallel to the vertical plane of the patient (Figure 20-2). The Veress needle cannula will retract twice, once as it punctures the fascia and again as it punctures the peritoneum. This "pop-pop" sensation is easy to perceive and reassures one of being in the peritoneal space. When following this approach, the contents of the left upper quadrant will bounce away from the needle or cannula tip, should they be hit. Realize that in this area the transverse colon and stomach each lie in relief, and their physical structure and composition are resilient (have you ever eaten tripe?). The spleen, except in cases of splenomegaly, is high and posterior in the recesses of the upper left abdomen, out of harm's way.

One might try an insertion of the needle through the cul-de-sac of Douglas, but that is time consuming. One foolproof way to ensure intraperitoneal placement of the needle may, to some, sound traumatic, when in reality it is benign. If you push the uterine manipulator and thus the uterine fundus up against the abdominal wall, a bulge created by the dome of the fundus can be seen or palpated. Next, place the Veress needle in the center of the bulge and plunge it into the fundus as the uterus is held stable with the manipulator (Figure 20-3). Once the fundus has been impaled, slowly draw the fundus back into the pelvis, dragging the needle with it. At this point, hold the needle stationary in one hand and withdraw the fundus away from the needle tip; the needle tip is now intraperitoneal. Any bleeding from the needle puncture in the uterine fundus will be scant and quickly stop.

Should there be concerns about the proper placement of the needle for insufflation, open laparoscopy is a reasonable alternative.

Large Trocars

All laparoscopists prefer sharp trocars. With today's disposable trocars, there is little reason to struggle with a dull

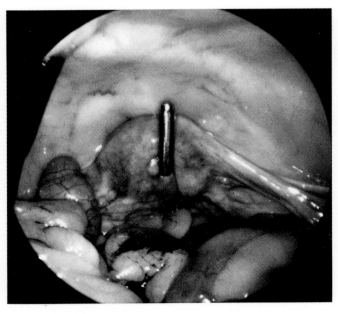

Figure 20-1 Uterine perforation during uterine manipulation. Bleeding usually stops spontaneously shortly after the manipulator is removed.

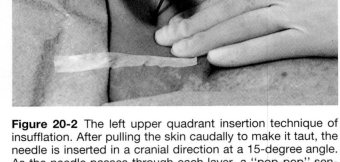

Figure 20-2 The left upper quadrant insertion technique of insufflation. After pulling the skin caudally to make it taut, the needle is inserted in a cranial direction at a 15-degree angle. As the needle passes through each layer, a ''pop-pop'' sensation is felt.

reusable trocar. If reusable trocars are to be used, good maintenance should be mandated as a department policy. With a sharp trocar, large or small, there is no need for a vigorous thrust during insertion. If one cups the handle of the trocar in the palm of one's hand and places two fingers of the other hand on the middle portion of the trocar sleeve shaft, overpenetration should not occur.

Some operators prefer to lift the abdominal wall with one hand during the insertion of the trocar and sleeve using the other hand (Figure 20-4). However, if the peritoneal cavity is adequately distended, all that can be lifted is the abdominal skin. Therefore, this technique eliminates the safety feature of the second hand from the insertion process; for those with small hands, the chance of overpenetration is thus increased.

When unipolar electrosurgery is used through the operating channel of an operating laparoscope, the laparoscope becomes a capacitor (a device capable of storing electrical energy through electrostatic physics) (Figure 20-5). This

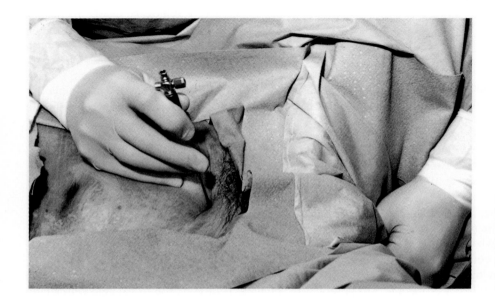

Figure 20-3 The suprapubic insertion technique of insufflation. Using the uterine manipulator to elevate the fundus against the abdominal wall, the needle is thrust into the fundus. Once the uterus is impaled, the uterus is withdrawn off the end of the needle ensuring intraabdominal placement.

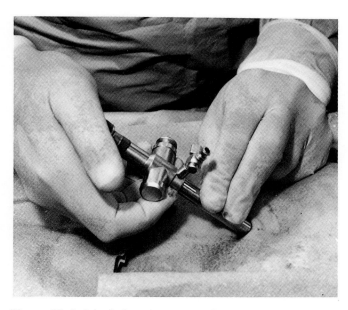

Figure 20-4 A technique to prevent deep penetration during the insertion of the umbilical trocar (closed technique). With adequate insufflation, the plane of the abdominal wall is elevated enough away from the great vessels so both hands can be used to insert the trocar with complete control.

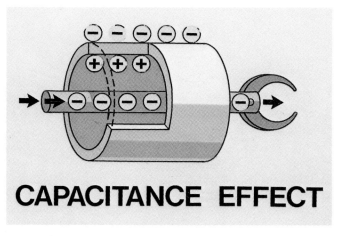

Figure 20-5 As energy passes through the insulated electrode which has been placed through the operating channel of the laparoscope, the laparoscope becomes a capacitor.

law of electrophysics places the patient at risk of injury if the trocar sleeve is nonconductive. In this situation, the laparoscope is not in contact with the patient; approximately 50% to 70% of the electrical energy passed through the active electrode in the operating channel of the laparoscope is induced into the metal shell of the scope. Because the laparoscope is isolated from any physical contact with the patient, the energy stored in its metal shell has no return pathway to ground; should a small portion of bowel or abdominal wall touch the shell, the energy will seek ground through the tissue, and a burn may occur. If the trocar sleeve is conductive, any capacitance effect will leak through the trocar sleeve to ground without harm. Because of this, the Food and Drug Administration (FDA) has advised manufacturers who produce nonconductive trocar sleeves above 7 mm in diameter to insert special warnings about capacitance with these sleeves. It should be emphasized that this risk occurs only during the activation of unipolar energy through the operating channel of an operating laparoscope.

With rare exceptions, the large trocar and sleeves should be inserted into the hollow of the pelvis without lateral deviation during the insertion process. If you hit the uterus, it will forgive you; iliac vessels will not! This requires a mental picture in the mind of the operating surgeon. If you place the patient in steep Trendelenburg position before insertion, your mental picture should compensate for this, as the sacral promontory and the bifurcation of the great vessels move, in a spatial sense, anteriorly (Figures 20-6 and 20-7).

On occasion, blood will be seen dripping from the tip of the laparoscope after one starts to view the pelvis. Usually,

this is from a lacerated vein in the periumbilical area. Should it persist, place a small endoscope (a cystoscope will do) through an accessory trocar sleeve and view the bleeding while the laparoscope and sleeve are in place. If necessary, place a third trocar sleeve and use a standard electrode to coagulate the bleeding vessel while viewing through the smaller endoscope. Sometimes, angling the trocar sleeve will compress the vessel and reduce or stop the flow.

Accessory Trocar Sleeves

All secondary or accessory trocar sleeves should be inserted under direct vision. Often, because the peritoneum will tent on the end of the trocar tip, a good view is not possible. If this occurs, a safe procedure is to aim at the top

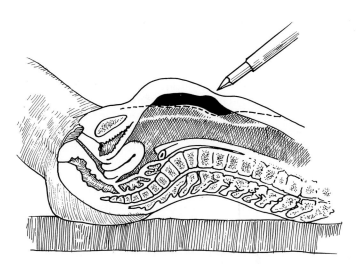

Figure 20-6 Trocar insertion with the operating table flat.

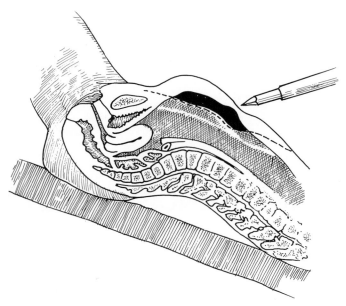

Figure 20-7 Position of the trocar and great vessels in steep Trendelenburg.

of the uterus. Here, should the fundus be punctured, its wound will be slight, and it will heal without consequence. Another trick is to withdraw the end of the laparoscope back into the midportion of the laparoscope's trocar sleeve. Under direct view, the tip of the accessory trocar can be directed into the end of the larger trocar sleeve. Once the tented peritoneum meets the distal rim of the large trocar sleeve, the increased resistance will permit an easy, safe, puncture of the peritoneal membrane. Be careful not to injure the laparoscope lens with the trocar tip.

Transilluminating the abdominal wall may help to reduce the laceration of superficial epigastric vessels during trocar insertion; it is not foolproof. Because the bleeding can be brisk, if such a laceration occurs, there is the temptation to enlarge the accessory trocar incision to find and place the suture. A simple alternative is to thread a long, thin, pediatric Foley catheter through the trocar sleeve in the abdomen. Once the bulb end can be seen through the laparoscope, inflate the bulb, and withdraw the trocar sleeve up the shaft of the catheter until the sleeve is outside the abdomen. Pull the inflated catheter bulb firmly against the abdominal wall peritoneum for a tamponade effect. Hold it in that position with a hemostat placed on the catheter as it exits the abdominal skin. One can then proceed with the planned procedure through other accessory trocar sleeves. By the end of the procedure, the catheter bulb can be deflated and removed. Usually, the vessels will have stopped bleeding; if not, unipolar coagulation frequently solves the problem.

An alternative to the catheter procedure is to tie the vessels through the trocar insertion site. If the patient is not too obese, use a large, curved, needle with absorbable suture.

Under endoscopic vision, remove the accessory trocar sleeve and place the needle tip into the trocar incision, placing the needle lateral to the punctured vessels. Once the needle tip penetrates the abdominal peritoneum, pass the curved needle under the vessels and continue the path of the needle back out through the abdominal wall skin medial to the trocar incision. Turn the needle 180° on the needle holder and reenter the needle's exit puncture wound. Here, pass the needle above the fascia and exit out of the trocar incision site next to the distal end of the suture (Figure 20-8). Once this suture loop has been completed, tie down the ligature and stop the bleeding. Thus there is no need to extend the trocar incision.

In recent years, as larger trocars have been used as accessory trocars, hernia formation has been reported, some which have lead to incarcerated bowel obstructions. Several suture devices, disposable and reusable, have been designed to expedite the fascial closure of trocar sites at risk of such hernia formations.

Laparoscope

Complications do not occur from the instrument itself, but a defective laparoscope can lead to complications. Poor maintenance will lead to misaligned lenses and broken fiberoptic bundles. A laparoscope that frequently fogs during an operative procedure is frustrating and may be dangerous. There is no excuse for the continued use of a defective laparoscope. If the image is blurry, or if the perimeter of the optical field appears to be oblong, indicating the lens is dislodged, send the instrument to the manufacturer for lens repair.

If the light transfer gives a dim view, remove the scope from the trocar sleeve and point the distal end at an over-

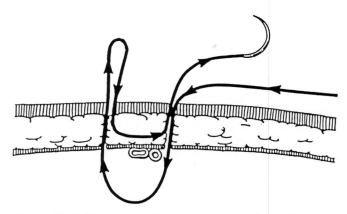

Figure 20-8 Through-and-through ligature. Under direct endoscopic view, pass the needle into the abdominal cavity, under the epigastric vessels, and take it out through the abdominal skin medial to the incision. Then reverse the needle and direct it back through the exit site, bringing it out through the trocar incision. Confirm placement and security endoscopically, once the ligation has been completed.

head light in the operating room. Disconnect the fiber light bundle from the laparoscope and inspect the fiberoptic nipple of the laparoscope. If 50% or more of the fibers appear black, it is time to replace the bundles.

To prevent fogging, laparoscope warmers are available; however, draping the distal end of the laparoscope with a warm, moist, towel may help. Commercial antifog solutions should be available in all operating rooms on request. During surgery, should the lens become fogged, the moisture can be swept away from the lens by touching the bowel serosa. Persistent fogging may indicate that moisture has leaked in behind the distal lens, and the instrument should be returned for repairs.

BLEEDING

General Considerations

A bleeding episode is a frequent event during operative laparoscopy. Even when an adhesion appears avascular, one might be surprised to see bleeding occur during the transection process. Here, patience is important. Such bleeders, as with laparotomy, will cease to bleed in a short period of time. A hasty attempt to coagulate a small bleeder in a retracted, severed, adhesion may increase the risk of burn beyond the area of desired coagulation. Here, a bipolar forcep can grasp and manipulate the bleeder before performing coagulation. Persistent bleeders can be clipped, coagulated,

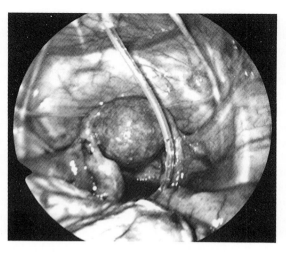

Figure 20-10 A 4-mm perforated suction drain in place after being threaded through a 5-mm trocar.

and ligated, depending on the experience of the surgeon. A few times, one may encounter a bleeding vessel that cannot be secured with any of the laparoscopic tools. A simple trick is to make a stab in the abdominal wall over the bleeding site and thread through the layers of the abdominal wall a long-nosed hemostatic clamp, of the type used during major laparotomy. View the peritoneal entry site and guide the forceps tip to the vessel and grasp the point of bleeding. Leave the clamp on the vessel for about 5 minutes (Figure 20-9). It is surprising to find that none of the intraabdominal gas will leak through the stab wound. When the clamp is removed, the crush effect will stop or slow up the bleeding so that electrocoagulation will be effective.

During a dissection procedure, pesky venous bleeding can develop. Place the patient in steep Trendelenburg position, which places the bleeding vein above the level of the heart; the venous pressure will drop, and the bleeding will slow up, or it may cease. The intraabdominal pressure will aid venous compression. Beware—if the bleeding ceases, be sure to check that area at the end of the laparoscopic procedure, after the patient has been placed flat, to be sure hemostasis is present.

As with laparotomy, applied hemostatic agents like Surgicel or Avitene might be considered. Unlike their use during laparotomy, external tamponade against the agent may be technically difficult or impossible. Bleeding vessels are best occluded rather than covered. If such agents are felt to be necessary, consider placing a small suction drain near the area. A small plastic suction drain with multiple perforations can be threaded through an accessory trocar sleeve and draped over the area that was oozing (Figure 20-10). Once the patient is transferred to the recovery room, hook the drain to low intermittent suction and monitor the fluid output, if any. If all goes well, at the time of patient discharge, disconnect the suction from the drain and gently

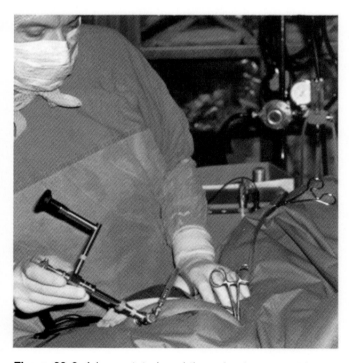

Figure 20-9 A hemostat placed through a trocar puncture to grasp and secure a bleeding vessel.

remove it. This is a useful monitoring device when performing a linear salpingostomy for an ectopic pregnancy.

Following an extensive operative laparoscopy, where postoperative bleeding is possible, get a hematocrit several hours later before deciding when to discharge the patient. Operative laparoscopy deserves the same respect as laparotomy in the monitoring protocols of the recovery period.

In 1991, I discovered the advantage of using glycine as an irrigant for operative laparoscopy where bleeding may be a problem. Glycine, a common distention medium for cystoscopic resectoscope procedures, is amino acetic acid, a nonelectrolytic solution. Its pH of 6.1 is physiologic, and it does not hemolyze blood. If, during laparoscopic procedures, this fluid is used for irrigation, electrocoagulation, either bipolar or unipolar, can be used *during* irrigation, or submerged in the fluid media. When persistent bleeders occur during laparoscopy, I flood the field with glycine and coagulate the bleeders during the irrigation. A particular advantage is that glycine will make the bleeding from open vessels stream through the medium, rather than blotching as seen with an electrolyte-rich solution. Thus the origin of bleeding can be seen and coagulated quickly. On occasion, I will fill the pelvis with glycine and search for bleeding under the fluid medium. Here, the bleeding sites extrude the blood in a snakelike formation, making pinpoint coagulation easy. Because of the electrolytes in saline and lactated Ringer's solution, electrosurgery energy cannot be activated with those media.

Perforation of Large Vascular Structures

A most devastating and life-threatening injury to occur during laparoscopy is laceration of a major abdominal blood vessel. The aorta, vena cava, common, right, and left iliac arteries and veins, superior mesenteric vessels, inferior epigastric, and patent umbilical veins, have all been perforated. The true incidence of great vessel injury is unknown since the majority of cases go unreported.

Patients at high risk for vascular injury include the thin, nulliparous woman with well-developed abdominal musculature. The aorta may lie less than an inch below the skin in these women. Obesity may play a role as the surgeon, in an effort to avoid properitoneal placement of the insufflating needle, overzealously thrusts the instrument in a perpendicular fashion and impales the retroperitoneal vessels against the sacral promontory. Morbid obesity can distort the surgeon's mental picture of the true anatomy. As complex operative laparoscopy becomes more common, intraoperative laceration may occur with increased frequency.

Several technical factors have been identified as contributing to injuries of the great vessels. Operator inexperience is an important factor. Most complications of any kind are known to occur in a surgeon's first 100 cases. Other factors are as follows:

1. a dull trocar
2. an inadequate pneumoperitoneum
3. a perpendicular or lateral insertion of the needle or trocar
4. a forceful thrusting motion for insertion
5. the failure to note anatomic landmarks and abnormal or inappropriate patient positioning
6. abnormal pelvic anatomy
7. inserting a trocar through a dense scar, which may cause a deflection

The aortic bifurcation occurs at the level of L-4 75% of the time. L-4 can be consistently located at the level of the summits of the iliac crests. Nine percent of the time the bifurcation will lie above L-4, and 11% of the time it will be below L4-5. Eighty percent of the time, however, the bifurcation will be within 1.25 cm above or below the iliac crests. Even in morbidly obese patients the iliac crests are usually palpable. The position of the umbilicus varies and should not be used to predict the location of the underlying great vessels. Trendelenburg position rotates the sacral promontory and the lower aorta into a location much closer to the umbilicus and changes the angle of safe insertion from 45° to a shallower angle (Figures 20-1 and 20-2). With the diminished margin of safety, a vascular injury will be more common. Be present in the operating room when the sterile drapes are being applied and the patient is positioned. Many anesthesiologists, in an effort to expedite the case, will place the patient in steep Trendelenburg. After the drapes are applied, it is difficult to ascertain the patient's true position.

Once the patient is placed in the supine position, prepared, and draped, palpate the superior aspect of the iliac crests and trace the aorta and its bifurcation by palpation. This maneuver allows you to assess the adequacy of general anesthesia and abdominal wall relaxation prior to initiating the procedure. During the superficial skin incision, make an effort to avoid peritoneal penetration. The superior mesenteric vein, presacral vein, and vena cava have been lacerated during the skin incision, one in a patient with a large rectus diastasis. The use of a curved No. 12 blade may help to avoid inadvertent incision of the peritoneum.

Before inserting the Veress needle, inspect and test it for proper function. On occasion, the operating personnel may reassemble the equipment improperly, i.e., forgetting the spring or combining a long needle with a short obturator. During insertion the stopcock valve must remain open. This allows room air to enter the abdominal cavity immediately upon peritoneal entry, thereby allowing the bowel to fall away from the needle tip. Many elevate the abdominal wall prior to needle insertion. This may be done manually or with towel clips, but this merely gives the illusion of safety. Since there is no space in the peritoneal cavity, the bowel is lifted as well. In the thin patient, vigorous bites with towel clips to attempt to raise the full thickness of the abdominal wall may perforate the bowel.

With the lower abdominal wall manually stabilized or elevated by the surgeon's nondominant hand, the Veress needle should be grasped at the hub, between the thumb and forefinger of the dominant hand like a pencil and firmly but gently guided at 45° toward the middle of the pelvic cavity or toward the fundus of the uterus. Place a syringe with 10 to 20 mL of saline on the hub of the needle. The fluid should drop freely into the peritoneal cavity. Inject and reaspirate the saline to test for properitoneal or intravascular placement. The return of small bowel or stomach contents demonstrates inappropriate placement. If blood returns from the needle, suspect a vascular, retroperitoneal injury unless a hemoperitoneum is known to preexist. Once proper intraperitoneal position is established, insufflation may begin. An intraperitoneal pressure greater than 15 or 20 mm Hg usually indicates that the needle is obstructed by the small bowel or the omentum. Lift and bounce the anterior abdominal wall manually. This will allow the impaled structure to fall off the needle tip. The Veress needle itself should not be moved from its plane of insertion. Several reports indicate that further vascular injury has occurred when the Veress needle was ''waggled'' after an increased insufflation pressure had been noted. Should the needle be inside the retroperitoneal space, further manipulation of the needle could cause a great vessel perforation or laceration. If the elevation of the abdominal wall does not decrease the insufflation pressure, the needle should be removed and replaced, using the same precautions.

Dull trocars contribute to vascular accidents. In addition, preperitoneal insufflation with consequent tenting of the peritoneum away from the abdominal wall, necessitating multiple attempts at trocar insertion, can be problematic. The force necessary to pass a sharp reusable trocar is twice as great as that needed for the disposable ones. The safety shield of the disposable trocar is designed to lock once the peritoneal resistance has been released. On occasion, it may get hung up before penetrating the peritoneum, necessitat-

ing several passes with the trocar. With either device, a smooth, steady, gentle pressure should be applied to the instrument. There are no data to suggest the safety shield of the disposable models provides additional protection.

A drop of saline can be placed in the insufflation port of the trocar sleeve with the stopcock closed. Using a ''Z'' technique, the trocar and the most distal end of the sleeve are tunneled horizontally under the skin for 1 to 2 cm (Figure 20-11). Some have argued that the Z technique may lead to iliac injury by making the operator unaware of his actual angle of insertion. In reality, burrowing 1 to 2 cm below the umbilicus should allow the trocar to begin its entry into the pelvic cavity well below the sacral promontory. Once the small insufflation ports of the trocar sleeve are subcutaneous, the stopcock is opened, allowing the saline to travel down the sleeve. When a gas-filled cavity is entered, saline will ''spit'' back from the port, a signal to the surgeon that the trocar sleeve is within the insufflation area.

Once the pneumoperitoneum has been established, no further elevation of the anterior abdominal wall can be accomplished. Rather than attempting to lift the abdominal skin, the surgeon's nondominant hand should be used to guide the depth of trocar insertion and steady the abdominal wall, ensuring the appropriate midline direction of insertion.

Using computer graphics, the great vessels of the lateral pelvic wall were measured to be at least a 30° deviation from the horizontal plane and a similar deviation from the sagittal plane recommended for primary trocar insertion. If resistance to penetration of the fascia is encountered, either due to a dull trocar, inadequate muscle relaxation, or scarred fascia from previous surgery, do not twist and thrust the trocar repeatedly; use a disposable or properly sharpened trocar. If additional equipment is unavailable, nick the fascia with a knife blade at the point of intended penetration, allowing a safe, gentle, and controlled entry of the trocar.

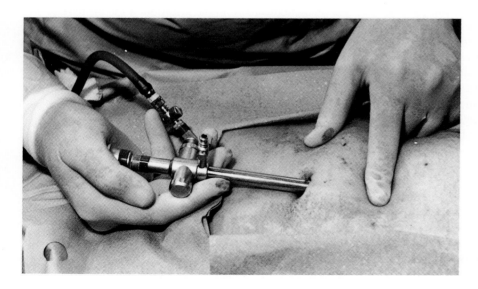

Figure 20-11 The ''Z'' technique of trocar insertion. This places the intraabdominal entry port several centimeters below the bifurcation of the great vessels and also reduces the risk of postoperative evisceration of the omentum.

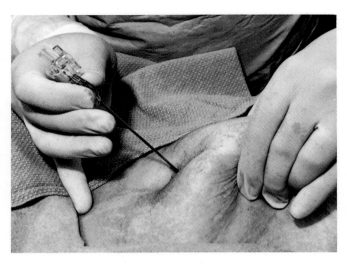

Figure 20-12 The insufflation needle should be inserted at a 45° angle into the hollow of the pelvic cavity. Most surgeons elevate the lower abdominal wall as shown. The insufflation valve is left open so room air will be sucked into the peritoneal cavity; thus the bowel will fall away from the tip of the needle.

Multiple passes with the trocar should be avoided. When the laparoscope is introduced through the trocar sheath and properitoneal fat is seen, insert a small atraumatic grasping forceps through the operating channel of an operating laparoscope and under direct vision enter the peritoneum.

Once a small opening has been made in the peritoneum, guide the laparoscope and trocar sleeve through the opening and insufflate the appropriate space through the trocar sleeve. Finally, place all additional trocars under direct vision.

Major vessel injury should be suspected whenever blood returns from the open insufflating needle. In addition, a sudden drop in blood pressure of a previously stable patient after needle or trocar insertion should alert all that a vascular accident has occurred, until proven otherwise. A large hematoma may accumulate in the retroperitoneal space before any intraperitoneal sign of hemorrhage is evident. Notify the anesthesiologist of the possibility of massive hemorrhage so that central lines can be placed and blood acquired. Perform a laparotomy immediately through a midline incision; adequate exposure of the retroperitoneal vessels cannot be accomplished via a Pfannenstiel incision. Control the large bleeding vessels with digital pressure or with sponge packs until the patient is stabilized and the appropriate surgical help has arrived. An additional anesthesiologist and a surgeon trained to manage vascular complications should be summoned immediately to the operating room. Once the patient has been stabilized, retractors can be placed for visualization, the peritoneum overlying the vessels incised, and the injuries repaired with vascular sutures, clips, or patches. Once a vascular repair has been accomplished, a thorough abdominal exploration should be done, searching for concomitant injuries, especially to the

bowel. Few sequelae have been reported when rapid and appropriate measures were initiated after vascular injury.

In summary, major vessel injuries during laparoscopy are, for the most part, preventable. The surgeon must palpate the abdomen and review the anatomy in each patient. The position of the patient should be verified and the equipment inspected. The Veress needle should be open to the air during insertion and directed at 45° toward the hollow of the pelvic cavity (Figure 20-12). Each trocar must be sharp and inserted at the proper angle, with careful, controlled descent. Finally, positive identification of the abdominal wall vessels and insertion of all additional trocars under direct vision will prevent most major vessel perforation.

ORGAN INJURIES

As with any operative procedure, an intraabdominal organ can be punctured, cut, or perforated. At times, these accidents are not preventable. A patient with severe scoliosis might make it difficult to know the probable location of a great vessel in the pelvis. However, trauma to the lateral iliac vessels in a normal patient should not occur without some unusual reason. With today's accessory instruments, a trained operative laparoscopist can manage many organ injuries without needing to perform a laparotomy, but it is neither a disgrace nor an admission of failure to resort to laparotomy. The following advice should be considered suggestions only, as each case may present differently.

Intestinal Complications

Injury to the small or large intestine is one of the most serious complications of operative endoscopy. While early reports implicated unipolar coagulation and high-voltage generators as the source of all injuries to the bowel, it is now clear that intestinal damage can and does occur by mechanical means from the insertion of the primary or secondary trocars, and with sharp dissection of adhesions. Thermal injuries may be caused by any laser or electrical instruments, unipolar or bipolar.

Inform all of your patients that bowel injuries do occur with laparoscopy, and obtain a consent for possible laparotomy. Patients who are at increased risk for intestinal perforation at the time of trocar insertion, i.e., those with histories of chronic bowel disease, pelvic inflammatory disease (PID), severe endometriosis, and especially those who have undergone multiple abdominal explorations in the past, are specifically advised about the possibility of open laparotomy and are "bowel-prepped" mechanically with Golytely. Open laparoscopy does not diminish the risk of intestinal injury but may permit better access to the peritoneal cavity under some conditions.

What should you do if a bowel injury is suspected? If, upon testing the patency of the Veress needle position, liquid green material is aspirated, the small bowel, most likely the distal ileum, has been entered. Withdraw the needle and either replace it in another location, i.e., left upper quadrant, transvaginally, adjacent to the first attempt, or proceed to open laparoscopy. Under most circumstances, the muscular wall of the intestine will self-seal the small opening and prevent longterm spillage. The contents of the small intestine are sterile, so lavage of the peritoneal cavity should be sufficient to prevent infection; antibiotic coverage is unnecessary. As usual, after recovery from anesthesia, discharge the patient with instructions to call immediately if she experiences a fever or increasing abdominal or pelvic pain. Send your patients home with pain pills such as ibuprofen for postoperative discomfort. Any need for increasing analgesia is a red flag to examine the patient.

To place the trocar into or through the intestine is more disconcerting. If recognized, the trocar must not be withdrawn, but left in place. Place a small laparotomy incision in proximity to the trocar insertion site. Gently pull the damaged bowel through the incision and place a pursestring suture around the damaged area. Slowly withdraw the trocar while closing the pursestring stitch (Figure 20-13). A reinforcing, interrupted, second-layer closure should be placed. Always check the contralateral side for a possible pinhole perforation. Copious, repeated peritoneal lavage is critical. In fact, small amounts of irrigating fluid repeated many times are better than large amounts repeated only a few times. Here, broad-spectrum antibiotic coverage is wise. The patient should be observed as with a standard laparotomy.

If you believe that laser, thermal, or electrical damage has been sustained by the bowel, the affected area should be excised. Merely touching the bowel with an electrical instrument, recently activated, cannot cause a burn. However, unipolar energy, inadvertently applied to the bowel wall while lysing adhesions or coagulating bleeders, can

Place no sutures within 4 cm of burned area

Resect intestinal burned area

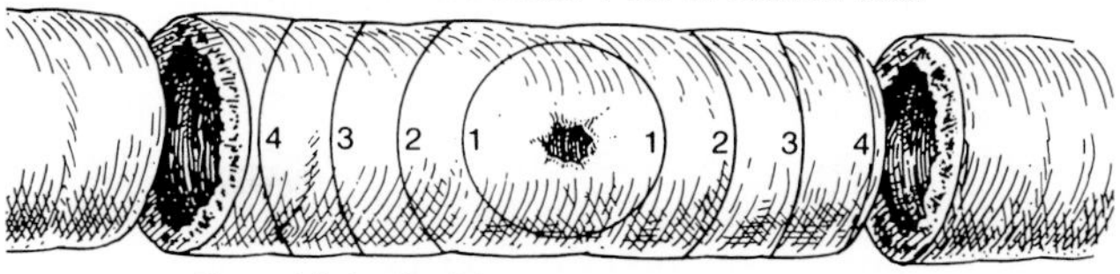

Figure 20-14 When an electrical burn of the bowel is suspected, always resect a generous segment on each side of the injury site.

create a large area of necrosis. If a persistent blanched area is found, a bowel resection of at least 5 cm surrounding the area should be performed (Figure 20-14).

Under most circumstances, however, direct application of energy to the bowel has not occurred. If there is concern about a possible injury to the bowel, observe the patient carefully. Any prolonged, persistent or increasing pelvic or abdominal pain, temperature elevation, or increasing abdominal distention and localized tenderness should prompt immediate evaluation and surgical exploration. Often the bowel injury goes unnoticed at the time of the initial procedure. A failure to recognize the classic signs and to react quickly to this medically urgent situation can be considered negligent even though the complications may be unpreventable. When a postoperative laparoscopy patient presents with prolonged, persistent or increasing pain, fever, and malaise, she should be seen immediately. Low-grade fever, tachycardia, and localized tenderness may be the only clues to a serious complication. Frequently, the white cell count is only slightly elevated, if at all; a left shift is usually present. This patient should be evaluated with a chest x-ray, and kidneys-ureters-bladder and upright films of the abdomen. When patients present early, intraabdominal CO_2 will still be present, and abdominal films are unrewarding. Usually, CO_2 and/or nitrous oxide used for insufflation is absorbed within 48 hours. Free air under the diaphragm beyond that time should prompt immediate exploration. When significant doubt exists, watersoluble contrast media might detect an opening in the gastrointestinal tract. Though ultrasound studies may reveal abscess formation, they are not conclusive; neither is free air always seen in cases of bowel perforation. If we suspect PID rather than a catastrophic complication, reexploration is still advisable. With localized peritonitis, laparoscopy can be used safely. It is much better to investigate early rather than observing a patient for several days. If managed early, bowel perforation will not be life-threatening; however, failure to recognize the complication and to treat it expeditiously has led to several deaths. *A patient who has persistent or increasing abdominal pain following laparoscopy has a bowel perforation until proven otherwise.*

Consult one of your general surgery colleagues, but you should remain actively involved in the management of your patient. When the decision is made to reexplore your pa-

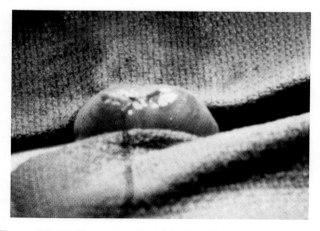

Figure 20-13 Through a "mini-lap" incision, a mechanical, small bowel perforation can be repaired with ease. (Courtesy of Daniel Martin, MD.)

tient, be sure you are available and present at the surgery. This is your best opportunity to assess the cause of the injury and protect yourself legally. Resect the area surrounding the bowel perforation in order to prove that traumatic perforation rather than thermal injury is what occurred. Traumatic perforations can be oversewn, but then no pathologic confirmation will be available.

In 1984, Soderstrom and Levy demonstrated that bowel injuries can be classified, via histology, as to their etiology. Thermal injuries destroy the full thickness of the bowel wall and lead to coagulation necrosis. The area of perforation will be surrounded by ''ghost cells,'' and white cells are conspicuously absent. In contrast, traumatic injuries of the bowel wall allow hemorrhage, increased vascularity, and infiltration by polymorphonuclear leukocytes. Thus the area of perforation, when viewed microscopically, will demonstrate hemorrhage and an acute inflammatory reaction with a heavy infiltration of neutrophils (Table 20-1). Hand-carry the specimen to your pathologist and discuss the case with him. He may be unaware of this research and may need some incentive to carefully review the slides. Staining the specimen with the Mallory Trichrome technique helps to highlight coagulated tissue. If a thermal injury is sectioned more than a few millimeters from the perforation site, the findings will mimic those found with traumatic injuries.

As always, the best way to manage a complication is to stay on top of things yourself. Though it is uncomfortable and depressing to see a sick patient every day, maintain close contact with your patient and control her management as one of the best defenses against malpractice litigation.

Bladder Perforation

When bladder perforation occurs, it is usually with insertion of the secondary trocar. The perforation is always in the dome of the bladder, and with an indwelling catheter placed for 1 week, it will heal spontaneously. Should you choose to repair the hole, the indwelling catheter is still necessary. Repair may be done by the proficient via operative laparoscopy techniques.

Table 20-1 *Features of puncture and electrical injuries*

Features of puncture injuries
- Limited noncoagulative-type necrosis, more severe in the muscle coat than the mucosa
- Rapid and abundant capillary ingrowth with rapid white cell infiltration
- Rapid fibrin deposition at the injury site followed by fibroblastic proliferation

Features of electrical injuries
- Absence of capillary ingrowth or fibroblastic muscle coat reconstruction
- Absence of white cell infiltration except in focal areas at the viable borders of injury
- An area of coagulation necrosis

Ureteral Injury

Where the bladder, should it be injured, is a resilient organ, the ureter is not. Ureters may be cut, burned with electrosurgery and lasers, or ligated. Removing ovaries with the Endoloop is not without a risk of ureter ligation. In the periuterosacral area, bipolar coagulation of endometriosis can coagulate the ureter as easily as unipolar coagulation. Lysis of adhesions at the pelvic rim carries with it an especial risk of sharp transection of the ureter, as does a tedious resection of endometrial implants on the posterior leaf of the broad ligament.

If the injury is suspected during the laparoscopic procedure, inject one ampule of indigo carmine intravenously; within 10 minutes, dye will spill from the injury site. If the hole is small, a urologist may be able to place, by cystoscopy, a ureteral stent to be removed several weeks later. Place a drain at the site of injury. If an extensive injury is evident, laparotomy and repair are required.

Ureteral injuries may not be evident for several days or weeks. Here, the patient usually presents with abdominal distention and/or ascites. Because of the diluent effect of the intraabdominal urine, an intravenous pyelogram may be nondiagnostic. Intravenous indigo carmine can be injected, and 1 hour later a paracentesis will make the diagnosis.

Tubal Laceration

Despite reasonable caution, the fallopian tube may start to bleed during organ manipulation. In the patient who wishes to preserve fertility, gross electrocoagulation is not appropriate. With the use of a microneedle electrode, drip glycine on the bleeding area and spot-coagulate the bleeders.

Ovarian Injury

The normal ovary is impervious to accidental injury, but functional ovarian cysts are not. Corpus luteum cysts, ruptured during pelvic examinations, have led to exploratory laparotomy or laparoscopy because of profound bleeding. Most of the time, should a functional cyst rupture, the bleeding will stop, but the amount of bleeding may be 100 mL or more before spontaneous hemostasis is accomplished.

If you find yourself inside of a large ovarian cyst when you insert the laparoscope, don't pull it out! Look carefully for signs of potential malignancy, and in cases of question, take a directed biopsy. Because you are in the cyst, so is the trocar sleeve. If you are using a diagnostic laparoscope, remove it and insert an operative laparoscope, and carefully suction (use low vacuum pressure) through the operative channel, keeping the distal end of the laparoscope in the cyst cavity until the cavity collapses, as determined by your direct observation through the bayonet eyepiece. Remove the laparoscope and send the fluid for a cytology examination. Once the cyst wall has collapsed, use a laparoscopic snare to amputate the collapsed cyst wall and retrieve it through the laparoscope trocar sleeve, pulling the operating scope, grasping forceps, and specimen, as a unit, through the trocar sleeve, and out of the abdominal cavity. Others may choose to use scissors with a multiple trocar approach.

CONCLUSION

As we advance to more complicated operative laparoscopy, the aforementioned complications may be accentuated, because new procedures have more problems in the early stage of the learning curve. The more extensive the tissue dissection, such as cul-de-sac resection of endometriosis, the more care is needed regarding the adjacent colon, rectum, and ureters. A methodical, cautious advance in each attempt at new complex procedures will reduce the possibility of injury. ''Prevention of complications is much better than the best management'' (CJL).

SUGGESTED READING

Borten M, ed. *Laparoscopic Complication—Prevention and Management.* Toronto: BC Becker, 1986.
Martin DC, ed. *Manual of Endoscopy.* Downey, IL: American Association of Gynecologic Laparoscopists, 1990.
Phillips JM, ed. *Laparoscopy.* Baltimore, MD: Williams & Wilkins, 1977.

Operative Laparoscopy, Second Edition
The Masters' Techniques in Gynecologic Surgery
Lippincott–Raven Publishers, Philadelphia © 1998.

21

Medicolegal Considerations

Richard M. Soderstrom

All operations have a complication rate. Laparoscopy is no exception, and specific complications should be known to the laparoscopist. Effective informed consent and good risk management involve informing patients of these specific complications. The physician and his or her support staff should also be alert to the warning signs of a possible complication. Once a complication is recognized, the proper and prompt management of the complication may make the difference between an incident and a lawsuit.

In addition to keeping their technical skills current, surgeons are required to have a working knowledge of their surgical instruments and equipment. In turn, hospitals have a fiduciary responsibility to provide an adequate array of laparoscopic tools, free of defect, to complete the proposed task. Proper maintenance of surgical equipment is the duty of the hospital. A surgeon's continued use of defective equipment, however, will also place the surgeon at risk for any related injury that the patient may suffer. Hospitals and surgeons should work together to ensure equipment is maintained at the highest level possible and to reduce operative complications.

PREOPERATIVE COUNSELING

Nothing can take the place of a discussion about a procedure or treatment between the physician and the patient. Informed consent is a process whereby the physician has a responsibility to make sure that the patient is fully informed in order to give a valid consent. Although not intended to replace the doctor-patient exchange of information, authoritative pamphlets are helpful tools in getting the information across to the patient. Audiovisual tapes can also serve the same purpose.

Unfortunately, with surgery that seems so simple as laparoscopy, patients and their families do not expect the rare complications associated with it. Terms like "Band-Aid surgery" performed in a "same-day surgical unit" foster a belief that all laparoscopic surgery is "simple" or "mi-nor," dispelling any thoughts of risk. A patient's recall, years later during legal discovery, may be void of any "consent" conversation. Thoughts such as "the doctor never mentioned my ureter could be injured" or "the physician guaranteed I could never become pregnant" are part of the spark that may result in the filing of a lawsuit. As a result, it is extremely important that physicians adequately document the informed consent process.

To record "I have discussed the benefits, risks, and alternatives with the patient" may not be enough; the notation should be as complete as possible. Additional documentation, such as a form detailing the risks and benefits of the procedure, signed by the patient, may prove beneficial in case of litigation. If a pamphlet is provided, remember to attach a copy of it to the medical record. If the patient views a videotape, note in the record which tape she viewed and consider the videotape part of the patient's record. You might want to consider having the patient sign a form that indicates that in addition to her discussion with the physician, she has reviewed a certain pamphlet or videotape on laparoscopy. Years later, if a suit occurs, you can share the pamphlet or videotape with the jury as additional evidence of the informed consent discussion.

With any discussion of informed consent, it is important to remember that the degree of disclosure for a valid consent varies from state to state. Some states use a "professional or reasonable physician standard" for disclosure. This standard is measured by the level of information physicians in the community usually provide their patients for the same procedure or treatment. Other states use the "materiality or patient viewpoint standard." With this standard, the information disclosed is based on what a reasonable person in the patient's position would want to know in similar circumstances. In addition, many states have specific informed consent laws that dictate what needs to be included in the consent form or detail specific information that must be told to patients before they consent to a procedure or treatment. A number of state courts have also held that a physician's duty to obtain informed consent cannot be delegated to a third party.

RISK MANAGEMENT

Next to abortion, laparoscopy is the most common gynecologic procedure performed today. Although the complications associated with it are infrequent, a thorough understanding of each is mandated. Thankfully, most complications come with warning signs that should alert the surgeon that something might be amiss. For instance, almost all patients who have an uncomplicated laparoscopy should improve with each postoperative hour. If a patient requires narcotic relief by injection the day after laparoscopy, something is wrong. Likewise, a patient who complains of continual and increased abdominal pain following discharge from the hospital should concern you. These patients need to be seen and examined by a physician familiar with laparoscopic complications. Since bowel injury is a known and serious complication of any laparoscopy, to delay in identifying and intervening in cases that may involve a possible bowel injury will make little sense to the jury.

Another risk, unique to laparoscopy, is the problem of weekend call. Laparoscopy is frequently scheduled before the weekend to reduce the patient's ''out of work'' time. It is not unusual for the surgeon to do a laparoscopy on Friday and immediately turn the weekend call over to a colleague. If you are not careful, this scenario could prove disastrous. Questions you should ask yourself include: Was the colleague told of any unusual occurrences during the procedure? Does the colleague realize that patients with increasing pain need to be seen? Will the patient be sent to an emergency room to be seen by an intern or another physician unfamiliar with laparoscopic complications? If you are not satisfied with the answers to these questions, steps need to be taken to change your procedures.

To know about complications is not enough; you must also know how to correct the problem. An accidental puncture of the dome of the bladder can be managed with an indwelling catheter for 7 days, rather than with an extensive incision, suture repair, and lengthy hospitalization. If you suspect both a bowel injury and electrical injury, the patient needs to be seen by someone with expertise in this combination of complications. This type of injury requires a bowel resection, not a simple closure of the perforation site.

Good record keeping is also essential to good risk management. Medical records must be legible, objective, and timely. They should also be comprehensive and contain complete details of the procedure. To say ''The tubes were coagulated'' is not enough. A complete description of the technique is needed. It is important to note whether electrosurgery was or was not used during the procedure, in case a bowel injury is later discovered. Although it is not essential to list all of the instruments used during the procedure, it may help you to remember the operation if you are asked about it years later. Imagine the jury's impression of a physician/defendant who does not know the tools that he or she used during a sterilization.

Good medical records are also an important part of communication between all members of the health care team. In addition, if you find yourself in a courtroom, a good medical record may prove to be your best defense.

WHEN A SUMMONS ARRIVES

Once a lawsuit is filed, you will be served with a summons and related papers informing you of the suit. Contact your professional liability insurance carrier immediately. Most insurance companies require timely notification of a lawsuit, or the insurance policy can be declared void. Some carriers even require notification if there is only a reasonable suspicion that a suit might be filed. It is important that you be aware of your obligations under your insurance contract.

After you have notified your carrier, you might be asked to review your records and prepare a written report recalling the events that led to the lawsuit. The carrier might also request a thorough analysis of the case for your attorney. If you are asked to furnish such a report, do not delay. Although it might take years for a case to come to trial, it is best to formulate your analysis when the events are fresh in your mind.

All documents related to a suit should be kept in a separate file, apart from the medical record. This is particularly true for any reports that you prepare for your insurance carrier or attorney. In order for these reports to be protected under the attorney ''work product privilege'' and not discoverable by the plaintiff, they must remain confidential between you and your attorney. If you have any questions about how to proceed, ask your attorney or insurance carrier for advice.

When preparing for litigation, if you discover a glaring mistake or omission in the records, remember: neither alter nor change. By the time a suit is filed, the plaintiff's attorney is well into his or her preparation and already has a copy of the patient's medical record. If the medical record is altered or supplemented, then the plaintiff's attorney will have a different set of records than the physician/defendant, which could only lead to trouble.

Laparoscopy is a complex surgical technique. Be sure your defense attorney does his or her homework and is prepared to handle the case. Educate your attorney on the medicine involved. Provide your attorney with an array of authoritative texts and articles. When possible, let your attorney attend an actual laparoscopy. A videotape of a laparoscopy may also help your attorney understand this not-so-simple operation.

Last, in defending your case, be sure you choose your experts well. A laparoscopist with experience and knowledge of recent work in the field is better than a witness with a prestigious academic title who may only have a peripheral contact with laparoscopy. Fortunately, laparoscopists in the United States have been an enthusiastic group eager to learn and teach, creating a large bank of qualified experts.

CASE 1

A large metropolitan hospital with an approved residency program was encouraged to switch from unipolar sterilization methods to the bipolar method. A directive from the chief of service was sent to the operating room supervisor to buy several Kleppinger bipolar forceps. Upon investigation, she learned that the forceps manufacturer insisted their forceps must be used with their bipolar generator and that if the instrument was modified for connection to another generator, the warranty was null and void and the hospital would assume all risk. Faced with the usual budgetary constraints, the supervisor sought counsel from a local electrogenerator representative who had served their existing electrogenerators. He stated that the existing generators could be used in the bipolar mode and there would be no difference if the Kleppinger bipolar forceps were modified.

During the following years, the ''modified'' Kleppinger bipolar forceps were used by an array of residents, frequently without direct observation or supervision. As with the unipolar method, the tube was grasped, coagulated in two adjacent places to a visual endpoint of coagulation. No records were kept as to the settings or current output of the electric generator. Isolated cases of failure began to surface, and after approximately 100 procedures, a failure rate above 10% was uncovered. Once the legal process began, the hospital, the generator manufacturer, and the medical staff became codefendants.

During discovery, it was shown that the hospital had voluntarily removed a plastic red tag that warned against modification. This tag had been welded onto the electrical cord attached to the Kleppinger forceps. The electrogenerator representative had no scientific evidence to support his claim that the Kleppinger forceps had been field-tested on human tubes when connected to his company's bipolar generator. It was shown that the output characteristics of the Kleppinger bipolar generator had a different waveform (cutting) than that used with the hospital's bipolar generator (coagulating). A coagulation waveform reduces the wattage output as much as fourfold.

Because of the limited destruction without lateral spread, a characteristic of bipolar technology, the length of tube coagulated (less than 2 cm) fell short of the necessary destruction described in the literature and that recommended by the inventor of the Kleppinger bipolar forceps. These facts raised serious questions regarding the quality of supervision provided by the institution.

CASE 2

On a Friday morning, a patient entered a same-day surgery facility for a laparoscopic sterilization. She had signed a consent form that stated that surgery is not a perfect art and results could not be guaranteed. The form went on to mention that sterilization failures, though rare, do occur; however, complications unique to laparoscopy were not listed. The form had been witnessed by the admitting clerk. A history and physical provided by the attending surgeon had all the check boxes marked normal with a single impression and disposition ''VTL'' (voluntary tubal ligation).

An uneventful procedure was completed by 8:15 A.M., and the patient was discharged at noon with 20 tablets of codeine for pain. At 5 P.M. the surgeon signed out to a colleague for the weekend. The patient called at 9 P.M. with complaints of increasing abdominal pain and was instructed to visit the emergency room. The emergency room physician explained that pain was expected after a laparoscopy, meperidine 100 mg was given intramuscularly, and the patient was sent home.

On Saturday, the answering service received and logged three separate phone calls to the weekend physician, each call with complaints of increasing abdominal pain. By Saturday evening, the patient admitted herself to the hospital. Her temperature was 37.4°C, her white blood cell count was 9000, and her hematocrit was the same as Friday morning—42%. Physical examination revealed a nervous patient, clutching the bedrails, with generalized abdominal pain and questionable rebound tenderness.

For the next 24 hours, meperidine 75 mg and hydroxyzine 50 mg were given every 3 to 4 hours while the patient was ''watched.'' A general surgeon was sought and a diagnosis of bowel injury entertained. On Monday morning, an exploratory laparotomy revealed a possible unipolar burn of the terminal ileum. The laparoscopic surgeon had patients in his office and chose not to be in attendance. The perforation (5 mm) was oversewn and the patient's abdomen closed. Five days later, she returned to the operating room where an intestinal perforation of 1.5 cm was found at the site of the original repair. After the second operation, multiple abscesses developed that required three separate trips to surgery for incision and drainage.

During discovery, the emergency room physician admitted he had never seen a laparoscopy. The weekend physician admitted that laparoscopic sterilization patients should improve and, if they don't, bowel injury should be strongly considered. He explained his delay on the grounds that she was ''highly nervous'' and the blood work was normal—a weak defense. The general surgeon was dropped from the case when it was shown that the management of suspected electrical bowel burns was clear in the gynecologic literature but was not available in the general surgical literature.

CASE 3

Two years following a Silastic ring sterilization, the patient became pregnant. She chose to carry the pregnancy but delivered a seriously handicapped child, secondary to fetal distress. At the time of the emergency cesarean section, each tube was removed and sent to pathology. The obstetric surgeon (and chairman of a prestigious medical school), who had never seen or performed a Silastic ring procedure, described the rings on the mesosalpinx next to the tube without any tubal separation on the left, but good separation on the right. The right ring was adherent to the tissue between the separation. He told the patient that the left Silastic ring had not been put on the left tube. Each tubal specimen was described by the pathologist as 8 cm in length, but no further studies were conducted. During discovery, the technical characteristics of the ring applicator and the ring method were analyzed by an expert witness familiar with Silastic ring use. It was shown that the ring is supposed to "fall off" once necrosis of the central knuckle of the tube is complete, but if tubal separation does not occur, a natural fistula is possible. The fact that each tube was of equal length supported the argument that a segment of each tube had been destroyed.

DISCUSSION

Case 1 exposes the need for adequate training, proper equipment, and a need to understand the interplay between different manufacturers' equipment. When one alters a rec-ognized method of sterilization, a new method of sterilization is born, the clock starts ticking, and the failure rate will not become evident until several years later.

Case 2 might be called the "beware of weekend complications" case. Because of the convenience of Friday surgery for laparoscopic sterilization, it is common to have an on-call physician who is not the primary surgeon. That physician should be familiar with the expedient management of laparoscopic complications; patients should only improve. If a consultant general surgeon is involved in subsequent surgery, the primary gynecologic surgeon should be present, and he or she should be familiar with the proper management of the complication.

Case 3 says don't jump to conclusions unless you know the facts. Be careful and be complete in your operative descriptions and communicate with all concerned before making a final diagnosis.

SUGGESTED READING

Medicolegal Forms with Legal Analysis. Chicago: AMA publications, 1991.

Corfman, Diamond, DeCherney (eds.). *Complications of Laparoscopy and Hysteroscopy.* Cambridge, MA: Blackwell Scientific, 1993.

Roberts DK, Shane JA, Roberts ML, eds. *Confronting the Malpractice Crisis.* Kansas City: Eagle Press, 1985.

Rozovsky FA. *Consent to Treatment, A Practical Guide,* 2nd ed. Boston: Little, Brown & Co., 1990.

Soderstrom RM. Bowel injury litigation after laparoscopy. *JAAGL* 1993; 1:74–7.

Operative Laparoscopy, Second Edition
The Masters' Techniques in Gynecologic Surgery
Lippincott–Raven Publishers, Philadelphia © 1998.

22

Documentation

22-1   Documentation for Endoscopy

Carl J. Levinson

As I perceive it, the purpose of documentation is to preserve information for subsequent review either by the surgeon or by others. It is particularly helpful since many patients have multiple procedures, and the decision regarding any one of these may be predicated on the findings of prior operations. Not only must the information be available, it must also be intelligible. It is toward this end that I will outline the techniques I use which have proven to be of value.

I include in the chart for surgery several forms (on $8\frac{1}{2}$-by-11-inch paper) containing diagrams of the pelvis and female genitalia. One form contains ''before'' and ''after'' diagrams (Figure 18-1.1). Immediately following the surgery (not a half hour later, not a week later), I will sit down with the hospital chart and complete the obligatory pages. On the diagrams I outline in two colors what was found and what was done. (For this purpose I have taped together a black and a red pen. It is kept in my locker; as I put my watch and ring into the locker, I take out the two-color pen.) These diagrams remain permanently in the patient chart, located behind the operative report. They serve as a visual aid for the referring physician when he is informed of the results of surgery. I find this technique most effective for subsequent review, as I refer to the diagram much more frequently than I do the operative report, especially during postoperative discussion with the patient.

Documentation *during the procedure* (real-time, real-life) is even better but more expensive and more cumbersome. Nevertheless, the use of photography and video are essential. The use of the video monitor has made it possible for several physicians and ancillary personnel to view the procedure as it is being performed, thereby providing efficient assistance. I prefer a three-chip charged, coupled device (CCD) video camera, along with a high-resolution video monitor.

The video monitor and camera are housed in a portable cabinet, one that will roll easily and can be made readily available in different operating rooms. The monitor sits atop the cabinet, which is 5 feet, 3 inches high. The camera is housed within the cabinet (along with a videocassette recorder [VCR], to be discussed later). The back of the cabinet should be open for ease of wiring and repairs. The monitor should be adjusted by a professional. Once adjusted for a given camera, there should be little need for changes during a procedure. Remember that adjusting the monitor during the procedure will change the image viewed by the operator but will not have any effect on the videotape that may be produced; thus it is best that all adjustments be made *before* the procedure is begun.

The ideal camera should (1) have a wide angle, (2) be easily focused, (3) provide clear detail at the periphery, and (4) have an internal lens adjustment that automatically narrows the lens as brightness increases, such as occurs in bringing the lens close to the white ovary. Some cameras can be soaked in antiseptic solution and therefore do not need to be covered. My operating room nurses insist that, unless the camera has just been soaked, we use a cover. I dislike the plastic cover as it is difficult to focus when the focus ring is below the plastic, especially if there is a rubber band in that area. Also, I believe that once the plastic has been removed from the tip and the camera applied to the eyepiece, true sterility no longer exists. Finally, statistics clearly show that infection is a rare complication of laparoscopic procedures (unless there is some inherent pelvic disease). The camera head must fit closely onto the telescope; it must be perfectly dry to prevent condensation on the camera lens, which will cause the monitor picture to be fuzzy (but if you look through the laparoscope, it will be clear).

The VCR is an integral part of documentation, since the visual image will vanish from the eye (in moments) and from the brain (in hours). The VCR should be of high grade and compatible with the monitor. It is possible to hook up two VCRs in series so as to make two tapes, one for the physician and one for the patient. At present I use one VCR but wish that I had two since either the patient or the referring physician would be pleased to receive a copy. (I have no idea how many times the patients review the tapes, nor whether they understand the imaging, nor whether they invite their friends in for

Name_____   Date_____

   #_____   Parity_____

Pre-Op Tubal Test

   HSG _____

           _____

   Endoscopy _____

           _____

Surgery (Tuboplasty):

   Classification _____

           _____

| Before | After |

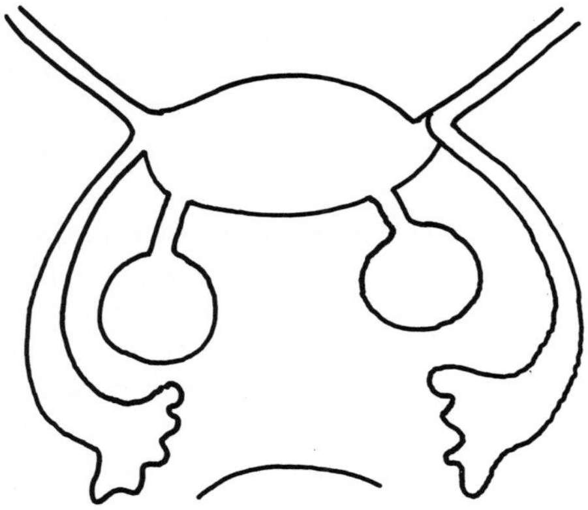

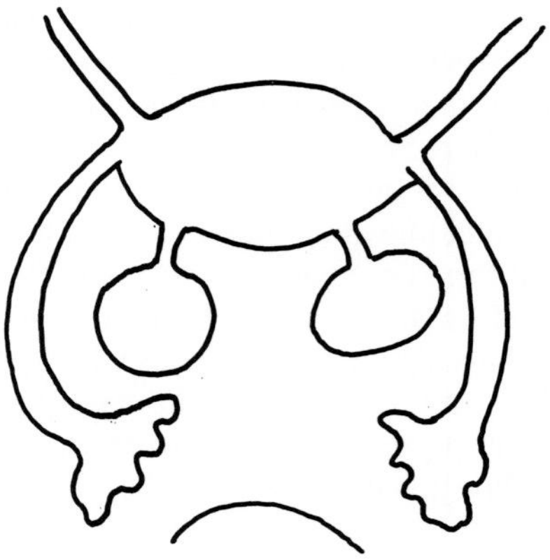

Magnification _____

Suture _____

Splint _____

UT Suspension _____

Medication _____

Miscellaneous _____

           _____

           _____

           _____

           _____

           _____

Figure 22-1.1 Documentation of the operative procedure to be superimposed over the sketch immediately following surgery.

an evening's entertainment.) Before the case begins, I put a piece of $\frac{1}{2}$-inch, thin pink tape on the videocassette itself and another on the outside of the box along the "binding" edge. On this are listed the date, the name of the patient, the procedure, and any special aspects (e.g., "s-ostomy plus Bruhat"), and I generally indicate the excellence of the recording by a designation of 1 + (worst) to 4 + (best). This gives me some idea of which tapes to use for demonstration or teaching. In general, I take the tape with me when I leave the operating room. Although I do not have a VCR and monitor in my office, I believe this would be an excellent method of demonstrating to the patient what procedure has been performed and its significance.

We have available in the operating theater a video printer that allows us to make an instant print of a frame on the video (i.e., an instant stop at a significant point in the operation). The picture is not of the highest quality, but it is possible to make a slide of these prints for teaching purposes (never as good as direct 35-mm slide photography, though). While the Polaroid picture is being projected from the machine, the images are being stored on a disc and may be reproduced (in better form) from the disc.

An almost ancient piece of equipment is a 35-mm camera specifically designed for the light source that I use. The camera is attached by a cord that can be plugged into the light source. Buttons enable me to adjust for the film speed. For many years this was my standard means of documentation. I would look through the laparoscope, ask for the camera, and take a picture at the beginning of the case. Although sterile plastic envelopes have been used for such cameras, I have found it simpler to take the pictures and then change gloves. (True, I may do this several times during the case.) At various points during the case, and when the operative procedure has been completed, more photographs are taken. In general, I have used slide film (ASA 400) on a regular basis, which allows for a fine collection of teaching slides. At one point, when I felt that I had a sufficient number of slides of every possible aspect of pelvic inflammatory disease, endometriosis, etc., I switched to ASA 400 print film. This was appreciated by the patient, as I would have a 4- by 6-inch print of her condition available at the time of the postoperative follow-up examination. Today, I use the video and the diagram for explanation to the patient. Although not as colorful, this has proven to be equally acceptable.

Not to be forgotten is the operative report. This should be dictated within 30 minutes of the termination of the procedure. Senior residents and fellows are quite capable of dictating an accurate report, although they are often too lengthy. (Sometimes minute details are dictated to excess, so that the big picture is lost!) Remember, the operative report becomes a focal point in any medicolegal situation, so the description must be complete, accurate, and significant, including important negative features. I always try to look ahead to future possibilities; for example, in an ectopic pregnancy one should always describe the opposite adnexum. Unfortunately, I am as guilty as most of not reading in great detail the operative description dictated by a trusted, albeit junior, colleague. When I do, there is almost invariably some wording or description that I would choose to change.

Written reports, diagrams, 35-mm slides, 35-mm prints, videotapes, operative reports, combined operative reports and photographs, instant printouts—all of these are available to the endoscopic surgeon. Superb documentation is available to us all (although it is expensive) and serves the needs that such documentation is meant to fulfill.

Operative Laparoscopy, Second Edition
The Masters' Techniques in Gynecologic Surgery
Lippincott–Raven Publishers, Philadelphia © 1998.

22-2   Documentation in Laparoscopy

Philip G. Brooks

VIDEO CAMERAS

From the earliest days of surgery, surgeons have sought to record their findings and results, first with handmade drawings and notations, then with dictated and typed records, and later with photographs. As early as 1879 there were attempts at placing small film cartridges in the tips of endoscopes to capture images of internal structures and pathology. Thus began the long struggle to develop what have become some of the most useful and exciting aspects of endoscopic surgery today. To understand the current state of the art of documentation, it is useful to note the major breakthroughs in technology in four separate areas: optics, illumination, instrumentation, and photographic equipment itself.

The first major breakthrough was the development of the Hopkins rod-lens system, a system that replaced multiple thin lenses separated by large columns of air with thick ''columns'' of lenses separated by smaller columns of air. This created an improved telescope with increased light transmission, better image quality, a larger viewing angle, the ability to alter the size of the image, and the ability to photograph through the telescope. The quest for increased illumination initially produced light sources that could generate far more power than the bulbs could handle, resulting in hot instrument tips and a lot of burned-out bulbs!

Another major breakthrough came around 1930 with the finding that light can be transmitted through a flexible instrument. Next, it was shown to be transmittable through fine glass fiber threads, with even greater intensity and brightness than ever before possible with existing telescopes. This change from hot and dangerous distal light bulbs to the current system of generating high-intensity light meant far less heat exposure for the area under investigation. The need for increased light for photographic purposes, and especially for video, was now met by developing high-intensity light systems. One such development, transmission through a quartz rod, allowed for the best color transmission but was far more cumbersome than the xenon arc globe, which contained compact globes and a housing that protected against explosion.

Once the light source and optical systems were adequate, it was fairly simple to develop or adapt the instrumentation to photographic needs. Fluid-filled cables replaced fibers (Figure 22-2.1), and telescopes with integrated cables were created to eliminate the junction between fiber bundles, thus

increasing light transmission even more. Color and image transmission improved noticeably. Photographs of internal structures were never clearer or more natural in color. Prism systems and intricate articulating arms were developed to allow simultaneous photography without interfering with the operator performing the procedure and retaining most of the available light for the camera.

What was left was the development of photographic equipment and a debate over still photography versus television for documentation. Numerous cameras were developed for still photography and then for movie photography, with various types of connectors and adaptors for endoscopes. Sixteen- and 35-mm film was used with reasonable success, and Polaroid instant film was promoted heavily for a time. The former didn't become popular because of the nuisance of developing the film and because of the bulk of the cameras; the latter did not succeed because of the poor quality and small size of the displayed image as compared to that of a transparency. While the need for less light for shorter periods of time made for less heat, and while the superb image and reasonable cost made still photography usable for even the novice, the requirement for larger trocars and the annoying delay in processing the film, sorting and labeling the pictures, and filing them for later retrieval for teaching or for patient care, made still photography documentation less than widely utilized.

It had become obvious that electronic imaging, with its instant display and relay capabilities, would likely be the method of choice in documentation if a camera could be developed with the size, performance, and optical characteristics to suit the operating needs of the profession. Early zeal for television filming and transmission of endoscopic procedures resulted in crowded operating rooms with cumbersome, impossible-to-keep-sterile equipment and poor-quality projection. In the past 25 years, there has been steady miniaturization of television cameras for this purpose. The first endoscope video camera was a black-and-white camera whose monochromatic display left much to be desired, but which showed that when color cameras were perfected, acceptable miniature equipment could be developed to be coupled to an endoscope without interfering with the routine of the operating room or the operator.

Dramatic changes in the past decade have resulted in progressive improvement in cameras, from the early image-tube cameras to the current high-resolution charged coupled device (CCD) chip cameras (Figure 22-2.2). At present,

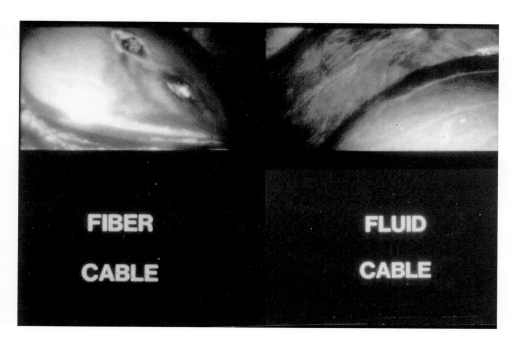

Figure 22-2.1 Image produced with fiber cables (left) versus more natural one produced using fluid-filled cables (right).

small (1-by-1-by-1.5 inch), lightweight (as light as 2 ounces) CCD cameras (Figure 22-2.3) are used routinely for virtually all endoscopic procedures, with a spring-loaded coupler that allows the camera to attach to telescopes of almost any manufacturer and for any specialty. Unlike their predecessors, which were heavy, bulky, and awkward to use, the chip cameras are mobile and do not detract from the ease of the procedure (Figure 22-2.4). In addition, most video cameras can be soaked in sterilizing liquids, thus eliminating cumbersome and annoying draping and not interfering with sterile technique.

Among the newest options available with endoscope cameras is a beam splitter; the surgeon can look through the telescope with one eye while projecting the image on the video monitor for assistants and others in the room to see. I seldom need to look through the telescope with one eye or through a beam splitter camera because of the great improvement in recent years in the resolution and color transmission of current cameras and video monitors. In general, resolution of cameras and monitors is expressed in the number of lines of transmission of the image in a specific space. Earlier standard monitors transmitted approximately 300 to 350 lines per inch, while current, high-resolution screens transmit over 500 lines per inch. It is important to note that it is essential that the resolution of the monitor should equal or exceed that of the camera.

For most of our procedures, working off of the monitor permits binocular viewing for easier and faster perception.

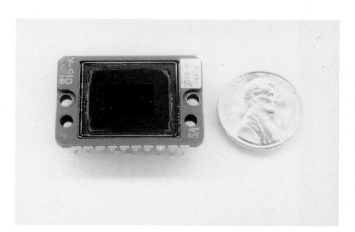

Figure 22-2.2 Charged coupled device (CCD) chip. Note miniature size.

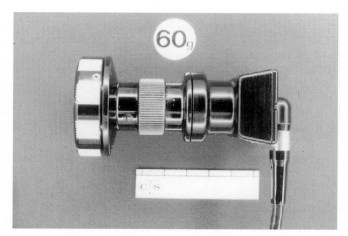

Figure 22-2.3 Miniature CCD chip endoscope camera and lens, attached to coupler for eyepiece of telescope.

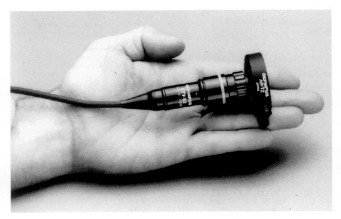

Figure 22-2.4 Laparoscope television camera. (Courtesy of Olympus Corporation.)

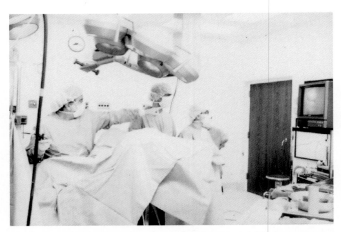

Figure 22-2.5 Working from a video monitor, demonstrating findings to students and nursing personnel in the operating room.

The image viewed is 20 to 30 times larger than when viewed directly through the laparoscope and allows for demonstration and description to all assistants, students, and nursing and anesthesia personnel in the room (Figure 22-2.5). If assistance is required, a far better coordination of motions is provided by the simultaneous viewing. The safety aspects of inserting accessory trocars or needles under direct visualization are even more fully ensured when the enlarged images are viewed by everyone involved. In addition, the use of video cameras provides for transmission of procedures to distant conference centers for concurrent demonstration and teaching (Figure 22-2.6).

A recent improvement in cameras has been the addition of a built-in zoom lens, which enlarges the image for even more precision. However, when you zoom in closer, enlarging the image, you lose a moderate amount of light intensity. It is always my practice first to zoom back all the way (widest field) and then zoom in if the light quality allows it.

Other recent improvements include automatic white balancing, an adjustment that allows for the best reproduction of color transmitted to the monitor, and the development of the "laparo-cam" (Figure 22-2.7), a one-piece telescope and camera combination that eliminates the significant amount of light lost at connection points between cables, telescopes, and cameras.

In addition, several manufacturers have created a new type of camera that has the best resolution, color sensitivity, and visual clarity ever developed, the three-chip camera (Figure 22-2.8). These cameras are better because each chip is dedicated to one color after separation of the colors into red, green, and blue.

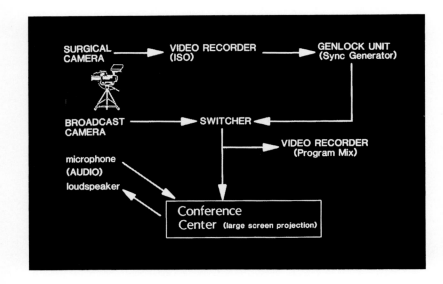

Figure 22-2.6 Diagram of use of video equipment for permanent recording and television to distant conference centers.

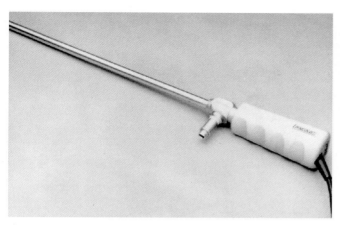

Figure 22-2.7 Television camera built into the telescope. (Courtesy of Karl Storz Co.)

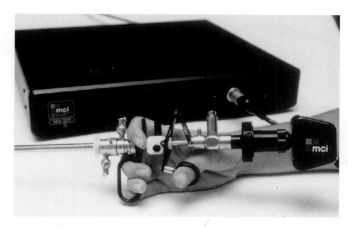

Figure 22-2.8 Three-chip video camera shown with telescope and control box.

While many physicians still prefer to perform endoscopic procedures without cameras, it is my preference to use cameras routinely and for all procedures, even for routine hysteroscopy (and especially for office hysteroscopy). Letting patients watch their own hysteroscopy on a video monitor provides significant distraction from any discomfort, and they can see any pathology as I do, building great understanding and confidence in the diagnosis and subsequent treatment plan. Cameras used in the office setting do not have to be soaked or otherwise sterilized. As a result, some manufacturers have developed cameras that are not sealed sufficiently to be soaked, thus lowering the price of the camera.

VIDEOTAPE

As anyone who has walked through an electronics store can certify, the development of video recorders has allowed even the home amateur to record on tape anything he or she sees on a videoscreen. And, unlike movie film, labeling to identify the patient, date, and any structure to be highlighted can be performed at the time of filming or at any future time using an electronic device called a character generator (Figure 22-2.9). Thus, once endoscopic video cameras were developed, the process of making permanent recordings on videotape was adapted for medical documentation. Clearly, viewing videotapes of operations became the best method for teaching and demonstrating anatomy, gross pathology, and operative techniques for students, and for patients and their families as well. Also, videotapes are used in medicolegal situations to define the steps and techniques used during a procedure more clearly than the written word or still photographs. In addition, I frequently use videotapes (both as sender and recipient) for referrals to and from other physicians for patients moving away or being referred for specialized procedures, such as in vitro fertilization or operative endoscopic procedures.

There are basically three types of videotape used for video documentation: three-quarter-inch tape, half-inch VHS tape, and 8-mm ("super 8") tape. Three-quarter-inch tape is used for commercial purposes or for making permanent teaching tapes. It has the best resolution and clarity, and copies placed onto narrower tape (i.e., half-inch) retain their clarity reasonably well (transfer from half-inch to three-quarter-inch results in too much loss of quality).

Half-inch tape is the most widely used and can be shown on any home or office video cassette recorder (VCR) and monitor, making it useful for routine documentation and patient/family demonstration. Depending on the length of the procedure, I usually get four to eight procedures on each cassette. However, because of the size and bulk of these cassettes, storage can get to be a significant problem, especially if you do a fair amount of videoendoscopy.

The newest and most convenient tape format is 8-mm tape, or super-8. This tape differs from the others in several

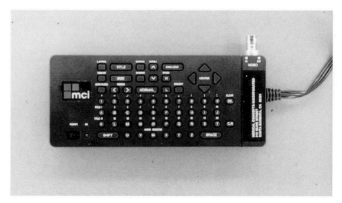

Figure 22-2.9 Character generator, an electronic device that allows labeling on the videotape at the time of the procedure.

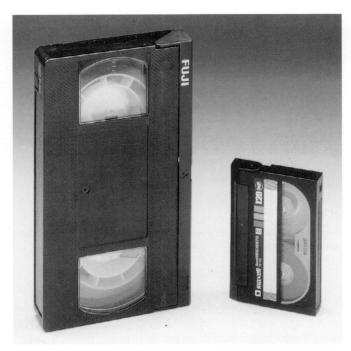

Figure 22-2.10 Half-inch tape cassette (left) and 8-mm tape cassette (right).

ways. Half-inch and three-quarter-inch tapes are coated with metal oxide, while 8-mm tape is painted with densely packed particles of pure metal, enabling the latter to record more information per square inch than can either of the other two. Despite the fact that the cassettes for 8-mm tape are much smaller (approximately the size of an audiotape cassette) (Figure 22-2.10), more information can be recorded because the recording drum is smaller and spins faster than with the larger tapes, and the reading head scans the tape in a diagonal way, rather than horizontally, as with the others, to handle even more information.

While the compactness of super-8 recorder and monitor combinations makes it useful for office procedures like hysteroscopy, most videolaparoscopy is done with the standard half-inch or three-quarter-inch recorders and large, 20- or 24-inch high-resolution video monitors.

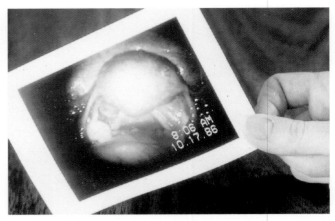

Figure 22-2.12 Print made during laparoscopic examination.

VIDEOPRINTERS

While the development of video cameras and recorders, along with the low cost of videotape, has resulted in their widespread use for endoscopic documentation, there are several drawbacks. Especially with tapes used for several patients' procedures, there are problems of bulk of storage, if the tapes are kept indefinitely, and the need for indexing in order to retrieve prior studies. Reproductions of pathology or procedures on tape are more difficult to send to referring or new physicians or even to keep filed with patients' regular records. The newest advances in endoscopic documentation, the development of high-quality video prints, has essentially solved these problems.

Video printers (Figure 22-2.11) are ingenious electronic devices that "freeze" or commit to memory one or more frames of video images that can be retrieved and printed immediately on photosensitive paper, so that one or more copies can be available to show the patient and/or her family right after the completion of the surgery or at a postoperative visit. In addition, copies can be affixed to patients' of-

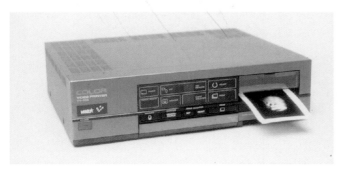

Figure 22-2.11 Video print emerging from printer.

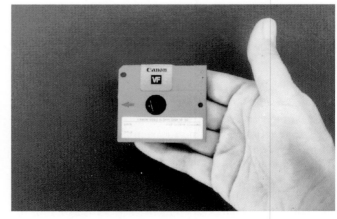

Figure 22-2.13 Two half-inch floppy disc used in video printers.

fice reports or mailed to the other physicians as desired (Figure 22-2.12). The images are memorized on small ($2\frac{1}{2}$-inch) floppy discs for later retrieval (Figure 22-2.13).

The process of converting a color video image to a print is complex. To begin with, the production of color, whether for television projecting or for color printing for books or for endoscopy, involves the separation of part or all of the colors in an image into the three primary colors, red, green, and blue. To make a color print, a printer must capture an image, sense the amounts and location of these three colors, and lay down a reproduction on photographic paper by one of three methods: the thermal method, the cathode ray tube (CRT) with instant-print method, and the multiple ink-jet method.

The earliest video printers, made by Sony and Canon, now greatly improved upon, used a system of many tiny ink jets to spray different colors of quick-drying ink onto the paper.

The Polaroid system, for a time widely promoted for medical documentation, is not preferred by most institutions because it takes the image off of a small internal CRT or television screen, separates the image into the three colors, and, using a color filter wheel, photographs the image three times and prints these onto Poloroid print paper, which results in a poor quality picture.

The thermal method, used by the Hitachi printer, has the most intricate system of memorizing the video image and converting it to a thermal signal. Paper is drawn around a spindle and rotated through a linear row of thermal heads. As the dye cartridge is drawn between the thermal heads and the print paper, each color is laid down separately on top of the previous one, and the print is made. The picture quality is good, but the method is very complex and expensive.

In conclusion, for many of us who now perform all endoscopic procedures from a video screen, it is difficult to imagine going back to working bent over, with one eye peering through a telescope and with no one else in the room able to see the procedure at the same time.

APPENDIX A

Color Atlas of Photographic Documentation

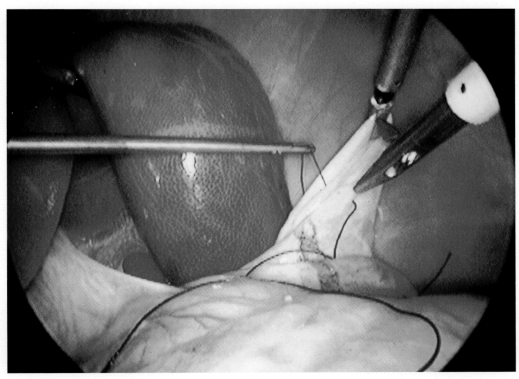

Figure 1 After a digitizing process, a three-chip video camera picture frame can be transferred to 35 mm. Ectachrome film provides remarkable clarity. (Courtesy of Professional Photo Laboratories.)

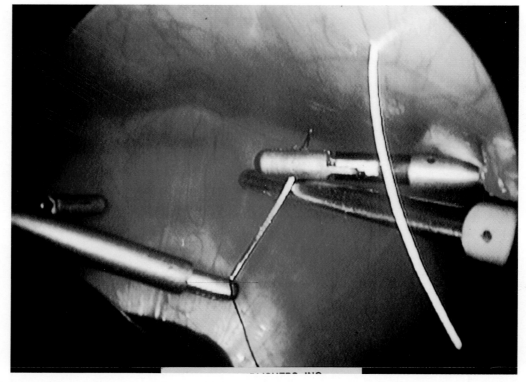

Figure 2 Advanced laparoscopic procedures, such as suturing, require multiple trocar insertions and qualified assistance. (Courtesy of Professional Photo Laboratories.)

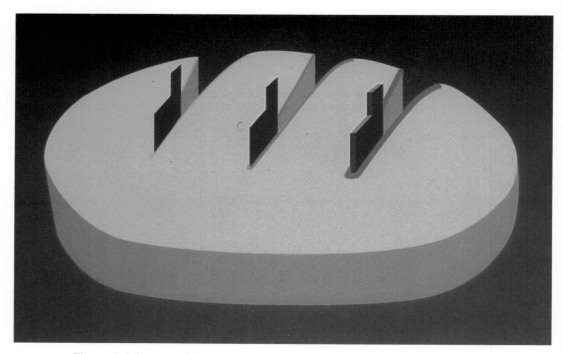

Figure 3 Influence of the shape of the electrode on the degree of coagulation.

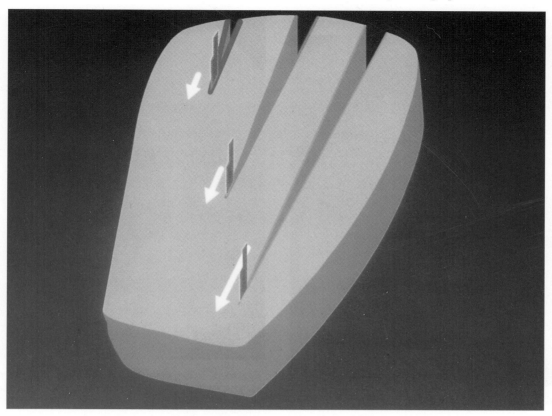

Figure 4 Influence of the speed of incision on the degree of coagulation.

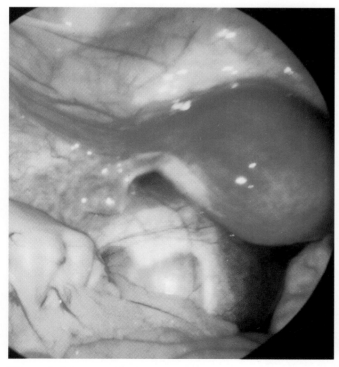

Figure 5 A large ovarian cyst nonresponsive to progestin therapy. Ultrasound criteria were declared benign and the CA125 was normal.

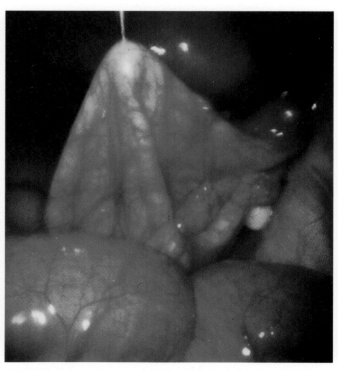

Figure 6 Same cyst as seen in previous figure during the aspiration process required to reduce its size for easy removal.

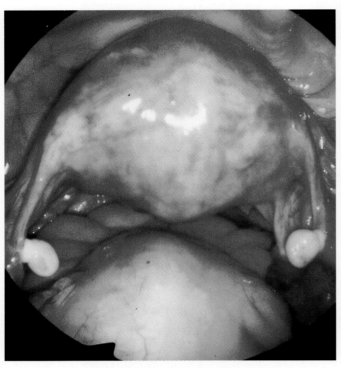

Figure 7 The proper application of the Falope rings for sterilization.

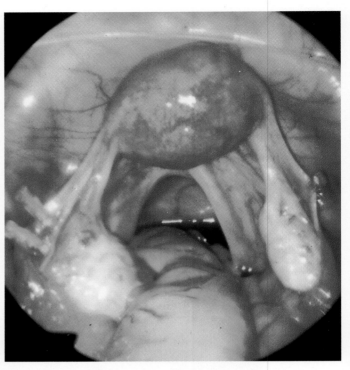

Figure 8 This patient was pregnant within one month of her Hulka clip sterilization. Though the clip was applied properly on the right tube, the left tube remained patent despite two clips which were applied distal to the isthmic portion of the tube.

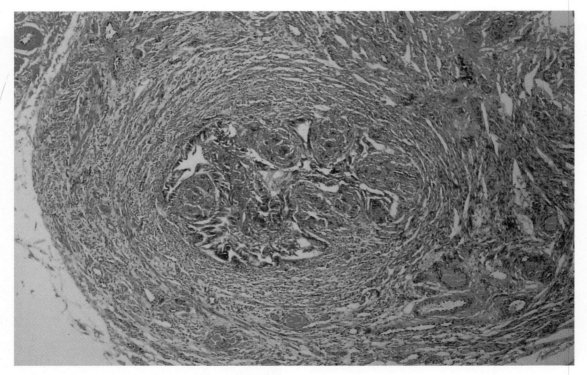

Figure 9 The histologic findings after a bipolar sterilization failure. Though the muscularis is coagulated, because a damped (coagulation) waveform was used instead of the recommended undamped (cutting) waveform, the endosalpinx mucosa shows only partial heat artifact.

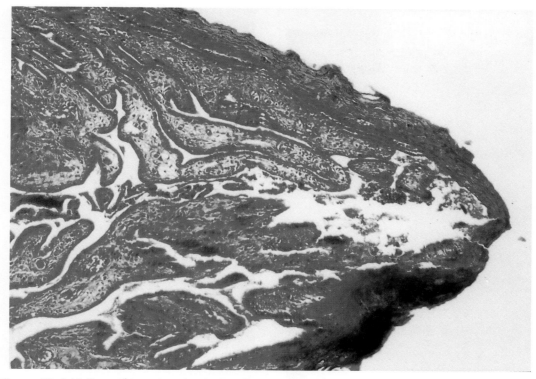

Figure 10 A Mallory trichrome stain highlights the coagulated muscularis of a tubal segment after a bipolar sterilization. The endosalpinx was spared because a damped waveform was used at 10 W of power. Always use an undamped waveform with bipolar procedures at 25 W or more.

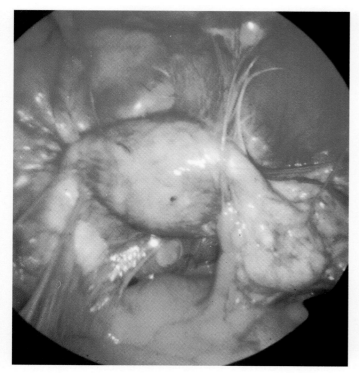

Figure 11 Chronic PID with dense adhesions. After laparoscopic lysis of adhesions this patient conceived an intrauterine pregnancy.

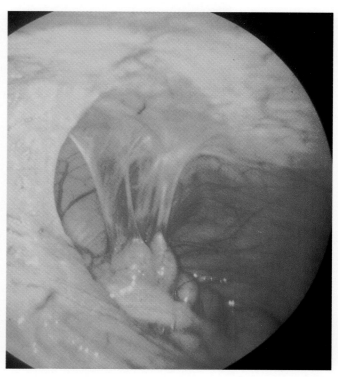

Figure 12 Vascular and avascular adhesions. The transparent areas can be cut without coagulation techniques. Beware of hidden structures behind dense adhesions.

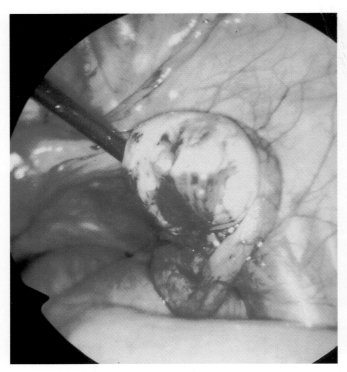

Figure 13 Enucleation of a dermoid cyst.

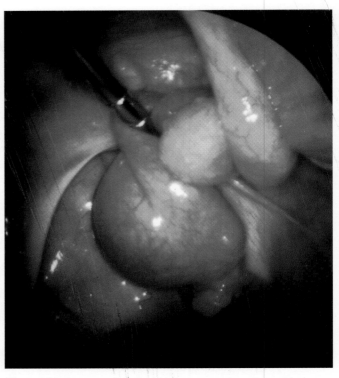

Figure 14 An unruptured ectopic pregnancy amenable to laparoscopic removal.

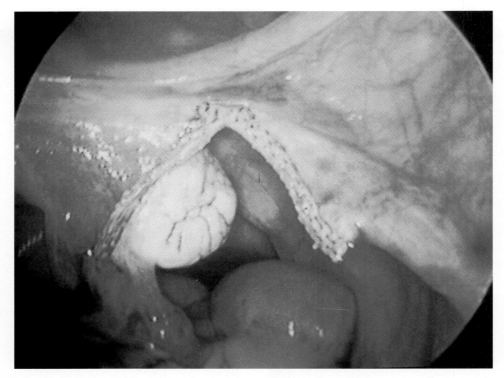

Figure 15 The infundibular ligament after staples have been applied and the ligament severed.

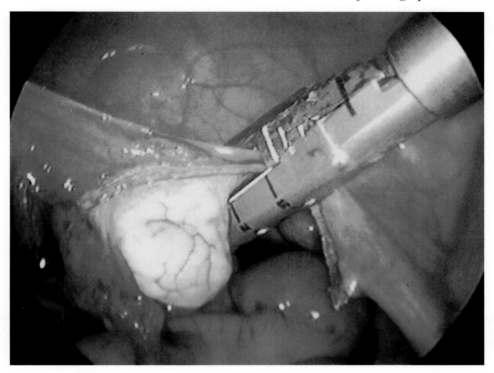

Figure 16 Applying more auto staples on the infundibular ligament. The stapling device secures and cuts the tissue simultaneously.

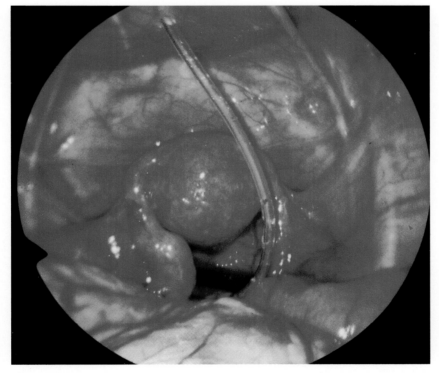

Figure 17 When postoperative bleeding occurs after extensive laparoscopic surgery, a suction drain can be placed through an accessory trocar sleeve and placed as desired.

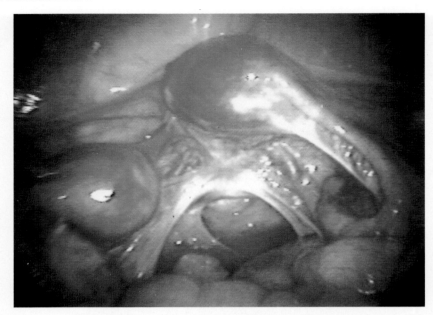

Figure 18 Despite the lack of endometriosis or hematometra, this patient conceived in the rudimentary uterine horn on the left. It is presumed that she conceived by cross fertilization from the right unicollis uterus. (Courtesy of Stephen Corson).

List of Manufacturers

Accurate Surgical & Scientific Instruments Corp.
300 Shames Drive
Westbury, NY 11590
(516) 333-2570

Advanced Surgical Corp.
23705 Van Owen Street, Suite 217
West Hills, CA 91307
(818) 883-5305

Allen Medical Systems
5198 Richmond Road
Bedford Heights, OH 44146
(216) 765-0990

American Surgical Instruments
901 East Sample Road, Suite C
Pompano, FL 33064
(800) 367-5694

American Medical Source/ L.A.S.E.R., Inc.
1803 Baker Drive
Tomball, TX 77375
(713) 351-4601

American Surgical Endoscope Division
1349 Biltmore Drive
Charlotte, NC 28207
(704) 373-1900

American V. Mueller/Baxter Healthcare Corporation
6600 Touhy Avenue
Niles, IL 60648
(312) 774-6800

Apple Medical
580 Main Street
Bolton, MA 07140-1306
(800) 255-2926

Applied Medical Resources
26051 Merit Circle, Building 104
Laguna Hills, CA 92653
(714) 582-6120

Aquintel
2680 Bayshore Parkway
Mountain View, CA 94043
(415) 938-3431

Aslan Medical Technologies
6376 Quain Run Drive
Kalamazoo, MI 49009
(616) 372-8222

Avalon Medical Corporation
6 Hurricane Lane
Williston, VT 05495
(802) 878-1110

Brun Medical Instruments, Inc.
1312 Vancouver Ave., P.O. Box 1629
Burlingame, CA 94010
(415) 343-1663

Cameron-Miller, Inc.
3949 South Racine Avenue
Chicago, IL 60609
(773) 523-6360
(800) 621-0142

Circon Corporation
6500 Hollister Avenue
Santa Barbara, CA 93117
(805) 685-5100

Cogent Light Technologies, Inc.
26145 Technology Drive
Santa Clarita, CA 91355
(800) 294-2989

Coherent Medical Group
3270 W. Bayshore Road
Palo Alto, CA 94303
(415) 852-3824

Computer Motion
130 Cremona Drive, Suite B
Goleta, CA 93117
(805) 685-3729

Conceptus, Inc.
1021 Howard Avenue
San Carlos, CA 94070
(415) 802-7255

Cone Instruments
5201 Naiman
Solon, OH 44139
(216) 248-1035

Conkin Surgical Instruments, Ltd.
P.O. Box 6707, Station A
Toronto, Ontario, Canada M5W 1X5
(416) 922-9496

Conmed Corporation
310 Broad Street
Utica, NY 13501
(315) 797-8375

Cook Ob/Gyn
1100 West Morgan Street, P.O. Box 271
Spencer, IN 47460
(812) 829-6500

Cooper Surgical
15 Forest Parkway
Shelton, CT 06484
(203) 929-6321
(800) 645-3760

Core Dynamics, Inc.
11222-4 St. John's Industrial Parkway
Jacksonville, FL 32246
(904) 641-6611

Cryomedical Sciences
1300 Piccard Drive, Suite 102
Rockville, MD 20850
(301) 417-7070

Cuda Products Corp.
6000 Powers Avenue
Jacksonville, FL 32217
(904) 737-7611

Davis & Geck, American Cyanamid Co.
Surgical Products Division
1 Casper Street
Danbury, CT 06813
(203) 743-4451

Davol, Inc.
100 Stockanossett, P.O. Box 8500
Cranston, RI 02920
(401) 463-7000

Dexide, Inc.
7509 Flagstone Drive
Fort Worth, TX 76181-5789
(800) 645-3378

Ellman International, Inc.
1134 Railroad Ave.
Hewlett, NY 11557-2316
(516) 569-1482
(800) 835-5355

Elmed Incorporated
60 West Fay Avenue
Addison, IL 60101
(630) 543-2792

Erbe, USA, Inc.
2225 Northwest Parkway, Suite 105
Marietta, GA 30067
(770) 955-4400

Ethicon, Inc.
Route 22, P.O. Box 151
Somerville, NJ 08876-0151
(908) 218-2465

Euro-Med, Inc.
8561 154th Avenue, N.E.
Redmond, WA 98052
(800) 848-0033

Everest Medical
13755 First Avenue North
Minneapolis, MN 55441
(612) 473-6262
(800) 852-9361

Fujinon
10 High Point
Wayne, NJ 07470
(800) 872-0196

Galileo Electro-Optics Corp.
Galileo Park, P.O. Box 550
Sturbridge, MA 01566
(508) 347-4318

General Surgical Innovations
3172A Porter Drive
Palo Alto, CA 94304
(415) 812-9730

W. L. Gore Associates, Inc.
1500 North Fourth Street
Flagstaff, AZ 86004
(520) 526-3030

Gynox, Inc.
40 North Grand Avenue, Suite 302
Ft. Thomas, KY 41075

Heraeus LaserSonics, Inc.
575 Cottonwood Drive
Milpitas, CA 95035
(408) 954-4210

American Heyer-Schulte (Mentor Corporation)
600 Pine Avenue
Goleta, CA 93117
(805) 681-6000

HGM Medical Laser Systems
3959 West 1820 South
Salt Lake City, UT 84104
(801) 972-0500

Imagyn Medical, Inc.
27651 La Paz Road
Laguna Niguel, CA 92677
(714) 362-2500

Inlet Medical, Inc.
9951 Valley View Road
Eden Prairie, MN 55344
(612) 942-5034

Innerdyne, Inc.
1244 Reamwood Avenue
Sunnyvale, CA 94089
(408) 745-6010

Jarit Surgical Instruments
9 Skyline Drive
Hawthorne, NY 10532
(914) 592-9050

Lasermatic
10575 Newkirk Street, Suite 740
Dallas, TX 75220
(214) 556-2555

Johnson & Johnson Medical, Inc.
2500 Arbrook Blvd.
Arlington, TX 76004-3130
(817) 784-5296

Kronner Medical
1443 Upper Cleveland Rapids Road
Roseburg, OR 97470
(541) 672-2543

Laser Photonics
12351 Research Parkway
Orlando, FL 32826
(407) 281-4103

Laserscope
3052 Orchard Drive
San Jose, CA 95134-2011
(408) 943-0636

Laurus Medical Corporation
30 Hughes, Suite 202
Irvine, CA 92718
(714) 859-6002

Leisegang Medical, Inc.
6401 Congress Avenue
Boca Raton, FL 33487
(561) 994-0202

Machida America, Inc.
40 Ramland Road
Orangeburg, NY 10962
(914) 365-0600

Marlow Surgical Technologies, Inc.
1810 Joseph Lloyd Parkway
Willoughby, OH 44094
(216) 946-2453
(800) 992-5581

Materials Conversion Corporation
2360B Egidi Drive
Wheeling, IL 60090
(847) 465-1194

Medical Concepts
175B Cremona Drive
Goleta, CA 93117-5502
(805) 968-5563

Medical Dynamics, Inc.
99 Inverness Drive East
Englewood, CO 80112
(303) 790-2990

Med Images, Inc.
9040 Executive Park Drive
Knoxville, TN 37923
(800) 366-7501

Mediflex—Division of Flexbar Machine Corp.
250 Gibbs Road
Islandia, NY 11752
(516) 582-8440

Megadyne Medical Products, Inc.
11506 South State Street
Draper, UT 84020
(801) 576-9669

Baxter V. Mueller
1500 Waukegan Road
McGaw Park, IL 60085
(708) 473-1500

New Eder Corporation
753 Edgewood
Wood Dale, IL 60191
(631) 860-8957

Nortech
600 Church Road
Elgin, IL 60123
(847) 608-8900

O.R. Direct
916 Main Street
Acton, MA 01720
(508) 635-0761

Origin Medsystems, Inc.
135 Constitution Drive
Menlo Park, CA 94025
(415) 617-5000

Pentax Endoscopic & Medical Instrument Corp.
23011 Moulton Parkway, Suite F-6B
Laguna Hills, CA 92653
(714) 830-5520

Premier Laser Systems
3 Morgan
Irvine, CA 92718
(714) 859-0656
(800) 544-8044

Pharmacia Laboratories
800 Centennial Avenue
Piscataway, NJ 08854
(800) 526-3619, ext 8110

Professional Photo Laboratory
13368 Beach Drive
Marina Del Rey, CA 90292
(800) 527-0206

R-Med, Inc.
3465 Navarre Avenue
Oregon, OH 43616
(419) 693-7481

Ranfac Corporation
30 Doherty Avenue
Avon, MA 02322
(508) 588-4400

Reznik Instruments, Inc.
7337 North Lawndale
Skokie, IL 60076
(312) 673-3444

Richard-Allan Medical—A Division of Urohealth
8850 M89, Box 351
Richland, MI 49083
(616) 629-5811

Seiler Instruments
170 East Kirkham
St. Louis, MO 63119
(800) 444-7952

Sharplan Lasers, Inc.
1 Pearl Court
Allendale, NJ 07401
(201) 327-1666
(800) 394-2000

Smith & Nephew, Inc.
160 Dascomb Road
Andover, MA 01810
(508) 470-2800

Snowden Penser DSP
5175 S. Royal Atlanta Drive
Tucker, GA 30084
(770) 496-0952

Solos Endoscopy
41 Brooks Drive
Braintree, MA 02184
(617) 356-4830

Karl Storz Endoscopy-America, Inc.
600 Corporate Pointe
Culver City, CA 90230
(310) 558-1500

Stryker Endoscopy
2590 Walsh Avenue
Santa Clara, CA 95051
(800) 624-4422

Surgical Lasers, Inc.
400 Lathrop, Suite 200
River Forest, IL 60305
(708) 771-2200

Surgikos
P.O. Box 130
Arlington, TX 76010
(817) 465-3141

Tahoe Surgical Instruments
954 Ponce De Leon Avenue, Suite 304
San Juan, PR 00907
(800) 824-5311

United States Surgical Corporation
150 Glover Avenue
Norwalk, CT 06856
(203) 845-4319

Utah Medical Products
7043 S. 300 W
Midvale, UT 84047
(800) 533-4984

Valleylab, Inc.
5920 Longbow Drive
Boulder, CO 80301
(800) 228-7507

Videomed, Inc.
5109 Ridge Road
Minneapolis, MN 55436
(800) 332-0633

Wave Form Systems, Inc.
P.O. Box 3195
Portland, OR 97208
(800) 332-8749

Weck Instruments
4174 W. Park Avenue
Chandler, AZ 85226
(800) 533-9325

WISAP/MARKET-TIERS, INC.
8305 Melrose Drive
Lenexa, KS 66214
(913) 492-5888

Richard Wolf Medical Instruments Corporation
353 Corporate Woods Parkway
Vernon Hills, IL 60061
(847) 913-1113
(800) 323-8653

Carl Zeiss, Inc.
1 Zeiss Drive
Thornwood, NY 10594
(914) 747-1800

Zinnati Surgical Instruments
21540 Prairie Street, Suite B
Chatsworth, CA 91311
(800) 223-4740

Subject Index

Page numbers in italic refer to figures; page numbers followed by "t" refer to tables.